Perspectives of Quorum Quenching in New Drug Development

Antibiotic resistance in pathogen microorganisms is a major global concern, especially the formation of biofilms. Quorum quenching has been practically used to control biofilm growth, and this indicates a promising hope for the development of new drugs for the control of biofilm-forming pathogens. This book provides a single source of information about two issues: the biology of quorum sensing and quorum quenching, and the perspectives of quorum quenching in new drug development. The text covers the latest literature from the last ten years and insights into quorum quenching and its need in medicine as an antivirulence strategy.

Features:

1. Exclusively focuses on quorum quenching and its ability to be used as an alternative to antibiotics in the control of multidrug-resistant pathogens.
2. Reviews the latest literature and case studies of the last ten years in the field of quorum sensing and quorum quenching.
3. Promotes a new approach to the development of the next generation of antibacterial drugs.
4. In the wake of rising antibiotic drug resistance, it is crucial to develop an alternative approach to control bacterial infection diseases and quorum quenching appears to be a promising strategy in the development of new medicines.

Perspectives of Quorum Quenching in New Drug Development

Edited By
Naga Raju Maddela
Venkataramana Thiriveedi
Rathna Silviya Lodi

CRC Press
Taylor & Francis Group
Boca Raton London New York

CRC Press is an imprint of the
Taylor & Francis Group, an **informa** business

First edition published 2024
by CRC Press
2385 Executive Center Drive, Suite 320, Boca Raton, FL 33431

and by CRC Press
4 Park Square, Milton Park, Abingdon, Oxon, OX14 4RN

CRC Press is an imprint of Taylor & Francis Group, LLC

Library of Congress Cataloging-in-Publication Data
Names: Maddela, Naga Raju, editor. | Thiriveedi, Venkataramana, editor. |
Lodi, Rathna Silviya, editor.
Title: Perspectives of quorum quenching in new drug development / edited by
Naga Raju Maddela, Venkataramana Thiriveedi, Rathna Silviya Lodi.
Description: First edition. | Boca Raton : CRC Press, 2024. | Includes
bibliographical references and index.
Identifiers: LCCN 2023051161 (print) | LCCN 2023051162 (ebook) | ISBN
9781032286457 (hbk) | ISBN 9781032286495 (pbk) | ISBN 9781003297826 (ebk)
Subjects: MESH: Drug Discovery--methods | Quorum Sensing | Biofilms--drug
effects | Drug Resistance, Bacterial--drug effects
Classification: LCC RM301.25 (print) | LCC RM301.25 (ebook) | NLM QV 745
| DDC 615.1/9--dc23/eng/20240124
LC record available at https://lccn.loc.gov/2023051161
LC ebook record available at https://lccn.loc.gov/2023051162

ISBN: 9781032286457 (hbk)
ISBN: 9781032286495 (pbk)
ISBN: 9781003297826 (ebk)

DOI: 10.1201/ 9781003297826

Typeset in Times
by Deanta Global Publishing Services, Chennai, India

Contents

Preface

In the constantly evolving drug discovery domain, endless efforts are made to fight infectious diseases, drug-resistant pathogens, and intricate microbial communities. One such endeavor, quorum quenching, has surfaced as an engrossing and promising path that could revolutionize medicine. In this book, we will explore the perspectives of quorum quenching in developing novel drugs, illuminating the significance of this innovative strategy. Quorum quenching is a biological occurrence that disrupts bacterial communication systems, specifically quorum sensing, a mechanism through which bacteria synchronize their actions based on population density. In quorum sensing, bacteria emit signaling molecules, like autoinducers, which instigate synchronized activities like expression of virulence factors or formation of biofilms upon reaching a certain threshold. Quorum quenching introduces a novel aspect in the fight against bacterial infections, as it specifically targets the fundamental communication systems that empower bacteria to organize and execute their deleterious activities. By impeding the quorum sensing process, researchers can neutralize the harmful effects of pathogens, thus reducing their virulence and enhancing their susceptibility to conventional antibiotic treatments.

The emergence of antibiotic-resistant bacteria poses a significant global health challenge. Quorum quenching offers a complementary strategy to traditional antibiotics by diminishing the pathogenic nature of bacteria. This approach can prolong the efficacy of existing antibiotics, thereby impeding the development of bacterial resistance. Bacterial biofilms are intricate structures that protect pathogens against immune responses and antimicrobial agents. Quorum quenching can disrupt the formation of biofilms, thereby rendering bacteria more susceptible to treatment and potentially paving the way for innovative therapies targeting chronic infections associated with biofilms. Quorum quenching can be customized to suit specific pathogens, rendering it a highly concentrated approach. This level of precision enables the development of therapies that aim to minimize any inadvertent harm endured by beneficial bacteria and host tissues, a notable obstacle encountered in conventional antibiotic treatments.

While quorum quenching is a promising avenue in drug development, it also brings forth specific challenges. The meticulous examination of the specificity of quorum quenching compounds and potential side effects is of utmost importance. Furthermore, the risk of inciting resistance to quorum quenching agents necessitates vigilant monitoring and mitigation. In the future, a more in-depth exploration of quorum quenching can be expected in the pursuit of developing groundbreaking drugs. This includes the design of synthetic quorum-sensing inhibitors and the discovery of natural compounds that exhibit properties conducive to quorum-quenching. Combining these endeavors with advancements in microbiome research may unveil novel therapeutic possibilities for various diseases.

Quorum quenching represents a cutting-edge approach with substantial potential to revolutionize drug development. By specifically targeting the communication systems that facilitate the coordination of harmful activities among bacteria, quorum quenching offers a distinctive method to combat infectious diseases, antibiotic resistance, and biofilm-related infections. Through ongoing research and innovation, this captivating avenue of exploration may shape medicine's future. As we embark on our foray into the unexplored realms of quorum quenching, the prospect of discovering novel and efficacious drugs for previously refractory infections beckons, evoking a sense of exhilaration and boundless possibilities.

The book consists of 12 chapters, which focus on the following topics: biofilms of pathogenic bacteria; biofilm regulation and quorum sensing in bacterial pathogens; quorum sensing in extremophiles; single- and dual-species biofilms of human pathogenic bacteria and the application of bacteriophages on biofilms; methods for extenuating biofilms-associated drug resistance by microtechnology and nanotechnology; ecological relevance of quorum quenching; quorum quenching in biofilm mitigation; the hypothalamic–pituitary–testicular axis in drug development for androgens across sex and lifespan; the GH–IGF1 axis and the hypothalamic–pituitary–testicular axis in drug development; reproductive endocrinology drug development hormones, metabolism, and fertility in female reproductive health; clinical trials and the approval process of novel drugs; and quorum quenching–based drug development. Forty contributors from eight different countries contributed to this book, which was edited by three subject experts.

Editors

Naga Raju Maddela earned his MSc (1996–1998) and PhD (2012) in microbiology from Sri Krishnadevaraya University, Anantapuramu, India. During his doctoral study in the area of environmental microbiology, he investigated the effects of industrial effluents/insecticides on soil microorganisms and their biological activities, and he has been working as a faculty member in microbiology since 1998, teaching undergraduate and postgraduate students. He received the Prometeo Investigator Fellowship (2013–2015) from Secretaría de Educación Superior, Ciencia, Tecnología e Innovación (SENESCYT), Ecuador; and a Postdoctoral Fellowship (2016–2018) from Sun Yat-sen University, China. He also received external funding from the China Postdoctoral Science Foundation in 2017; internal funding from Universidad Técnica de Manabí in 2020; worked in the area of environmental biotechnology; participated in 20 national/international conferences; and presented research data in China, Cuba, Ecuador, India, and Singapore. Since 2018, he has been working as a full professor at the Facultad de Ciencias de la Salud, Universidad Técnica de Manabí, Portoviejo, Ecuador. He has published 15 books, 40 chapters, and 80 research papers.

Venkataramana Thiriveedi completed his PhD (2018) at the University of Hyderabad, India. During his doctoral program, he focused on the biology of the electron transport chain in mitochondria. He identified an essential role for glutathionylated hMia40 (CHCHD4) in mitochondrial electron transport chain biogenesis. His studies shed light on a previously unknown posttranslational modification of hMIA40 that impacts reactive oxygen species levels and cellular redox homeostasis. He received the Indian Council of Medical Research–Senior Research Fellowship (ICMR-SRF), India. He also received an Award of Research Proficiency from the University of Hyderabad in recognition of publishing the research article in *Redox Biology*. He published four research papers during his doctoral program, participated in ten national and international conferences, presented research data in India and the USA, and presented his research data in Ecuador as an invited speaker. Currently, he is working as a postdoctoral associate at Duke University Medical Center, USA. During his postdoctoral training, he focused on how the commensal microbiota regulates intestinal stem cell function in epithelial tissue.

Ratna Silviya Lodi earned her BSc, MSc, and PhD in microbiology in the years 2009, 2011, and 2017, respectively, in India. During her doctoral thesis, she worked on molecular detection and evaluation of *Candida* sp, (albicans and non-albicans) from oral infections of diabetic patients. She finished her first postdoctoral research at Jiangsu University, China, during 2019–2021, where she investigated how GDF-15 promotes colorectal cancer development by upregulating the immune checkpoint TIGIT/CD-155. She has hands-on experience in microbiological and molecular biological techniques, particularly in the medical field. Currently, she is working as a postdoctoral research fellow at Shandong Academy of Agricultural Sciences, Jinan, Shandong Province, China, studying diversity, composition, antimicrobial, and anticancer activity of culturable microbial endophytes in *Panax quinquefolius* (American ginseng). To her credit, she has around 20 scientific publications and presented her data at more than ten international conferences.

Contributors

Babatunde Hadiyatullahi Ajao
Department of Animal Production,
University of Ilorin, Nigeria

Ulelu Jessica Akor
Faculty of Agriculture, University of
Abuja, Nigeria

S. Anju
Department of Microbiology, Bhavan's
Vivekananda College of Science,
Humanities and Commerce, Telangana,
India

Y. Aparna
Department of Microbiology, Bhavan's
Vivekananda College of Science,
Humanities and Commerce, Telangana,
India

Sevcan Aydin
Division of Biotechnology, Biology
Department, Faculty of Science,
Istanbul University, Turkey

Ebunoluwa Elizabeth Babaniyi
Biology Department, Obafemi Awolowo
University, Ife, Nigeria

Gabriel Gbenga Babaniyi
Department of Agricultural
Development and Management,
Agricultural and Rural Management
Training Institute (ARMTI), Nigeria

Jeongdong Choi
Department of Environmental
Engineering, Korean National
University of Transportation, Chungju,
South Korea

Mahmoud A. Elfaky
Department of Natural Products,
Faculty of Pharmacy, King Abdulaziz
University, Jeddah, Saudi Arabia
and
Centre for Artificial Intelligence in
Precision Medicines, King Abdulaziz
University, Jeddah, Saudi Arabia

Lucía I. Castellanos de Figueroa
PROIMI, CONICET (Planta Piloto de
Procesos Industriales Microbiológicos),
Tucumán, Argentina
and
Faculty of Biochemistry, Chemistry and
Pharmacy, Microbiology Department,
National University of Tucumán,
Argentina

Sabrin R. M. Ibrahim
Department of Chemistry, Batterjee
Medical College, Jeddah, Saudi Arabia
and
Department of Pharmacognosy, Faculty
of Pharmacy, Assiut University, Egypt

Ramkumar J
Department of Chemistry, Panimalar
Engineering College, Tamilnadu, India

SenthilKannan K
Department of Physics,
Saveetha School of Engineering,
SIMATS, Tamilnadu, India

Radha K S
Department of Chemistry,
R.M.D Engineering College,
Tamilnadu, India

Srinivasan Kameswaran
Department of Botany, Vikrama
Simhapuri University College,
Andhra Pradesh, India

Rasineni Karuna
Department of Internal Medicine,
University of Nebraska Medical Center,
Omaha, Nebraska, USA

Fawzeia Khamis
Department of Physics, Faculty of
Science, University of Tripoli, Libya

Shashank Kumar
Molecular Signaling & Drug
Discovery Laboratory, Department of
Biochemistry, Central University of
Punjab, India

Mariano J. Lacosegliaz
PROIMI, CONICET (Planta Piloto de
Procesos Industriales Microbiológicos),
Tucumán, Argentina

Vimalan M
Department of Physics, Saveetha School
of Engineering, SIMATS, Tamilnadu,
India

Balamurugapandian N
Department of Chemistry, Velammal
Engineering College, Tamilnadu, India

Carlos G. Nieto-Peñalver
PROIMI, CONICET (Planta Piloto de
Procesos Industriales Microbiológicos),
Tucumán, Argentina
and
Faculty of Biochemistry, Chemistry and
Pharmacy, Microbiology Department,
National University of Tucumán,
Argentina

Najla A. Obaid
Department of Pharmaceutics,
College of Pharmacy,
Umm Al-Qura University,
Mecca, Saudi Arabia

Sasikumar P
Department of Physics, Saveetha School
of Engineering, SIMATS, Tamilnadu,
India

Durbaka Vijaya Raghava Prasad
Department of Chemistry, Sogang
University, Seoul, South Korea

Divya R
Department of Physics, S.T. Hindu
College, Tamilnadu, India

Krishnaveni R
Visiting Scientist, Phoenix Group,
Tamilnadu, India

Bellemkonda Ramesh
Department of Internal Medicine,
University of Nebraska Medical Center,
Omaha, Nebraska, USA

Pallavali Roja Rani
Department of Environmental
Engineering, Korean National
University of Transportation, Chungju,
South Korea

Guda Dinneswara Reddy
Department of Chemistry, Sogang
University, Seoul, South Korea

Şuheda Reisoglu
Division of Biotechnology,
Biology Department,
Faculty of Science,
Istanbul University, Turkey

J. Sarada
Department of Microbiology, Bhavan's
Vivekananda College of Science,
Humanities and Commerce, Telangana,
India

J. Swathi
Biology Lab, IISER,
Thiruvananthapuram, India

Mariela A. Torres
PROIMI, CONICET (Planta Piloto de
Procesos Industriales Microbiológicos),
Tucumán, Argentina

Alejandra L. Valdez
PROIMI, CONICET (Planta Piloto de
Procesos Industriales Microbiológicos),
Tucumán, Argentina
and

Faculty of Biochemistry, Chemistry and
Pharmacy, Microbiology Department,
National University of Tucumán,
Argentina

Degati Vijayalakshmi
Department of Chemistry, Sogang
University, Seoul, South Korea

Carolina M. Viola
PROIMI, CONICET (Planta Piloto de
Procesos Industriales Microbiológicos),
Tucumán, Argentina

Reham Wasfi
Department of Microbiology and
Immunology, Faculty of Pharmacy,
October University for Modern Sciences
and Arts, Giza, Egypt

1 Biofilms of Pathogenic Bacteria

*Mahmoud A. Elfaky, Sabrin R. M. Ibrahim,
Najla A. Obaid, and Reham Wasfi*

1.1 BIOFILM: AN OVERVIEW

Biofilms are organized microbial communities that include cells embedded in an extracellular matrix (Flemming and Wuertz 2019). Biofilms are often generated to help microorganisms survive in tough conditions (Flemming et al. 2016). The biofilm lifestyle differs from that of free-living bacterial cells due to social and physical interactions between cells, as well as the matrix's features. As a result, biofilm communities exhibit emergent features that differ from free-living bacterial cells (Konopka 2009). Among these emergent features, the role of the self-produced extracellular polymeric substances (EPS) matrix, which is primarily composed of polysaccharides, proteins, lipids, and extracellular DNA (eDNA), and responsible for the formation of physical and social interactions, an increased rate of gene exchange, and an increased antimicrobial resistance (Flemming and Wingender 2010). The production of biofilm has been linked to chronic infections in plants and animals, including humans (Costerton et al. 2003), as well as the contamination of medical equipment and implants.

In some circumstances, matrix structural components may have other functions that help the biofilm. For instance, the curli protein, which, along with cellulose, contributes to the biofilm's desiccation tolerance, is the main structural component of the matrix in *Escherichia coli* biofilms, and the proteins called hydrophobins, used by *Bacillus subtilis* to form highly hydrophobic biofilms that float at the air–liquid interface (Hobley et al. 2015). The EPS matrix self-assembles into a liquid crystal structure in *Pseudomonas aeruginosa* biofilms by entropic interactions between polymers. Finally, external membrane vesicle-packaged enzymes in gram-negative bacteria can contribute to the matrix's degrading potential (Schooling and Beveridge 2006). As a result, the matrix is not merely an amorphous gel made up of polysaccharides, but rather a highly heterogeneous mixture of biopolymers that are responsible for its function and emergent properties (Hobley et al. 2015).

1.2 BIOFILM FORMATION AND ANTIBIOTIC RESISTANCE

One of the most important emerging features of biofilms is increased resistance or tolerance to antibiotics and other antimicrobial agents as compared to free-living bacterial cells (Flemming et al. 2016). Tolerance in biofilms might be a result of the

DOI: 10.1201/9781003297826-1

biofilm matrix's features, such as antimicrobial trapping or inactivation, as well as the slow microbial growth that can occur in biofilms. The EPS matrix could appear to be a diffusion barrier at first glance. Antimicrobials that do not interact with EPS molecules, on the other hand, have been found to diffuse easily through biofilms (Daddi Oubekka et al. 2012), thus the diffusion barrier alone is not nearly responsible for biofilms' reduced antibiotic sensitivity.

Quenching of the activity of antimicrobials is mediated by diffusion–reaction inhibition, which can involve complex formation by chelation or enzymatic degradation of antimicrobials (Daddi Oubekka et al. 2012).

Resistance due to biofilm is substantially greater than planktonic bacteria's antibiotic resistance (Hoyle and Costerton 1991). Biofilm-related infections are thus more difficult to treat and more likely to recur (Cerqueira and Peleg 2011). Biomedical experts are very interested in the link between biofilm and antibiotic resistance. Several studies have shown that small dosages of some antibiotics can cause biofilm development (Kaplan 2011), suggesting that biofilm regulation may play a role in the overall response to external stresses, such as antibiotics.

According to reports, biofilm-mediated antibiotic resistance may be due to the following factors (Figure 1.1) (Høiby et al. 2010): (a) a polymeric matrix that restricts antibiotic diffusion, (b) antibiotic interaction with a polymeric matrix that reduces antibiotic activity, (c) enzyme-mediated resistance such as β-lactamase, (d) alteration of metabolic activity within the biofilm, (e) genetic modification of target cells or hiding target sites, (f) efflux of antibiotics by efflux pumps, and (g) the existence of an outer membrane structure in gram-negative organisms (S. Singh et al. 2017).

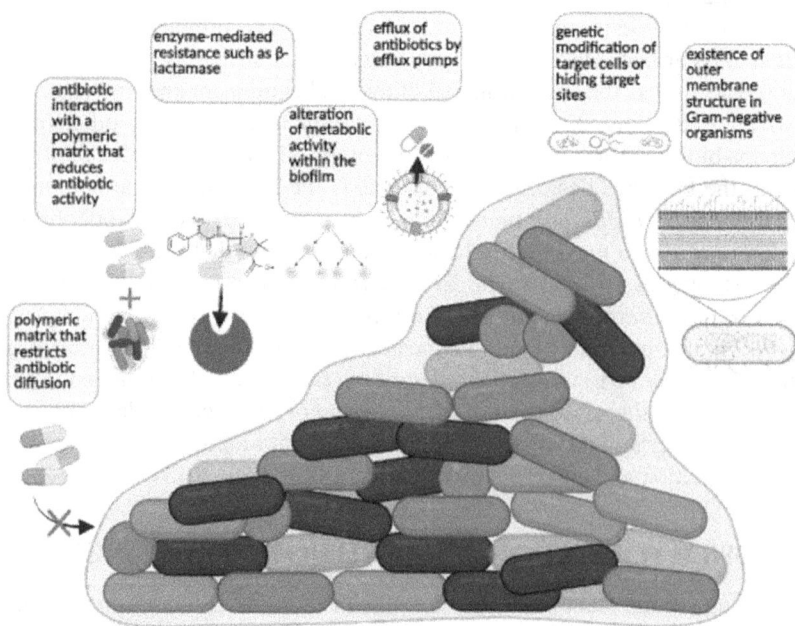

FIGURE 1.1   Mechanisms of biofilms-mediated antibiotic resistance.

The uptake of resistance genes through horizontal gene transfer (Mah 2012) is one way to increase the antimicrobial resistance of cells in biofilms. Biofilms have been claimed to provide an optimal environment of characteristics for successful horizontal gene transfer, including the uptake of resistance genes, due to their high cell density, greater genetic competence, and accumulation of mobile genetic elements (Fux et al. 2005). The matrix also serves as a source of DNA in the form of eDNA (Madsen et al. 2012) and offers a stable physical environment for cell-to-cell interaction, which is essential for various gene transfer methods. Plasmid conjugation is a frequent method of horizontal gene transfer in biofilms. In dual-species biofilms of *Pseudomonas putida* and *E. coli* (Meervenne et al. 2014), for example, plasmids carrying genes conferring antibiotic resistance were easily transferred. In general, conjugation in biofilms has been demonstrated to be 700 times more effective than in free-living bacterial cells (Król et al. 2013). Other research on *S. aureus* found that conjugal plasmid transfer was observed in biofilms but not in cultures of free-living bacterial cells (Savage et al. 2013), demonstrating yet another example of biofilm behavior that is not feasible in free-living bacterial cells.

The biofilm matrix could become the target of potential antimicrobial drugs if researchers can figure out how the biofilm produces and maintains its structural integrity (Hobley et al. 2015). For example, using the fundamental understanding of polysaccharides and adhesins required for biofilm formation, much effort is being put toward developing new vaccines for *Staphylococcus aureus* (Jansen et al. 2013).

1.3 MICROBIAL BIOFILMS ASSOCIATED WITH CHRONIC INFECTIONS

Biofilm formation is an essential survival mechanism for bacteria in almost any environment including the human host. This phenotype provides bacteria within its matrix with protection against the immune defense and antimicrobial treatment (Fazeli-Nasab et al. 2022). Biofilms are dynamic and responsive to their environment. Thus, they can adapt to changes in their environment in the host body and in the hospital environment (Paula et al. 2020). Over 80% of microbial infections in the body are caused by biofilm, according to the US National Institutes of Health. Therefore, biofilms are resistant to antimicrobial treatment (Kolpen et al. 2022).

It was thought a long time ago that acute infections were usually caused by planktonic bacteria and therefore susceptible to treatment, while chronic infections were due to biofilm formation and therefore resistant to treatment (Bjarnsholt et al. 2013). Recent research has shown that microscopic analysis of specimens taken from acute and chronic infections contain biofilm, which was evidence of the existence of biofilm phenotypes in both acute and chronic infections. The difference between bacteria in both phenotypes was the metabolic rate (Kolpen et al. 2022; Chakraborty et al. 2020). Chronic infections associated with biofilm include but are not limited to cystic fibrosis, infective endocarditis, diabetic foot ulcers, chronic wounds, catheter-associated infections, and eye infections.

1.3.1 Cystic Fibrosis

Cystic fibrosis (CF) is a progressive genetic disease caused by mutations in the cystic fibrosis transmembrane conductance regulator (CFTR) gene. This mutation makes the CFTR protein dysfunctional and thus unable to move chloride to the cell. Mucus in various organs become thick and sticky due to a deficiency in chloride on the cell surface, which hinders water attraction to the cell (Brown et al. 2017). CF lung disease is characterized by inflammation overlaid with a chronic bacterial infection in the biofilm form (Martin et al. 2021). More than 70,000 people worldwide suffer from cystic fibrosis ("About Cystic Fibrosis | Cystic Fibrosis Foundation" 2022). Biofilms in the CF lung are very resistant to antibiotic treatment, which contributes to the overall economic impact of CF and reaches an annual cost of $7500 million a year (Cámara et al. 2022). The two most common pathogens complicating CF are *Pseudomonas aeruginosa* and *Staphylococcus aureus*, in addition to other organisms such as *Burkholderia* spp., non-tuberculous *Mycobacteria* (NTM) spp., *Stenotrophomonas maltophilia*, *Achromobacter* spp., as well as fungi such as *Aspergillus* spp. The presence of bacteria in biofilm form in the CF lung is supported by several pieces of evidence including the observation of clusters of bacterial cells, similar to microcolonies of biofilm in immunostaining studies performed on the lung tissue (Baltimore et al. 2012) and sputum of CF patients. Additional evidence is the presence of quorum-sensing molecules in CF sputum in the same ratio for their detection in bacterial biofilm (P. K. Singh et al. 2000). Quorum-sensing inhibitors became a promising alternative for the treatment of CF lung infections (Scoffone et al. 2019).

1.3.2 Infective Endocarditis

Infective endocarditis (IE) includes infection of the inner surface of the heart (the endocardium, especially heart valves) or those residing on implanted cardiac devices (Lerche et al. 2021). The incidence of infective endocarditis is rising with an estimated annual economic impact of $16 billion globally (Cámara et al. 2022). The mortality rate of patients with IE is considerably high, reaching 25% and more than one-third of patients die within a year (Holland et al. 2016; Østergaard et al. 2019). Microlesions in the endocardium initiate microbial adherence and biofilm formation, while intact endothelium is resistant to microbial colonization. Such colonization can occur by opportunistic bacteria. This infection is usually caused predominately by bacteria including gram-positive bacteria such as *Staphylococcus* sp., *Streptococcus* sp., and *Enterococcus* spp. accounting for more than 80% of cases (Østergaard et al. 2019). Less frequently, endocardium could be infected by gram-negative bacteria such as the HACEK group (*Aggregatibacter* [formerly *Haemophilus*] *aphrophilus/paraaphrophis*, *Aggregatibacter actinomycetemcomitans*, *Cardiobacterium hominis*, *Eikenella corrodens*, and *Kingella* spp.), while infection by fungi is rare (Liesman et al. 2017). The inflammatory response induced by established infection results in further damage to the heart valve, thus worsening the condition (Werdan et al. 2013).

1.3.3 CHRONIC WOUND INFECTIONS

Chronic wounds (CWs) is the term used to describe non-healing injuries such as diabetic foot ulcers, venous leg ulcers, and nonhealing surgical site infections. Caring for chronic wounds in the UK creates a financial burden of US$3.4–4.6 billion a year, while in the USA the spending on wound care reached $35.3 billion in 2014, of which $26.3 billion was spent on infections and chronic ulcers (Gupta et al. 2017). Deep injuries are usually associated with infections due to the intrusion of bacteria into deeper layers and the colonization of deep tissues, which initiates the formation of biofilm. Biofilms have been reported to be in 80% of chronic wounds (Kim et al. 2019). The poor oxygenation of deep wound tissues in addition to the adherence of microorganisms to the wound bed surface facilitates the development of biofilm in the wound (Kim et al. 2019). The exopolysaccharide matrix of biofilm protects the bacteria within the biofilm from the attaching of macrophages and dendritic cells as well as antimicrobial treatment thus delaying the healing process and developing chronic wounds (Mendoza et al. 2019). Biofilm delays the healing of wounds because it creates persistent inflammation and impairs epithelization and granulation. Chronic wounds can be colonized by numerous bacterial species, that belong to the *Enterobacteriaceae* family, *Staphylococcaceae* family, or *Pseudomonadaceae* family.

1.3.4 INDWELLING MEDICAL CATHETERS

Indwelling medical catheters have become part of modern medical practice to save lives, however, they are risk factors for the development of healthcare-associated infections (HAIs). They account for two of the main HAIs, namely, catheter-associated urinary tract infections (CAUTIs) and central venous line catheter bloodstream infections (Neoh et al. 2017). The global annual cost of infections due to central venous line catheters and urinary catheters has been estimated to be $11.5 billion and $1 billion, respectively (Cámara et al. 2022). Catheters connect the normally sterile, hydrated body site to the outside world; therefore, they could transfer microorganisms that migrate along their surface to the inside of the body (Trautner and Darouiche 2004). Microorganisms colonizing catheters could be originating from the host normal flora (e.g., from the flora of the skin or mucosal membrane) or from exogenous sources such as other patients or health care personnel and contaminated fomites (Gastmeier et al. 2005). Colonizing microorganisms on the central line catheter depend on the source of contamination, and they belong to four groups as follows: coagulase-negative staphylococci, *Staphylococcus aureus*, enteric gram-negative bacilli, and *Candida* spp. (Gominet et al. 2017), while various bacterial and yeast strains can lead to CAUTIs. Adsorbed protein on the catheter surface facilitates the binding of microorganisms to catheters forming a biofilm. Colonization of the medical catheters is initiated as early as 24 hours after catheterization (Mermel 2011). Biofilms are known to have a role in catheter blockage, commonly caused by the presence of urease-producing bacteria such as *Proteus mirabilis*, *Proteus vulgaris*, and *Providencia rettgeri* (Wasfi et al. 2020). Interestingly, catheter blockage can also occur by bacteria that do not produce crystals such as *Klebsiella pneumoniae* and *Pseudomonas aeruginosa*. Consequently, they can cause the same problems associated with halted bladder drainage (Stickler 2014).

Catheter encrustation can cause numerous unfavorable outcomes for patients. Encrusted catheters become blocked, leading to urine retention that is not just painful for the patient but also constitutes a medical emergency (Feneley et al. 2015).

1.3.5 BIOFILM IN EYE INFECTIONS

Biofilm infections can present in the eye and eyelids, but also because of contact lenses and artificial lenses introduced during cataract surgery (Bispo et al. 2015). The annual global cost of eye conditions associated with biofilms is in the region of $759.3 million (Cámara et al. 2022). The introduction of eye lenses can lead to many ocular infections that can progress into permanent sequelae of impaired vision or loss of sight (Bispo et al. 2015). Eye surgeries could also introduce microorganisms to the eye causing infections such as endophthalmitis. Normal flora residing on the ocular surface include gram-positive organisms, with coagulase-negative staphylococci, followed by *Propionibacterium acnes*, *Corynebacterium* spp., and *S. aureus* (Willcox 2013). Cataract surgery could result in infection of the anterior chamber ranging from 2% to 46% and is usually caused by gram-positive commensal organisms found on the ocular surface, most frequently *S. epidermidis* (Bausz et al. 2006).

Contact lens (CL) wear is the most important risk factor for bacterial keratitis infections (Fleiszig and Evans 2010). Wearing contact lenses is associated with changes in the ocular microbiota and predisposition to microbial keratitis. *Pseudomonas* spp. is the predominant cause of CL-related microbial keratitis (El-Ganiny et al. 2017), followed by *Staphylococcus* spp. and *Serratia* spp. (Willcox et al. 2012). In addition to bacteria, fungi and *Acanthamoeba* spp. are also capable of causing contact lens-associated keratitis (Szentmáry et al. 2019).

1.4 PHENOTYPIC AND GENOTYPIC DETECTION OF BIOFILM FORMATION

The development of biofilms is a dynamic process that is likely an innate behavioral mechanism shared by most bacterial species (O'Toole et al. 2000). However, this process is brought on by many factors, mainly environmental stressors and genetic attributes of each bacterial species. Biofilm inducers include nutrient availability, physical stress, immune response (Walker et al. 2005), and antibiotics (Abdallah et al. 2014). The main aspect inside a living thing is the defense mechanism and the host's immune system against any irritant. The formation of a biofilm inside host tissue significantly enhances the acquisition of immune cells that are resistant. The acquisition of nutrients, defense against the immune system and antibiotics/disinfectants, stationary growth, protected communities as sources for detachment, metabolic cell connecting, and genetic material exchange are all factors that increase or decrease the formation of biofilms. Since nutrients are abundant inside living things, they are not a major factor inside a living organism. Nutrient deprivation could be a major effector to the biofilm formation on abiotic (nonliving) surfaces but not for the biofilm formed on biotic surfaces (living tissues).

In a biofilm, bacteria may disengage, thereby providing an ability for protected forms to be retained while simultaneously allowing the species to spread and explore new niches. Also, when environmental conditions favor dispersal (e.g., nutrient deprivation, antibiotic insult) (Rumbaugh and Sauer 2020), many bacterial species initiate a programmed response of detachment where some bacteria are dispersed from the biofilm and are able to find more favorable conditions while possessing bacterial-resistance phenotypes (Rumbaugh and Sauer 2020).

Many approaches used to detect biofilm are based on the identification of dispersed cells that migrate from the biofilm core to understand the behavior of the biofilm that caused the problems related to biofilms such as antimicrobial resistance and immune cell confliction. To discuss the behavior of the biofilm, we need to understand the factors that controlled the formation of biofilm such as the phenotypic (biofilm formation ability) and genotypic (quorum-sensing signaling) determinants (Guzmán-Soto et al. 2021). Microscopy, cell infection models, and more contemporary molecular, cellular, and immunological assays are examples of traditional microbiological in vitro techniques (Balouiri et al. 2016). Different components of bacterial culture media can affect bacterial phenotypes, including early adhesion on the surface, biofilm development, or gene expression (Kostakioti et al. 2013). To understand these factors and assist in detecting biofilm and to be more efficient in translating the result to the clinical situation regarding the biofilm infection, we need to select effective assays that replicate the biological condition. These assays may be performed both in vitro and in vivo to overcome any factors that can affect the phenotype of the isolated microorganism and reduce the ability to detect the biofilm formation that caused biofilm-associated infection (BAI).

1.4.1 In Vitro Protocols and In Vivo Study of Biofilm

It is important to study the microorganism that causes BAI to identify a biofilm from a clinical sample. The accurate and rapid diagnosis of the BAI benefits the rapid identification of the cause of infection and therefore rapid treatment. According to Parsek–Singh criteria, biofilm infection has to be associated with a surface (Parsek and Singh 2003). Examination of the site of infection shows an aggregation of cells enclosed within a matrix, confined to a particular site in the host, recalcitrance to antibiotic treatment, culture-negative results, and ineffective host clearance (Hall-Stoodley and Stoodley 2009; Jahan et al. 2022). In addition to these criteria, studies also suggest insufficient diagnosis based only on culture and conventional diagnostic sampling (Hall-Stoodley and Stoodley 2009; Hall-Stoodley et al. 2012). Thus using genotypic approaches to amplify bacterial DNA in the sample such as the polymerase chain reaction (PCR) technique and the nucleic acid amplification test (NAAT) (Barken et al. 2007) provide evidence of the presence of bacteria forming a biofilm although if the culture results were negative. Amplification of the bacterial DNA or mRNA in a sample and using sequencing by whole-genome shotgun sequencing (WGSS) provide strong evidence of unculturable and biofilm-associated infection (Weaver et al. 2019; Ponraj et al. 2022).

1.4.2   MOLECULAR AND CELLULAR VIABILITY METHODS TO DETECT BIOFILM

A diagnostic method was proposed earlier by Costetron (2012), which is the detection of antigens related to biofilm infection by using immune staining. Multiplex is the combination of the PCR and immune test which was introduced and provides benefits for BAI (Costerton 2012). The combination of PCR and immunofluorescence staining was then progressed and the interest in this method of detecting biofilm (Tang et al. 2020).

Also, microscopy was determined as a superior technique to diagnose BAI according to Hall-Stoodley et al. (2012). The surface-associated biofilm structure has been extensively studied using microscopy for the structural and ultrastructural composition of the biofilm. Destructive and nondestructive methods have been applied in recent years to investigate the formation of biofilm on abiotic and biotic surfaces. For example, confocal microscopy using a laser provides a precise identification of bacterial cluster cells and differentiates the live/dead cells using specific fluorescence probes (Wilson et al. 2017; Hall-Stoodley et al. 2012). Viable quantification of dead/live cells and determination of the viable cell count in the biofilm is considered as one of the direct observations to detect biofilm. The colony-forming unit (CFU) is a standard method to detect the presence of viable cells that form the structure of biofilm (Wilson et al. 2017). Colonies on the plates are enumerated, and the number of cells per milliliter (cfu/mL) is determined after incubation (often 24–72 hours) (Wilson et al. 2017). Optical density (OD) is measured prior to plating to produce a calibration curve used to connect cell quantity with absorbance. This enumeration is a particularly helpful quantification technique in pure cultures. Thus, the absorbance of a sample with an unknown cell number can be evaluated in subsequent studies to calculate the cell concentration (Wilson et al. 2017).

1.4.3   IMAGING TECHNIQUES FOR DETECTION OF BIOFILM

As discussed in the previous section, the traditional culture method of the sample mainly gives a false negative. Therefore, other advanced techniques for faster diagnosis of BAI include fluorescence in situ hybridization assay (FISH) (Hardy et al. 2015), immunoblotting and separation of immunogens by two-dimensional gel electrophoresis (2DG) (Tang et al. 2020), and matrix-assisted laser desorption ionization–time of flight (MALDI-TOF), which are also separation techniques used for identification of proteins such as antigens of specific bacterial cells to ensure the colonization of cells as the cause of infection (Silva et al. 2021). However, these biofilm detection methods may not be applied in the routine diagnostic laboratory to identify biofilm from clinical samples because these protocols are expensive and demand highly qualified technical expertise.

Imaging of the device-associated infection (DAI) by using magnetic resonance imaging (MRI) and computed tomography (CT) scan help to investigate and detect the infection to conclude with the other microbiological investigations that biofilm could be the cause of infection. These methods currently used for the diagnosis of biofilm-related infection are still not providing a quick diagnosis and practitioners need a faster method.

It has been demonstrated that low-intensity ultrasonication by ultrasonic bath with subsequent sonicate culturing increases culture sensitivity (Hall-Stoodley et al. 2012). Ultrasonication releases bacteria that would otherwise stay connected to the surface and break away associated biofilm, increasing the sensitivity of the culture (Miller et al. 2018). However, because sonication is carried out with a saline buffer, it is possible that it may also affect the physiology of released bacteria, converting them to be more easily culturable planktonic phenotype (Trampuz et al. 2007). To avoid the culture method issues, sonication can help to disturb the biofilm matrix and allow the cells to grow in traditional media and become easily identifiable and countable. However, this method would not be helpful in some cases with issues in sampling and contamination of other microorganisms from the site of infection.

1.4.4 In Vivo Study of Biofilm

Animal models are frequently employed to further assess potential candidates discovered through the use of in vitro models. The in vivo models using animals or part of tissues are not as straightforward, affordable, or high throughput as in vitro studies. The existence of the host immune system is the primary distinction between in vivo and in vitro models (Guzmán-Soto et al. 2021). It is crucial that these models mimic in vivo biological conditions to enhance our understanding of the virulence of biofilms since biofilm infection is mostly related to chronic infection (Bjarnsholt et al. 2013).

However, it is challenging to duplicate the prolonged inflammatory response and extensive antibiotic therapy of chronic biofilm infection in animal models (Bjarnsholt et al. 2013). Animal models using precolonized implants to grow biofilm models are favored because these models have the benefit of being able to manage the inoculum on the implant prior to insertion. Some studies used silicone implant models using precolonized silicone tubes to observe how immune cells and the biofilm interact (van Gennip et al. 2012). These models are also very beneficial in studying the effect of antibiofilm materials on the formation of biofilm on the surfaces of implants after loading bacteria prior to implanting them into the animal models (Manav et al. 2020). However, in terms of spatial aggregation imaging of biofilm, the in vivo biofilm appears smaller in aggregate diameter than the in vitro biofilm when studying chronic biofilm models (Bjarnsholt et al. 2013). Therefore, when linking in vitro data to in vivo biofilms, it is crucial to understand the limitations of the present in vitro systems and to formulate the appropriate questions.

Animal models usually encounter many difficulties such as ethics approval, which is time-consuming, and sometimes the experiments are not approved and then have to be discontinued. Therefore, there have been recent studies of biofilm using other biological systems such as the nematode model (*Caenorhabditis elegans*) (Lima et al. 2020), and using these models to investigate the effect of antibiofilm and quorum-sensing inhibitors for different gram-negative biofilm-forming bacterial species (Liu et al. 2020). Some other models were also adopted to study the virulence of bacterial and biofilm formation in the *Drosophila melanogaster* model (Wongsaroj et al. 2018). The advantages of these models are the simplicity of handling and the low costs of such an approach. Additionally, the models' small size makes them simple,

making them a useful approach for comprehending the interaction between pathogens and hosts.

Based on the consistency between results from in vitro biofilm (e.g., microtiter
plate assay) and from in vivo observations in representative animal models, we can
conclude a link between in vitro and infectious biofilms. The differences between in
vivo models and some in vitro models with flow cells are related to the discrepancies
between the host and the flow cell's microenvironment, or the substrate and mass
transfer limitations from the biofilm structure (Bjarnsholt et al. 2013). Optimization
of the in vitro flow cell study to mimic the in vivo experimental conditions is the
most important advice given in the literature by biofilm experts in the last decade
to improve the biofilm chronic infection investigations (Bjarnsholt et al. 2013). This
optimization of in vitro flow cell studies is possible by developing imaging techniques and improving microfluidic techniques to study biofilm formation that aid in
better detection of biofilm infection. The microfluidic flow system in vitro study is
discussed in the following section.

1.4.5 TRADITIONAL METHODS OF IN VITRO VERSUS MICROFLUIDIC METHODS

Traditional biofilm detection methods are conducted by performing experiments
to confirm the biofilm formation, quantifications, and assessments on the development of biofilm. These in vitro experiments are based on qualitative and quantitative
characterization of biofilm usually by staining of the biofilm material (EPS) after
growing this material into tools such as polystyrene microplate wells or glass tubes
(Christensen et al. 1985). These methods have been developed over the last three
decades to investigate the biofilm formation and slime production of bacterial cells,
and to explore the effect of antibiofilm agents (Boudarel et al. 2018). The in vitro
models are categorized into two main groups based on the status of the fluid and
nutrients. Static or closed systems and dynamic or open systems create the main
scheme of the in vitro biofilm. The static model is mainly with limited nutrients
and oxygen supplying the biofilm structure and should be renewed and resupplied
(Guzmán-Soto et al. 2021). A summary diagram (Figure 1.2) shows the comparison
between the biofilm analysis approaches.

1.4.6 STAINING ASSAYS BY USING STATIC AND FLOW METHODS

Qualitative and quantitative detection methods for biofilm adherence were evaluated
and compared to establish a relatively easy and inexpensive in vitro static approach
(Mathur et al. 2006). The Congo Red Agar (CRA) method, microtiter plate (MTP)
assay, tube method (TM), and bioluminescent assay were evaluated using clinical
isolates that indicated that MTP assay was superior in terms of quantitation and reliability compared to the other qualitative methods (Hassan et al. 2011; Stepanović
et al. 2007; Silva et al. 2021). MTP assay may be one of the most reliable assays
useful for phenotypic diagnostic detection of biofilm for BAI (Bhardwaj et al. 2018;
Kuinkel et al. 2021). These assays are considered static methods and the main drawback for them is the need for resupplementing the nutrients to reach optimum biofilm

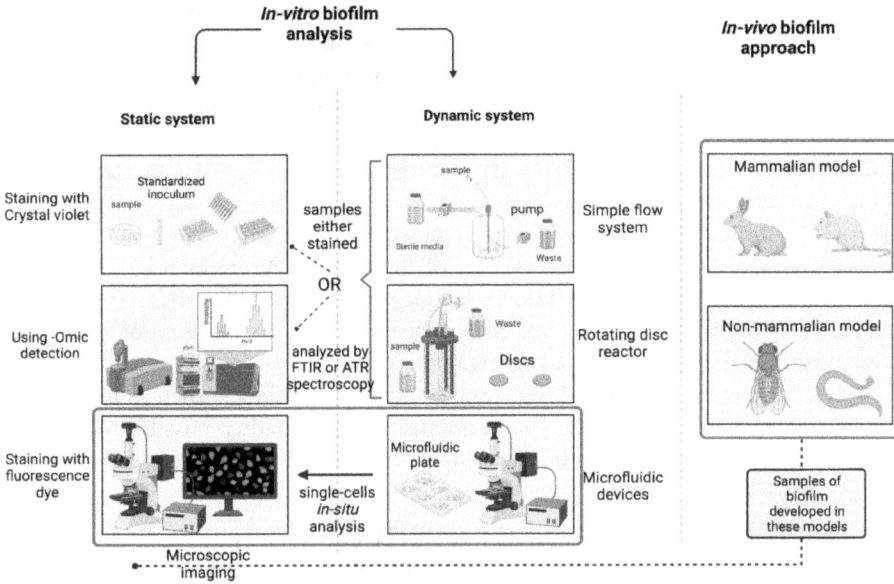

FIGURE 1.2 An overview of in vitro and in vivo approaches to study biofilm, and to detect in situ, investigate biofilm formation, or detect biofilm structure.

growth. Polystyrene makes up the majority of the adhering surfaces employed in static models when glass predominates in a contentious manner utilized for dynamic assays (Pouget et al. 2021).

Detecting biofilm formation with dynamic methods is performed by the flow cell assays. The flow system, also called the open system, focuses and depends on the ability of the microbial cells to adhere and form biofilm on the surfaces of a device or other biological cell lines. The amount of fluid and the sheer force of the flow may determine the degree of biofilm adherence, thus the biofilm formed on the surface. One system introduced in the mid-1990s was developed by Xu et al. (1998) who applied a "drip-flow reactor" to study the spatial physiological patterns of biofilms. Another system was developed in the early 2000s called the "rotating disc reactor". This system involved the flow of nutrients and the introduction of inoculated bacteria onto discs, which were then subjected to spatial imaging to visualize the formation of biofilm (Pitts et al. 2001). Another reactor was developed to compose several discs immersed in a 500 ml container to aid in the nutrient flow and formation of biofilm. This reactor is called the "CDC biofilm reactor" with coupons containing metallic discs that are used for analysis by attenuated total reflectance (ATR) Fourier transform infrared (FTIR) spectroscopy (Donlan et al. 2004).

1.4.7 MICROFLUIDIC METHODS

Microfluidic devices were introduced in the field of biofilm formation by using biochip microchannels with different sheer flow velocities (Lee et al. 2008). Biomedical companies then started to develop microfluidic devices to apply more control and to help the investigators. One of the systems introduced in the 2010s was the BioFlux device (Fluxion Biosciences) for the viability screening of flow biofilm (Benoit et al. 2010). This microfluidic system offers a high-throughput ability for flow cells with a micro volume of fluid including the nutrient supplies and the microbial inoculum, and is compatible with single-cells in situ analysis (Azeredo et al. 2016). This enables follow-up with converted light microscopy and a microplate for 24 replicates (Azeredo et al. 2016). Hence this device is very useful for screening biofilm-inhibitory substances, antibodies, or other substances. The high operating cost of the BioFlux system is the only disadvantage of the system (Azeredo et al. 2016). The general applicability of microfluidic techniques in the flow cell assays has some difficulties in being widely applied because of the complexity of the technology and the prerequisite skills for successful employment.

The achievement of new and improved hardware techniques, such as microfluidics flow techniques and high-resolution microscopy, has made it possible to examine the physiology of cells and the interactions within a biofilm with many details.

1.5 NATURAL COMPOUNDS INHIBITING BIOFILM FORMATION

Various cultures have employed herbal remedies and natural metabolites for centuries to counteract and treat infectious illnesses (Anand et al. 2019; Dhama et al. 2018; Lau and Plotkin 2013). Plants, fungi, and marine organisms revealed their potential as wealthy pools of new metabolites for fighting versus biofilms formation by different bacterial strains (Lu et al. 2019). Many of these metabolites have proven to prohibit quorum sensing (QS) and regulate the formation of biofilm (Asfour 2018; Kouidhi et al. 2015; Artini et al. 2012). It was reported that natural metabolites could prohibit biofilm formation through various aspects, including prohibiting polymer matrix formation and peptidoglycan synthesis, ECM (extracellular matrix) generation interruption, attachment, and cell adhesion repression, damaging the structure of the microbial membrane, and the reduction of virulence-factors production, therefore blocking QS network and developing of biofilm (Mu et al. 2018; Asfour 2018; Artini et al. 2012). Fortunately, some of them have revealed substantial capacity for ameliorating or preventing various infectious illnesses in clinical and preclinical assessments. Increasing the biofilm-derived microbial resistance necessitates a need for developing new antibiofilm from natural sources. In the current work, a brief account of some of the recently reported natural biofilm inhibitors was given. These metabolites could serve as effective therapeutic agents for improving the anti-infectious efficiency versus biofilm-linked infections (Figures 1.3 and 1.4).

Essential oils, phenolics, terpenoids, alkaloids, lectins, polyacetylenes, and polypeptides possessed significant antibiofilm potential (Yong et al. 2019). Among the phenolics, tannins, particularly condensed tannins, revealed antibiofilm capacity (Trentin et al. 2011).

Recently, increasing oral candidiasis incidence has contributed to the increase in the prevalence of HIV infection, organ transplantation, and diabetes, as well as the use of dentures, and anti-cancer, corticosteroid, and broad-spectrum antibiotics

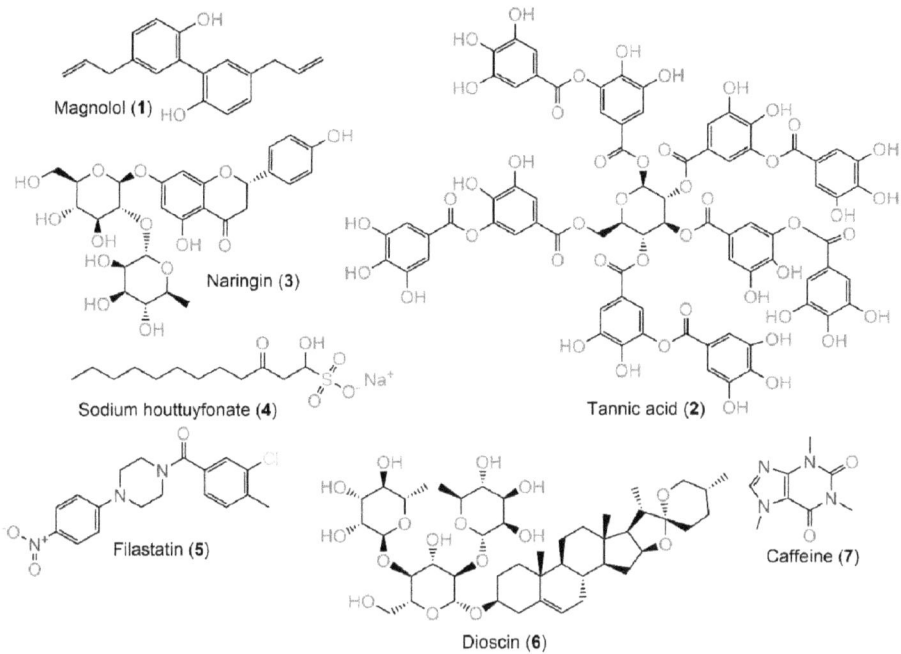

FIGURE 1.3 Chemical structures of antibiofilm natural metabolites.

usage (Chanda et al. 2017). Its management represents a remarkable problem due to the potential toxicity of clinically utilized antifungals and drug resistance development. The reported polyphenol from *Magnolia officinalis bark*, magnolol was assessed versus various oral and standard *Candida* spp. isolates. It was revealed that magnolol demonstrated marked antifungal (MICs 16.0–64.0 μg/mL) and antibiofilm potential versus four tested strains with an average of 69.5% inhibition. It also caused plasma membrane and cell wall rupture, intracellular content release, and cell wall swelling. Additionally, it had less hemolytic effectiveness (%lysis = 11.9%) versus red blood cells compared to amphotericin B (%lysis = 25.4%). Its effect was due to interaction with fungal cell wall ergosterol as evidenced by the molecular docking study (Behbehani et al. 2017). Further, it revealed notable inhibition on yeast hyphal transition, adhesion, and biofilm forming by *C. albicans* (L. Sun et al. 2015). It also displayed synergism with azoles versus *C. albicans* (L. M. Sun et al. 2015).

In 2018, Dong et al. proved that tannic acid, a phenolic compound, had a remarkable antibiofilm effectiveness at sub-minimum inhibitory concentrations (MICs) versus *S. aureus* by targeting peptidoglycan, destroying the cell wall integrity. Hence, it could be an effective potential candidate for treating infections caused by multidrug-resistant *S. aureus* (Mu et al. 2018). Another study by D. Wu et al. (2010) verified that it also prohibited FabG (β-ketoacyl-ACP-reductase), a substantial enzyme in the bacterial synthesis of fatty acids.

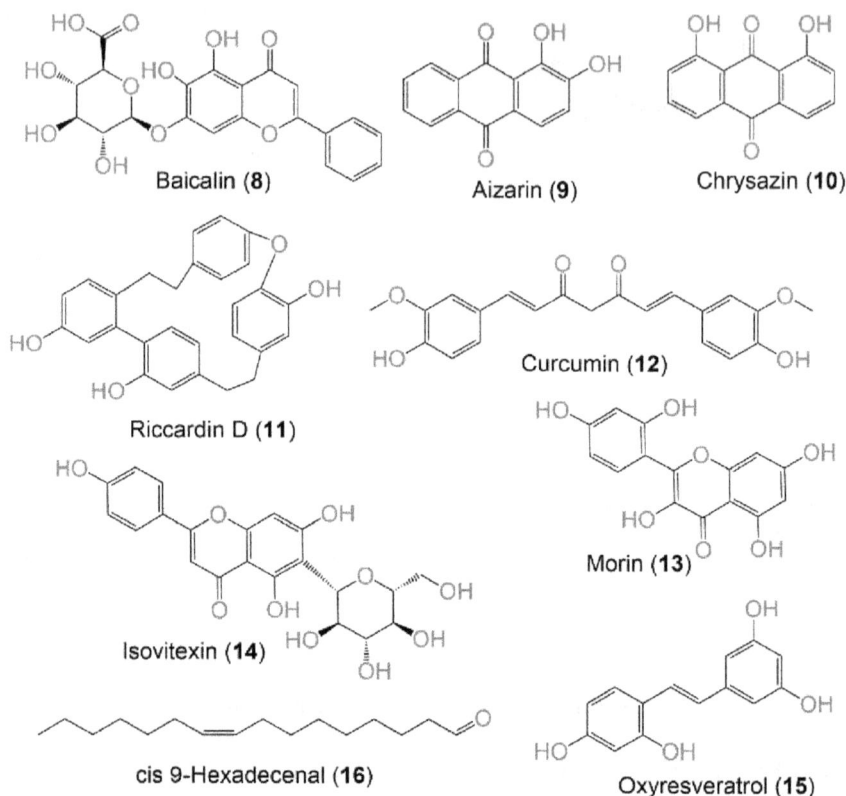

FIGURE 1.4 Chemical structures of antibiofilm natural metabolites.

The flavanone glycoside, naringin separated from grape and citrus fruits demonstrated more efficient biofilms influence versus *P. aeruginosa* compared to tetracycline and ciprofloxacin (Dey et al. 2020). It was found to deplete EPS biofilm, accelerate antimicrobial diffusion, lessen pellicle formation, and diminish the bacteria flagellar movement on catheter surfaces (Dey et al. 2020). Its combination with antibiotics could be beneficial for emerging efficacious topical antimicrobials, as well as in catheter wrapping to counteract biofilm-accompanied infection because of catheterization (Dey et al. 2020).

Additionally, sodium houttuyfonate biosynthesized by *Houttuynia cordata* promisingly prohibited the motility and biofilm formation of *P. aeruginosa*. Also, it notably hindered *S. epidermidis* and *C. albicans* biofilm formation (Shao et al. 2012; Shao et al. 2013) and acted synergistically with levofloxacin and Na_2-EDTA versus biofilm formation (Shao et al. 2012; M. Zhao et al. 2015). In in vitro study, it efficiently hindered *P. aeruginosa* biofilm dispersion and the main biofilm regulator BdlA (biofilm-dispersion-locus A) gene and protein expression. Therefore, it penetrated *P. aeruginosa* biofilm, resulting in the repression of the life cycle of biofilm (Thi Viet Huong et al. 2019).

It is noteworthy that diverse metabolites biosynthesized by various actinomycetes species revealed antibiofilm potential via interrupting the cell wall and interaction among cells (Azman et al. 2019).

Fazly et al. (2013) stated that filastatin prohibited the yeast-to-hyphal transition and impeded the fungal cells' adhesion to various biomaterials through repression of *HWP1*, a hyphal-specific promoter. Interestingly, its combination with fluconazole safeguarded *Caenorhabditis elegans* versus infection of *C. albicans* in vivo. It also suppressed biofilm development in vulvovaginal *Candida*-infected mice.

Dioscin, a natural saponin, separated from *Dioscorea panthaica* compound repressed *C. albicans* virulence factors, extracellular phospholipase production, yeast-to-hyphal transition, adherence to abiotic surfaces, and biofilm production. It even reduced the preformed biofilm viability at high concentrations (Yang et al. 2018).

Caffeine displayed marked antimicrobial capacity (MIC 200 µg/mL) versus *P. aeruginosa*. It revealed significant repression (conc. 40 and 80 µg/mL) of *P. aeruginosa* biofilm developing through interfering with *P. aeruginosa* QS by swarming motility targeting as it was found to interact with QS proteins (LasI and LasR), as well as it diminished the virulence-factors secretion. Nevertheless, it can be further developed as an antibiofilm agent for controlling *P. aeruginosa*–produced infection (Chakraborty et al. 2020).

Baicalin is one of the major flavones purified from *Scutellaria baicalensis* root (Q. Zhao et al. 2016). It minimized the expression of H-NS (histone-like nucleoid-structuring) and rpoS (RNA polymerase sigma S) genes via AI-2 (autoinducer-2) production prohibition, leading to QS system suppression (Guan et al. 2015). It also disturbed curli pili development by interference with the curli-particular genes (csgB and csgA), which negatively influenced bacterial binding and biofilm formation (Peng et al. 2019). In another study, it was established to suppress type 1 pili production through the reduction of fimB gene expression. The *Burkholderia cepacian* gene, *CepI*, boosts the AHL (N-acyl-homoserine lactone) signaling molecule production, C8-HSL (N-octanoyl-homoserine lactone) and C6-HSL (N-hexanoyl-homoserine lactone) (Brackman et al. 2009), whereas these molecules enhanced the QS system by complex formation with their receptors (Slachmuylders et al. 2018). *CepI* inhibition by baicalin repressed biofilm developing by QS system suppression, preventing the bacterial cells from binding to body surfaces (Slachmuylders et al. 2018).

Manoharan et al. (2017) stated that the anthraquinone derivatives alizarin (1,2-dihydroxyanthraquinone) and chrysazin (1,8-dihydroxyanthraquinone) had antibiofilm potential versus *C. albicans* due to a C1 hydroxyl group with toxic influence. It downregulates the expression of various biofilm-related and hyphal-specific genes (e.g., *ECE1*, *ALS3*, *RBT1*, and *ECE2*). Also, they (conc. 2 mg/mL) capably hampered yeast-to-hyphal formation and raised the *C. albicans*–infected *C. elegans* survivability (Manoharan et al. 2017).

A natural macrocyclic-bisbibenzyl derivative, riccardin D, reported from *Dumortiera hirsuta* had shown in vitro antibiofilm effectiveness. It possessed therapeutic and prophylactic capacity versus *C. albicans* biofilm production based on XTT (2,3-bis(2-methoxy-4-nitro-5-sulfo-phenyl)-2H-tetrazolium-5-carboxanilide) reduction assay results utilizing a CVC (central venous catheter)-infected rabbit model (Y. Li et al. 2012). This compound downregulated hypha-linked genes (e.g., *ALS3*, *ALS1*, *EFG1*, *ECE1*, *CDC35*, and *HWP1*), revealing that the hypha formation retardation was attributable to Ras–cAMP–Efg pathway suppression, resulting in biofilm maturity imperfection. Further, its riccardin D-fluconazole combination demonstrated raised antifungal potential (Y. Li et al. 2012).

Some pathogenic bacteria affect host tissues and cells via pili proteins and/or surface proteins that display pivotal function during infection (Asadi et al. 2018). Sortase A enzyme (Srt-A) is utilized by Staphylococcal species for adhering surface proteins to their cell walls (Thappeta et al. 2020). Therefore, prohibition of *S. aureus* Srt-A produces remarkable mitigation of bacterial virulence, involving binding capacity to IgG, fibrinogen, and fibronectin, additionally lowered biofilm establishment stages in some Staphylococcal species (Thappeta et al. 2020). Hu et al. (2013) assessed the inhibition potential of curcumin on *S. mutans* biofilm. It was proven that curcumin suppressed purified *S. mutans* Srt-A with (IC_{50} 10.2 µM/L). It also (conc. 15 µM/L) released the Pac protein and reduced *S. mutans* biofilm production. Therefore, curcumin exhibited its anticaries effectiveness via an antiadhesion-induced process (Hu et al. 2013). The flavonoid morin was established to possess potential Srt-A inhibition on *S. aureus*. Huang et al. demonstrated that it also exhibited inhibition influence versus *S. mutans* SrtA (IC_{50} 27.2 µM) with no influence on bacteria survival and growth. At conc. 30 µM, it partially boosted the Pac-protein release and reduced *S. mutans* biofilm mass without affecting the viability. These results indicate that morin might be important as a new agent to prevent caries (Huang et al. 2014). Further, the flavonoid-C-glucoside isovitexin showed notable Srt-A inhibition (IC_{50} 28.98 µg/mL) capacity, leading to a reduced quantity of SpA (staphylococcal-protein A) on the cell surface, suggesting its possible utilization as an antiinfection agent versus *S. aureus* (Mu et al. 2018).

In 2020, Wu et al. assessed the effectiveness of oxyresveratrol separated from *Artocarpus lakoocha* heartwood versus *S. mutans*. The results established that this compound (conc. 250 µg mL) lessened the bacteria survival rate, hindered H_2O-insoluble glucans synthesis, disturbed biofilm development, and noticeably repressed *gtfB* (glucosyl-transferase-I) and *gtfC* (glucosyltransferase-SI) expression. On the other hand, it upregulated the *atpD* expression of (ATP synthase subunit beta) and *ldh* (lactate dehydrogenase). It also boosted *gtfD* (glucosyltransferase S) expression and promoted the synthesis of H_2O-soluble glucan. It activated *liaR*, *vicR*, *comE*, and *comD*, which enhanced the self-protecting process (J. Wu et al. 2020).

Aspergillus fumigatus is a pathogenic fungus accountable for diverse dangerous lung disorders, including aspergilloma, allergic-bronchopulmonary aspergillosis, and invasive-pulmonary aspergillosis in hypersensitive immunocompromised individuals (Tseung and Zhao 2016). This fungus was found to produce a hydrophobic biofilm consisting of many coiled hyphae wrapped with ECM in the lungs (Tseung and Zhao 2016). Cis-9-hexadecenal (palmitole-aldehyde) was found in *Pentaclethra macrophylla*, *Myristica fragrans*, *Cuminum cyminum*, and *Thuja orientalis* (Hoda et al. 2020). At 0.078 mg/mL, it prohibited 90% of *A. fumigatus* planktonic growth in the broth micro-dilution assay (Hoda et al. 2020). In vitro, its combination with amphotericin B possessed enhanced efficacy versus *A. fumigatus* in the checker-board assay. It had a 0.156 mg/mL MBEC80 (minimal-biofilm-eradicating concentration 80) versus *A. fumigatus* in the MTT assay with an observed absence of tangled hyphae and ECM in cis 9-hexadecenal–treated biofilm in scanning electron microscopy (Hoda et al. 2020). It was nontoxic up to 0.62 mg/mL to L-132 (normal human lung epithelial cell line) in the cytotoxicity assay, therefore, it could be a remarkable therapeutic agent for *A. fumigatus*–related diseases (Hoda et al. 2020).

1.6 RECENT ADVANCES IN BIOFILM CONTROL

So far, three primary techniques for controlling biofilm formation or targeting distinct phases of biofilm growth have been addressed. The first strategy is to prevent bacteria from adhering to biofilm-forming surfaces from the beginning, lowering the possibilities of biofilm formation. The second strategy aims to disrupt the biofilm throughout the maturation phase (Kalia and Purohit 2011). The third option involves interfering with the way the bacteria communicate, also known as the quorum-sensing system, which coordinates biofilm development and growth in bacterial pathogens (Wright et al. 2004).

Biocides and antiseptic solutions, which create toxic by-products, and antibiotics, which have limited efficiency on bacterial resistance and slow-growing, persistent bacteria, are now the most common biofilm management options. Alternative medicines have been attempted to eliminate or suppress biofilms due to the inability of conventional antibiotics to treat them. Many natural compounds block QS, have anti-adhesin activity, and limit biofilm formation. Other treatments include bacteriophages, which are viruses that target specific bacteria, or enzymes that break down the extracellular biofilm matrix (Sahli et al. 2022).

1.6.1 BACTERIOPHAGES

The use of bacteriophages, viruses that selectively infect bacteria, is the basis of phage treatment. Because these viruses do not infect eukaryotic cells, the danger of opportunistic infections is reduced. Their usual size is 25 to 200 nm, and they are made up of a protein capsid that protects their genome (which contains nucleic acid), a variable-length tail (through which genetic material is delivered), and tail fibers that ensure host recognition (pili can be receptors) ("Bacteriophage" 2022). Bacteriophages can disrupt polysaccharides in biofilms by utilizing enzymes called depolymerases, which are found at the extremities of the tail fibers (Pires et al. 2016), allowing them to diffuse deeper into the biofilm matrix and therefore increase their efficiency. Furthermore, bacteriophages can readily move across the biofilm's water channels (Sutherland et al. 2004). Bacteriophages are quite specific to a species and population. The Soviet Union (USSR) invested in bacteriophages to cure bacterial diseases during the 20th century. Because it couldn't afford antibiotics, which were mostly produced in Western countries, the USSR turned to alternate methods of treating its people. As a result, the Eliava Institute in Georgia, which was once part of the USSR, currently boasts one of the largest collections of bacteriophages, having begun its studies in 1923 ("Phages: Bacterial Eaters from Georgia to Fight Antibiotic Resistance | Science | In-Depth Reporting on Science and Technology | DW | 21.11.2019" 2022). Phage-resistant subtypes can form within the biofilm community, just as they can in planktonic cultures (Fu et al. 2010). Due to mutations in the genes encoding the phage receptors, phage-resistant mutants of *P. aeruginosa* biofilm emerge following treatment with anti-pseudomonas bacteriophages (Oechslin et al. 2017). QS is linked to bacteriophage resistance in biofilms: in response to AHL detection signals, *E. coli* lowers the number of receptors on the cell surface, causing a twofold decrease in the rate of phage adsorption (Høyland-Kroghsbo et al. 2013).

1.6.2   BIOFILM-DISPERSING ENZYMES

The biofilm matrix is an appealing target for antibiofilm treatment due to its porous nature and exposure to the surrounding environment. The polymers in the biofilm matrix can be degraded by certain enzymes. This stops them from forming, softens the matrix that forms on a surface, and makes bacteria in biofilms more sensitive to anti-bacterials (Sahli et al. 2022). Deoxyribonuclease I (DNase I) is one of these enzymes with antibiofilm activity against gram-positive bacteria (*Enterococcus faecalis, Staphylococcus aureus, Staphylococcus epidermidis, Staphylococcus haemolyticus, Streptococcus intermedius, Streptococcus mutans, Streptococcus pneumoniae,* and *Streptococcus pyogenes*) as well as gram-negative bacteria (*Acinetobacter baumannii, Aggregatibacter actinomycetemcomitans, Bdellovibrio bacteriovorus, Campylobacter jejuni, Comamonas denitrificans, E. coli, Haemophilus influenzae, Klebsiella pneumoniae* and *P. aeruginosa*) (Kaplan 2009). It prevents the production of biofilms in 7 of the 17 species examined, may partially or completely remove biofilms from 15 of the 17 species, and renders 7 of the 17 species antibacterial sensitive. *A. actinomycetemcomitans* produces dispersin B naturally. This enzyme hydrolyzes poly-(-1,6)-N-acetylglucosamine (PNAG), an extracellular polysaccharide generated by various bacteria, including *S. epidermidis, S. aureus,* and several gram-negative Proteobacteria. The biofilm matrix degradation causes it to disperse, resensitizing remnant bacteria to antibiotic activity (Izano et al. 2008).

1.6.3   NANOTECHNOLOGY AGAINST BIOFILMS

New technologies have evolved alongside traditional ways of treating bacterial biofilms. Nanotechnology is the study and design of materials at the nanoscale, generally between 1 and 1000 nm. The nanoscale character results in distinct physicochemical and biological features. This is owing to their high surface-to-volume ratios, which give them features that are distinct from the bulk. Nanotechnologies have a wide range of applications, including health, energy, defense, environment, and information storage (Khan 2020; Hussein 2015; Saleem and Zaidi 2020; Juang and Bogy 2005). Because biofilm pore diameters average around 50 nm, nanomaterials with sizes smaller than this can readily penetrate through the biofilm matrix and reach microorganisms in the biofilm's interior regions. Encapsulated medications have

TABLE 1.1

Application of nanotechnology in biofilm inhibition

Nanomaterial	Mode of action	Bacteria	Biofilm impact	Reference
Liposomes	Hydrophilic, lipophilic, amphiphilic	*S. aureus, P. gingivalis*	Slow down, growth inhibition	(M. Li et al. 2019)
SLNs	Prolonged release: hydrophilic, lipophilic	*S. aureus*	Growth inhibition	(Paliwal et al. 2020)
QSIs	Anti-agglomeration, anti-aggregation	*P. aeruginosa, V. fischeri*	Eradication, growth inhibition	(Nafee et al. 2014)
PNPs	Hydrophilic, hydrophobic	*E. coli, S. mutans, S. aureus, P. aeruginosa, E. cloacae*	Matrix disruption, eradication, growth inhibition	(Wang et al. 2020)
Dendrimers	Hydrophilic, hydrophobic	*S. aureus, E. coli*	Antimicrobial	(Svenson and Tomalia 2005)
Cyclodextrins	Hydrophobic	*C. albicans, S. aureus, P. aeruginosa, E. faecalis, P. vulgaris*	Adhesion inhibition, eradication	(Gharbi et al. 2012)
Hydrogels	Bacteriophage, hydrophilic, hydrophobic	*P. aeruginosa, S. aureus, MRSA, Acinetobacter baumannii*	Biofilm eradication, wound healing	(Xia Li et al. 2021)
SLNs	Prolonged release: hydrophilic, lipophilic	*S. aureus*	Growth inhibition	(Paliwal et al. 2020)
QSIs	Anti-agglomeration, anti-aggregation	*P. aeruginosa, V. fischeri*	Eradication, growth inhibition	(Nafee et al. 2014)
PNPs	Hydrophilic, hydrophobic	*E. coli, S. mutans, S. aureus, P. aeruginosa, E. cloacae*	Matrix disruption, eradication, growth inhibition	(Wang et al. 2020)

(Continued)

TABLE 1.1 (CONTINUED)
Application of nanotechnology in biofilm inhibition

Nanomaterial	Mode of action	Bacteria	Biofilm impact	Reference
Dendrimers	Hydrophilic, hydrophobic	*S. aureus, E. coli*	Antimicrobial	(Svenson and Tomalia 2005)
Cyclodextrins	Hydrophobic	*C. albicans, S. aureus, P. aeruginosa, E. faecalis, P. vulgaris*	Adhesion inhibition, eradication	(Gharbi et al. 2012)
Hydrogels	Bacteriophage, hydrophilic, hydrophobic	*P. aeruginosa, S. aureus,* MRSA, *Acinetobacter baumannii*	Biofilm eradication, wound healing	(Gharbi et al. 2012)
SPIONs	Magnetic disturbance, ROS generation, thermal therapy, drug delivery	*P. aeruginosa, H. pylori, M. tuberculosis, S. aureus, S. mutans*	Oxidative stress, cell lysis, colonization prevention	(Van de Walle et al. 2020)
Ag-NPs	ROS generation, antibacterial, drug carrier	*P. aeruginosa, E. coli, S. aureus, K. pneumoniae, S. flexneri, S. mutans*	Oxidative stress, inhibition, genetic mutation, structural alteration	(Xia Li et al. 2021)
Au-NPs	Thermal and photodynamic therapies, photosensitizer	*S. aureus, P. aeruginosa, E. coli, C. albicans*	Matrix disruption, growth prevention,	(Pham et al. 2021)
Other inorganic NPs	Photocatalysis, ROS generation, antimicrobial, antioxidant	*E. coli, S. aureus, P. aeruginosa, S. epidermidis*	Matrix disruption, growth inhibition	(Mohanta et al. 2020)

distinct biokinetics from free drugs, concentrating antibiotic activity on the biofilm while limiting human cell exposure (Peulen and Wilkinson 2011). Diffusion inside the biofilm is also influenced by the surface properties of nanomaterials. Positively charged nanomaterials enter biofilms with a negatively charged matrix better, while hydrophobic particles distribute better inside biofilms than hydrophilic particles. Furthermore, nanoparticles' physical characteristics can be used to combat biofilm. Some inorganic nanoparticles' intrinsic bacterial toxicity, or the ability of some nanomaterials to locally create heat, can be used to kill bacteria (Xiaoning Li et al. 2015). To inhibit bacterial biofilms, many nanomaterials have been developed and evaluated. They are classified into two categories: (1) organic nanoparticles (NPs), such as liposomes, polymeric nanoparticles (PNPs), dendrimers, cyclodextrins (CDs), QS-inhibitor (QSI) nanoparticles and solid-lipid nanoparticles (SLN); and (2) inorganic nanoparticles (IONPs), such as metallic nanoparticles (MNPs) (gold Au-NPs, silver Ag-NPs, silica, copper, etc.), metal oxides (iron oxide, aluminum oxide, etc.), quantum dots, fullerenes, and organic-inorganic mixtures. Bactericidal action is attributed to the type of nanomaterial or nanocarrier in some systems. Others allow a medicine to be encapsulated, shielding it from enzymatic inactivation as well as environmental factors (lack of oxygen, pH) and the bacteria's defensive mechanisms (P. Singh et al. 2021). Table 1.1 summarizes the results linked to the use of nanotechnology in biofilm inhibition.

1.6.4 NEW APPROACHES

Unlike traditional treatments, which involve simply giving a drug and waiting for its effect, innovative strategies use a magnetic field or laser irradiation to stimulate an NP, which may be associated with a drug, in order to generate a local temperature rise, release the drug, and/or mechanically destabilize the biofilm. The effectiveness of drugs is significantly improved when they are associated with NPs that have been activated in this manner (Sahli et al. 2022).

REFERENCES

Abdallah, Marwan, Corinne Benoliel, Djamel Drider, Pascal Dhulster, and Nour Eddine Chihib. 2014. "Biofilm Formation and Persistence on Abiotic Surfaces in the Context of Food and Medical Environments." *Archives of Microbiology* 196 (7): 453–472. doi:10.1007/S00203-014-0983-1/TABLES/1.

"About Cystic Fibrosis | Cystic Fibrosis Foundation." 2022. Accessed August 29. https://www.cff.org/intro-cf/about-cystic-fibrosis.

Anand, Uttpal, Nadia Jacobo-Herrera, Ammar Altemimi, and Naoufal Lakhssassi. 2019. "A Comprehensive Review on Medicinal Plants as Antimicrobial Therapeutics: Potential Avenues of Biocompatible Drug Discovery." *Metabolites* 9: 258. doi:10.3390/METABO9110258.

Artini, M., R. Papa, G. Barbato, G. L. Scoarughi, A. Cellini, P. Morazzoni, E. Bombardelli, and L. Selan. 2012. "Bacterial Biofilm Formation Inhibitory Activity Revealed for Plant Derived Natural Compounds." *Bioorganic & Medicinal Chemistry* 20 (2): 920–926. doi:10.1016/J.BMC.2011.11.052.

Asadi, Arezoo, Shabnam Razavi, Malihe Talebi, and Mehrdad Gholami. 2018. "A Review on Anti-Adhesion Therapies of Bacterial Diseases." *Infection* 47 (1): 13–23. doi:10.1007/ S15010-018-1222-5.

Asfour, Hani Z. 2018. "Anti-Quorum Sensing Natural Compounds." *Journal of Microscopy and Ultrastructure* 6 (1): 1. doi:10.4103/JMAU.JMAU_10_18.

Azeredo, Joana, Nuno F. Azevedo, Romain Briandet, Nuno Cerca, Tom Coenye, Ana Rita Costa, Mickaël Desvaux, Giovanni Di Bonaventura, Michel Hébraud, Zoran Jaglic, Miroslava Kačániová, Susanne Knøchel, Anália Lourenço, Filipe Mergulhão, Rikke Louise Meyer, George Nychas, Manuel Simões, Odile Tresse, and Claus Sternberg. 2016. "Critical Review on Biofilm Methods." *Critical Reviews in Microbiology* 43 (3): 313–351. doi:10.1080/1040841X.2016.1208146.

Azman, Adzzie Shazleen, Christina Injan Mawang, Jasmine Elanie Khairat, and Sazaly AbuBakar. 2019. "Actinobacteria—A Promising Natural Source of Anti-Biofilm Agents." *International Microbiology* 22 (4): 403–409. doi:10.1007/S10123-019-00066-4/ TABLES/1.

"Bacteriophage." 2022. Accessed May 27. https://www.microbiologybook.org/mayer/phage.htm.

Balouiri, Mounyr, Moulay Sadiki, and Saad Koraichi Ibnsouda. 2016. "Methods for in Vitro Evaluating Antimicrobial Activity: A Review." *Journal of Pharmaceutical Analysis* 6 (2): 71–79. doi:10.1016/J.JPHA.2015.11.005.

Baltimore, R. S., C. D. C. Christie, and G. J. Walker Smith. 2012. "Immunohistopathologic Localization of Pseudomonas Aeruginosa in Lungs from Patients with Cystic Fibrosis: Implications for the Pathogenesis of Progressive Lung Deterioration." *American Review of Respiratory Disease* 140 (6): 1650–1661. doi:10.1164/AJRCCM/140.6.1650.

Barken, Kim B., Janus A. J. Haagensen, and Tim Tolker-Nielsen. 2007. "Advances in Nucleic Acid-Based Diagnostics of Bacterial Infections." *Clinica Chimica Acta* 384 (1–2): 1–11. doi:10.1016/J.CCA.2007.07.004.

Bausz, Mária, Eszter Fodor, Miklós D. Resch, and Katalin Kristóf. 2006. "Bacterial Contamination in the Anterior Chamber after Povidone–Iodine Application and the Effect of the Lens Implantation Device." *Journal of Cataract & Refractive Surgery* 32 (10): 1691–1695. doi:10.1016/J.JCRS.2006.05.019.

Behbehani, Jawad, Sheikh Shreaz, Mohammad Irshad, and Maribassapa Karched. 2017. "The Natural Compound Magnolol Affects Growth, Biofilm Formation, and Ultrastructure of Oral Candida Isolates." *Microbial Pathogenesis* 113 (December): 209–217. doi:10.1016/J.MICPATH.2017.10.040.

Benoit, Michael R., Carolyn G. Conant, Cristian Ionescu-Zanetti, Michael Schwartz, and A. Matin. 2010. "New Device for High-Throughput Viability Screening of Flow Biofilms." *Applied and Environmental Microbiology* 76 (13): 4136–4142. doi:10.1128/AEM.0306 5-09/ASSET/663CFC28-FF56-4A17-A87A-402506D4B9EE/ASSETS/GRAPHIC/ZA M9991010750005.JPEG.

Bhardwaj, Ashwani, Amit C. Kharkwal, and Versha A. Singh. 2018. "A Comparative Appraisal of Detection of Biofilm Production Caused by Uropathogenic Escherichia Coli in Tropical Catheterized Patients by Three Different Methods." *Asian Journal of Pharmaceutics (AJP)* 12 (4): 1445. doi:10.22377/AJP.V12I04.2949.

Bispo, Paulo J. M., Wolfgang Haas, and Michael S. Gilmore. 2015. "Biofilms in Infections of the Eye." *Pathogens* 4 (1): 111–136. doi:10.3390/PATHOGENS4010111.

Bjarnsholt, Thomas, Oana Ciofu, Søren Molin, Michael Givskov, and Niels Høiby. 2013. "Applying Insights from Biofilm Biology to Drug Development — Can a New Approach Be Developed?" *Nature Reviews Drug Discovery* 12 (10): 791–808. doi:10.1038/nrd4000.

Boudarel, Héloïse, Jean Denis Mathias, Benoît Blaysat, and Michel Grédiac. 2018. "Towards Standardized Mechanical Characterization of Microbial Biofilms: Analysis and Critical Review." *NPJ Biofilms and Microbiomes* 4 (1): 1–15. doi:10.1038/s41522-018-0062-5.

Brackman, Gilles, Ulrik Hillaert, Serge Van Calenbergh, Hans J. Nelis, and Tom Coenye. 2009. "Use of Quorum Sensing Inhibitors to Interfere with Biofilm Formation and Development in Burkholderia Multivorans and Burkholderia Cenocepacia." *Research in Microbiology* 160 (2): 144–151. doi:10.1016/J.RESMIC.2008.12.003.

Brown, Sheena D., Rachel White, and Phil Tobin. 2017. "Keep Them Breathing: Cystic Fibrosis Pathophysiology, Diagnosis, and Treatment." *Journal of the American Academy of Physician Assistants* 30 (5): 23–27. doi:10.1097/01.JAA.0000515540.36581.92.

Cámara, Miguel, William Green, Cait E. MacPhee, Paulina D. Rakowska, Rasmita Raval, Mark C. Richardson, Joanne Slater-Jefferies, Katerina Steventon, and Jeremy S. Webb. 2022. "Economic Significance of Biofilms: A Multidisciplinary and Cross-Sectoral Challenge." *NPJ Biofilms and Microbiomes* 8 (1): 1–8. doi:10.1038/s41522-022-00306-y.

Cerqueira, Gustavo M., and Anton Y. Peleg. 2011. "Insights into Acinetobacter Baumannii Pathogenicity." *IUBMB Life* 63 (12): 1055–1060. doi:10.1002/IUB.533.

Chakraborty, P., D. G. Dastidar, P. Paul, S. Dutta, D. Basu, S. R. Sharma, S. Basu, R. K. Sarker, A. Sen, A. Sarkar, and P. Tribedi. 2020. "Inhibition of Biofilm Formation of Pseudomonas Aeruginosa by Caffeine: A Potential Approach for Sustainable Management of Biofilm." *Archives of Microbiology* 202 (3): 623–635. doi:10.1007/S00203-019-01775-0/FIGURES/7.

Chanda, Warren, Thomson P. Joseph, Wendong Wang, Arshad A. Padhiar, and Mintao Zhong. 2017. "The Potential Management of Oral Candidiasis Using Anti-Biofilm Therapies." *Medical Hypotheses* 106 (September): 15–18. doi:10.1016/J.MEHY.2017.06.029.

Christensen, Gordon D., W. A. Simpson, J. J. Younger, L. M. Baddour, F. F. Barrett, D. M. Melton, and E. H. Beachey. 1985. "Adherence of Coagulase-Negative Staphylococci to Plastic Tissue Culture Plates: A Quantitative Model for the Adherence of Staphylococci to Medical Devices." *Journal of Clinical Microbiology* 22 (6): 996–1006. doi:10.1128/JCM.22.6.996-1006.1985.

Costerton, J. W. 2012. "Tackling Bacterial Biofilms." *Chemistry & Industry* 76 (2): 30–32. doi:10.1002/CIND.7602_9.X.

Costerton, J. W., K. J. Cheng, G. G. Geesey, T. I. Ladd, J. C. Nickel, M. Dasgupta, and T. J. Marrie. 2003. "Bacterial Biofilms in Nature and Disease." *Annual Review of Microbiology* 41 (November): 435–464. doi:10.1146/ANNUREV.MI.41.100187.002251.

Daddi Oubekka, S., R. Briandet, M. P. Fontaine-Aupart, and K. Steenkeste. 2012. "Correlative Time-Resolved Fluorescence Microscopy to Assess Antibiotic Diffusion-Reaction in Biofilms." *Antimicrobial Agents and Chemotherapy* 56 (6): 3349–3358. doi:10.1128/AAC.00216-12/SUPPL_FILE/MOVIES1.MOV.

Dey, Pia, Debaprasad Parai, Malabika Banerjee, Sk Tofajjen Hossain, and Samir Kumar Mukherjee. 2020. "Naringin Sensitizes the Antibiofilm Effect of Ciprofloxacin and Tetracycline against Pseudomonas Aeruginosa Biofilm." *International Journal of Medical Microbiology* 310 (3): 151410. doi:10.1016/J.IJMM.2020.151410.

Dhama, K., K. Karthik, R. Khandia, A. Munjal, R. Tiwari, R. Rana, S. K. Khurana, S. Ullah, R. U. Khan, M. Alagawany, and M. R. Farag. 2018. "Medicinal and Therapeutic Potential of Herbs and Plant Metabolites / Extracts Countering Viral Pathogens – Current Knowledge and Future Prospects." *Current Drug Metabolism* 19 (January). doi:10.2174/1389200219666180129145252.

Donlan, R. M., J. A. Piede, C. D. Heyes, L. Sanii, R. Murga, P. Edmonds, I. El-Sayed, and M. A. El-Sayed. 2004. "Model System for Growing and Quantifying Streptococcus Pneumoniae Biofilms in Situ and in Real Time." *Applied and Environmental Microbiology* 70 (8): 4980–4988. doi:10.1128/AEM.70.8.4980-4988.2004/ASSET/B255AA96-5605-4EA8-B3A3-C622B595EDB3/ASSETS/GRAPHIC/ZAM0080446590009.JPEG.

El-Ganiny, Amira M., Ghada H. Shaker, Abeer A. Aboelazm, and Heba A. El-Dash. 2017. "Prevention of Bacterial Biofilm Formation on Soft Contact Lenses Using Natural Compounds." *Journal of Ophthalmic Inflammation and Infection* 7 (1): 1–7. doi:10.1186/ S12348-017-0129-0/FIGURES/2.

Fazeli-Nasab, Bahman, R. Z. Sayyed, Laleh Shahraki Mojahed, Ahmad Farid Rahmani, Mehrangiz Ghafari, Sarjiya Antonius, and Sukamto. 2022. "Biofilm Production: A Strategic Mechanism for Survival of Microbes under Stress Conditions." *Biocatalysis and Agricultural Biotechnology* 42 (July): 102337. doi:10.1016/J.BCAB.2022.102337.

Fazly, Ahmed, Charu Jain, Amie C. Dehner, Luca Issi, Elizabeth A. Lilly, Akbar Ali, Hong Cao, Paul L. Fidel, Reeta P. Rao, and Paul D. Kaufman. 2013. "Chemical Screening Identifies Filastatin, a Small Molecule Inhibitor of Candida Albicans Adhesion, Morphogenesis, and Pathogenesis." *Proceedings of the National Academy of Sciences of the United States of America* 110 (33): 13594–13599. doi:10.1073/PNAS.1305982110/ SUPPL_FILE/PNAS.201305982SI.PDF.

Feneley, Roger C. L., Ian B. Hopley, and Peter N. T. Wells. 2015. "Urinary Catheters: History, Current Status, Adverse Events and Research Agenda." *Journal of Medical Engineering & Technology* 39 (8): 459–470. doi:10.3109/03091902.2015.1085600.

Fleiszig, Suzanne M. J., and David J. Evans. 2010. "The Pathogenesis of Contact Lens-Associated Microbial Keratitis." *Optometry and Vision Science: Official Publication of the American Academy of Optometry* 87 (4): 225. doi:10.1097/OPX.0B013E3181D408EE.

Flemming, Hans Curt, and Jost Wingender. 2010. "The Biofilm Matrix." *Nature Reviews Microbiology* 8 (9): 623–633. doi:10.1038/nrmicro2415.

Flemming, Hans Curt, and Stefan Wuertz. 2019. "Bacteria and Archaea on Earth and Their Abundance in Biofilms." *Nature Reviews Microbiology* 17 (4): 247–260. doi:10.1038/ s41579-019-0158-9.

Flemming, Hans Curt, Jost Wingender, Ulrich Szewzyk, Peter Steinberg, Scott A. Rice, and Staffan Kjelleberg. 2016. "Biofilms: An Emergent Form of Bacterial Life." *Nature Reviews Microbiology* 14 (9): 563–575. doi:10.1038/nrmicro.2016.94.

Fu, Weiling, Terri Forster, Oren Mayer, John J. Curtin, Susan M. Lehman, and Rodney M. Donlan. 2010. "Bacteriophage Cocktail for the Prevention of Biofilm Formation by Pseudomonas Aeruginosa on Catheters in an in Vitro Model System." *Antimicrobial Agents and Chemotherapy* 54 (1): 397–404. doi:10.1128/AAC.00669-09/ASSET/9109678A-BD65-4BDA-B0E1-600C2795A20F/ASSETS/GRAPHIC/ZAC001108700004B.JPEG.

Fux, C. A., J. W. Costerton, P. S. Stewart, and P. Stoodley. 2005. "Survival Strategies of Infectious Biofilms." *Trends in Microbiology* 13 (1): 34–40. doi:10.1016/J.TIM.2004.11.010.

Gastmeier, Petra, Sabine Stamm-Balderjahn, Sonja Hansen, Frauke Nitzschke-Tiemann, Irina Zuschneid, Katrin Groneberg, and Henning Rüden. 2005. "How Outbreaks Can Contribute to Prevention of Nosocomial Infection: Analysis of 1,022 Outbreaks." *Infection Control and Hospital Epidemiology* 26 (4): 357–361. doi:10.1086/502552.

Gharbi, Aïcha, Vincent Humblot, Frédéric Turpin, Claire Marie Pradier, Christine Imbert, and Jean Marc Berjeaud. 2012. "Elaboration of Antibiofilm Surfaces Functionalized with Antifungal-Cyclodextrin Inclusion Complexes." *FEMS Immunology and Medical Microbiology* 65 (2): 257–269. doi:10.1111/J.1574-695X.2012.00932.X.

Gominet, Marie, Fabrice Compain, Christophe Beloin, and David Lebeaux. 2017. "Central Venous Catheters and Biofilms: Where Do We Stand in 2017?" *APMIS* 125 (4): 365–375. doi:10.1111/APM.12665.

Guan, Jingyuan, Xiao Xiao, Shengjuan Xu, Fen Gao, Jianbo Wang, Tietao Wang, Yunhong Song, Junfeng Pan, Xihui Shen, and Yao Wang. 2015. "Roles of RpoS in Yersinia Pseudotuberculosis Stress Survival, Motility, Biofilm Formation and Type VI Secretion System Expression." *Journal of Microbiology* 53 (9): 633–642. doi:10.1007/ S12275-015-0099-6.

Gupta, S., C. Andersen, J. Black, J. de Leon, C. Fife, JC, L.I., J. Niezgoda, R. Snyder, B. Sumpio, W. Tettelbach, and T. Treadwell. 2017. "Management of Chronic Wounds: Diagnosis, Preparation, Treatment, and Follow-Up." *Wounds : A Compendium of Clinical Research and Practice* 29 (9): S19–S36. https://europepmc.org/article/med/28862980.

Guzmán-Soto, Irene, Christopher McTiernan, Mayte Gonzalez-Gomez, Alex Ross, Keshav Gupta, Erik J. Suuronen, Thien Fah Mah, May Griffith, and Emilio I. Alarcon. 2021. "Mimicking Biofilm Formation and Development: Recent Progress in in Vitro and in Vivo Biofilm Models." *IScience* 24 (5): 102443. doi:10.1016/J.ISCI.2021.102443.

Hall-Stoodley, Luanne, and Paul Stoodley. 2009. "Evolving Concepts in Biofilm Infections." *Cellular Microbiology* 11 (7): 1034–1043. doi:10.1111/J.1462-5822.2009.01323.X.

Hall-Stoodley, Luanne, Paul Stoodley, Sandeep Kathju, Niels Høiby, Claus Moser, J. William Costerton, Annette Moter, and Thomas Bjarnsholt. 2012. "Towards Diagnostic Guidelines for Biofilm-Associated Infections." *FEMS Immunology & Medical Microbiology* 65 (2): 127–145. doi:10.1111/J.1574-695X.2012.00968.X.

Hardy, Liselotte, Vicky Jespers, Nassira Dahchour, Lambert Mwambarangwe, Viateur Musengamana, Mario Vaneechoutte, and Tania Crucitti. 2015. "Unravelling the Bacterial Vaginosis-Associated Biofilm: A Multiplex Gardnerella Vaginalis and Atopobium Vaginae Fluorescence In Situ Hybridization Assay Using Peptide Nucleic Acid Probes." *PLOS ONE* 10 (8): e0136658. doi:10.1371/JOURNAL.PONE.0136658.

Hassan, Afreenish, Javaid Usman, Fatima Kaleem, Maria Omair, Ali Khalid, and Muhammad Iqbal. 2011. "Evaluation of Different Detection Methods of Biofilm Formation in the Clinical Isolates." *Brazilian Journal of Infectious Diseases* 15 (4): 305–311. doi:10.1590/S1413-86702011000400002.

Hobley, Laura, Catriona Harkins, Cait E. MacPhee, and Nicola R. Stanley-Wall. 2015. "Giving Structure to the Biofilm Matrix: An Overview of Individual Strategies and Emerging Common Themes." *FEMS Microbiology Reviews* 39 (5): 649–669. doi:10.1093/FEMSRE/FUV015.

Hoda, Shanu, Lovely Gupta, Jata Shankar, Alok Kumar Gupta, and Pooja Vijayaraghavan. 2020. "Cis-9-Hexadecenal, a Natural Compound Targeting Cell Wall Organization, Critical Growth Factor, and Virulence of Aspergillus Fumigatus." *ACS Omega* 5 (17): 10077–10088. doi:10.1021/ACSOMEGA.0C00615.

Høiby, Niels, Thomas Bjarnsholt, Michael Givskov, Søren Molin, and Oana Ciofu. 2010. "Antibiotic Resistance of Bacterial Biofilms." *International Journal of Antimicrobial Agents* 35 (4): 322–332. doi:10.1016/J.IJANTIMICAG.2009.12.011.

Holland, Thomas L., Larry M. Baddour, Arnold S. Bayer, Bruno Hoen, Jose M. Miro, and Vance G. Fowler. 2016. "Infective Endocarditis." *Nature Reviews. Disease Primers* 2 (September). doi:10.1038/NRDP.2016.59.

Høyland-Kroghsbo, Nina Molin, Rasmus Baadsgaard Mærkedahl, and Sine Lo Svenningsen. 2013. "A Quorum-Sensing-Induced Bacteriophage Defense Mechanism." *MBio* 4 (1). doi:10.1128/MBIO.00362-12.

Hoyle, B. D., and J. W. Costerton. 1991. "Bacterial Resistance to Antibiotics: The Role of Biofilms." *Progress in Drug Research* 37: 91–105. doi:10.1007/978-3-0348-7139-6_2.

Hu, Ping, Ping Huang, and Min Wei Chen. 2013. "Curcumin Reduces Streptococcus Mutans Biofilm Formation by Inhibiting Sortase A Activity." *Archives of Oral Biology* 58 (10): 1343–1348. doi:10.1016/J.ARCHORALBIO.2013.05.004.

Huang, Ping, Ping Hu, Su Yun Zhou, Qian Li, and Wei Min Chen. 2014. "Morin Inhibits Sortase A and Subsequent Biofilm Formation in Streptococcus Mutans." *Current Microbiology* 68 (1): 47–52. doi:10.1007/S00284-013-0439-X/FIGURES/3.

Hussein, Ahmed Kadhim. 2015. "Applications of Nanotechnology in Renewable Energies—A Comprehensive Overview and Understanding." *Renewable and Sustainable Energy Reviews* 42 (February): 460–476. doi:10.1016/J.RSER.2014.10.027.

Izano, Era A., Irina Sadovskaya, Hailin Wang, Evgeny Vinogradov, Chandran Ragunath, Narayanan Ramasubbu, Saïd Jabbouri, Malcolm B. Perry, and Jeffrey B. Kaplan. 2008. "Poly-N-Acetylglucosamine Mediates Biofilm Formation and Detergent Resistance in Aggregatibacter Actinomycetemcomitans." *Microbial Pathogenesis* 44 (1): 52–60. doi:10.1016/J.MICPATH.2007.08.004.

Jahan, Fahmida, Suresh V. Chinni, Sumitha Samuggam, Lebaka Veeranjaneya Reddy, Maheswaran Solayappan, and Lee Su Yin. 2022. "The Complex Mechanism of the Salmonella *Typhi* Biofilm Formation That Facilitates Pathogenicity: A Review." *International Journal of Molecular Sciences* 23 (12): 6462. doi:10.3390/IJMS23126462.

Jansen, Kathrin U., Douglas Q. Girgenti, Ingrid L. Scully, and Annaliesa S. Anderson. 2013. "Vaccine Review: 'Staphyloccocus Aureus Vaccines: Problems and Prospects.'" *Vaccine* 31 (25): 2723–2730. doi:10.1016/J.VACCINE.2013.04.002.

Juang, Jia Yang, and David B. Bogy. 2005. "Nanotechnology Advances and Applications in Information Storage." *Microsystem Technologies* 11 (8–10): 950–957. doi:10.1007/S00 542-005-0563-Z/FIGURES/12.

Kalia, Vipin Chandra, and Hemant J. Purohit. 2011. "Quenching the Quorum Sensing System: Potential Antibacterial Drug Targets." *Critical Reviews in Microbiology* 37 (2): 121–140. doi:10.3109/1040841X.2010.532479.

Kaplan, Jeffrey B. 2009. "Therapeutic Potential of Biofilm-Dispersing Enzymes." *The International Journal of Artificial Organs* 32 (9): 545–554. doi:10.1177/039139880903200903.

Kaplan, Jeffrey B. 2011. "Antibiotic-Induced Biofilm Formation." *International Journal of Artificial Organs* 34 (9): 737–751. doi:10.5301/ijao.5000027.

Khan, F.A. 2020. "Major Nano-based Products: Nanomedicine, Nanosensors, and Nanodiagnostics." In Khan, F. (eds), *Applications of Nanomaterials in Human Health*. Springer, Singapore. doi:10.1007/978-981-15-4802-4_11.

Kim, Jane H., Benjamin Yang, Amanda Tedesco, Elyson Gavin D. Lebig, Paul M. Ruegger, Karen Xu, James Borneman, and Manuela Martins-Green. 2019. "High Levels of Oxidative Stress and Skin Microbiome Are Critical for Initiation and Development of Chronic Wounds in Diabetic Mice." *Scientific Reports* 9 (1): 1–16. doi:10.1038/s41598-019-55644-3.

Kırmusaoğlu, Sahra. 2022. "The Methods for Detection of Biofilm and Screening Antibiofilm Activity of Agents." *Books.Google.Com*. Accessed August 29. https://books.google.com /books?hl=en&lr=&id=AGb8DwAAQBAJ&oi=fnd&pg=PA99&dq=KIRMUSAOĞL U,+S.+2019.+The+methods+for+detection+of+biofilm+and+screening+antibiofilm+act ivity+of+agents.+Antimicrobials,+antibiotic+resistance,+antibiofilm+strategies+and+a ctivity+methods,+1-17.&ots=q-94NRgNqx&sig=1Lah5UQQBp61-_S_L6_Peu4pzPQ.

Kolpen, Mette, Kasper Nørskov Kragh, Juan Barraza Enciso, Daniel Faurholt-Jepsen, Birgitte Lindegaard, Gertrud Baunbæk Egelund, Andreas Vestergaard Jensen, Pernille Ravn, Inger Hee Mabuza Mathiesen, Alexandra Gabriella Gheorge, Frederik Boëtius Hertz, Tavs Qvist, Marvin Whiteley, Peter Østrup Jensen, and Thomas Bjarnsholt. 2022. "Bacterial Biofilms Predominate in Both Acute and Chronic Human Lung Infections." *Thorax* 77: 1015–1022. doi:10.1136/THORAXJNL-2021-217576.

Konopka, Allan. 2009. "What Is Microbial Community Ecology?" *The ISME Journal* 3 (11): 1223–1230. doi:10.1038/ismej.2009.88.

Kostakioti, Maria, Maria Hadjifrangiskou, and Scott J. Hultgren. 2013. "Bacterial Biofilms: Development, Dispersal, and Therapeutic Strategies in the Dawn of the Postantibiotic Era." *Cold Spring Harbor Perspectives in Medicine* 3 (4): a010306. doi:10.1101/ CSHPERSPECT.A010306.

Kouidhi, Bochra, Yasir Mohammed A. Al Qurashi, and Kamel Chaieb. 2015. "Drug Resistance of Bacterial Dental Biofilm and the Potential Use of Natural Compounds as Alternative for Prevention and Treatment." *Microbial Pathogenesis* 80 (March): 39–49. doi:10.1016/J.MICPATH.2015.02.007.

Król, Jaroslaw E., Andrzej J. Wojtowicz, Linda M. Rogers, Holger Heuer, Kornelia Smalla, Stephen M. Krone, and Eva M. Top. 2013. "Invasion of E. Coli Biofilms by Antibiotic Resistance Plasmids." *Plasmid* 70 (1): 110–119. doi:10.1016/J.PLASMID.2013.03.003.

Kuinkel, Susmita, Jyoti Acharya, Binod Dhungel, Sanjib Adhikari, Nabaraj Adhikari, Upendra Thapa Shrestha, Megha Raj Banjara, Komal Raj Rijal, and Prakash Ghimire. 2021. "Biofilm Formation and Phenotypic Detection of ESBL, MBL, KPC and AmpC Enzymes and Their Coexistence in Klebsiella Spp. Isolated at the National Reference Laboratory, Kathmandu, Nepal." *Microbiology Research* 12 (3): 683–697. doi:10.3390/MICROBIOLRES12030049.

Lau, Denny, and Balbina J. Plotkin. 2013. "Antimicrobial and Biofilm Effects of Herbs Used in Traditional Chinese Medicine." *Natural Product Communications* 8 (11): 1617–1620. doi:10.1177/1934578X1300801129.

Lee, Joung Hyun, Jeffrey B. Kaplan, and Woo Y. Lee. 2008. "Microfluidic Devices for Studying Growth and Detachment of Staphylococcus Epidermidis Biofilms." *Biomedical Microdevices* 10 (4): 489–498. doi:10.1007/S10544-007-9157-0.

Lerche, Christian Johann, Franziska Schwartz, Marie Theut, Emil Loldrup Fosbøl, Kasper Iversen, Henning Bundgaard, Niels Høiby, and Claus Moser. 2021. "Anti-Biofilm Approach in Infective Endocarditis Exposes New Treatment Strategies for Improved Outcome." *Frontiers in Cell and Developmental Biology* 9 (June): 1363. doi:10.3389/FCELL.2021.643335/XML/NLM.

Li, Mingyuan, Chunyang Du, Na Guo, Yuou Teng, Xin Meng, Hua Sun, Shuangshuang Li, Peng Yu, and Hervé Galons. 2019. "Composition Design and Medical Application of Liposomes." *European Journal of Medicinal Chemistry* 164 (February): 640–653. doi:10.1016/J.EJMECH.2019.01.007.

Li, Xia, Ya Nan Fu, Lifei Huang, Fang Liu, Thomas Fintan Moriarty, Lei Tao, Yen Wei, and Xing Wang. 2021. "Combating Biofilms by a Self-Adapting Drug Loading Hydrogel." *ACS Applied Bio Materials* 4 (8): 6219–6226. doi:10.1021/ACSABM.1C00540.

Li, Xiaoning, Yi Cheun Yeh, Karuna Giri, Rubul Mout, Ryan F. Landis, Y. S. Prakash, and Vincent M. Rotello. 2015. "Control of Nanoparticle Penetration into Biofilms through Surface Design." *Chemical Communications (Cambridge, England)* 51 (2): 282–285. doi:10.1039/C4CC07737G.

Li, Yan, Yukui Ma, Li Zhang, Feng Guo, Lei Ren, Rui Yang, Ying Li, and Hongxiang Lou. 2012. "In Vivo Inhibitory Effect on the Biofilm Formation of Candida Albicans by Liverwort Derived Riccardin D." *PLOS ONE* 7 (4): e35543. doi:10.1371/JOURNAL.PONE.0035543.

Liesman, Rachael M., Bobbi S. Pritt, Joseph J. Maleszewski, and Robin Patela. 2017. "Laboratory Diagnosis of Infective Endocarditis." *Journal of Clinical Microbiology* 55 (9): 2599–2608. doi:10.1128/JCM.00635-17/ASSET/A59362EE-9C74-4BFD-868D-D07B73B358E3/ASSETS/GRAPHIC/ZJM9990956270002.JPEG.

Lima, Soraia Lopes, Luana Rossato, and Analy Salles de Azevedo Melo. 2020. "Evaluation of the Potential Virulence of Candida Haemulonii Species Complex and Candida Auris Isolates in Caenorhabditis Elegans as an in Vivo Model and Correlation to Their Biofilm Production Capacity." *Microbial Pathogenesis* 148 (November): 104461. doi:10.1016/J.MICPATH.2020.104461.

Liu, Wugao, Hongjia Lu, Xinyu Chu, Tianzheng Lou, Ning Zhang, Bao Zhang, and Weihua Chu. 2020. "Tea Polyphenols Inhibits Biofilm Formation, Attenuates the Quorum Sensing-Controlled Virulence and Enhances Resistance to Klebsiella Pneumoniae Infection in Caenorhabditis Elegans Model." *Microbial Pathogenesis* 147 (October): 104266. doi:10.1016/J.MICPATH.2020.104266.

Lu, Lan, Wei Hu, Zeru Tian, Dandan Yuan, Guojuan Yi, Yangyang Zhou, Qiang Cheng, Jie Zhu, and Mingxing Li. 2019. "Developing Natural Products as Potential Anti-Biofilm Agents." *Chinese Medicine (United Kingdom)* 14 (1): 1–17. doi:10.1186/S13020-019-0232-2/TABLES/4.

Madsen, Jonas Stenløkke, Mette Burmølle, Lars Hestbjerg Hansen, and Søren Johannes Sørensen. 2012. "The Interconnection between Biofilm Formation and Horizontal Gene Transfer." *FEMS Immunology & Medical Microbiology* 65 (2): 183–195. doi:10.1111/J.1574-695X.2012.00960.X.

Mah, Thien Fah. 2012. "Biofilm-Specific Antibiotic Resistance." *Future Microbiology* 7 (9): 1061–1072. doi:10.2217/FMB.12.76.

Manav, Safa, M. Sühan Ayhan, Erkan Deniz, Esra Özkoçer, Çiğdem Elmas, Meltem Yalinay, and Erdem Şahin. 2020. "Capsular Contracture around Silicone Miniimplants Following Bacterial Contamination: An in Vivo Comparative Experimental Study between Textured and Polyurethane Implants." *Journal of Plastic, Reconstructive & Aesthetic Surgery* 73 (9): 1747–1757. doi:10.1016/J.BJPS.2020.02.049.

Manoharan, Ranjith Kumar, Jin Hyung Lee, Yong Guy Kim, and Jintae Lee. 2017. "Alizarin and Chrysazin Inhibit Biofilm and Hyphal Formation by Candida Albicans." *Frontiers in Cellular and Infection Microbiology* 7 (October): 447. doi:10.3389/FCIMB.2017.00447/BIBTEX.

Martin, Isaac, Valerie Waters, and Hartmut Grasemann. 2021. "Approaches to Targeting Bacterial Biofilms in Cystic Fibrosis Airways." *International Journal of Molecular Sciences* 22 (4): 2155. doi:10.3390/IJMS22042155.

Mathur, T., S. Singhal, S. Khan, D. J. Upadhyay, T. Fatma, and A. Rattan. 2006. "Detection of Biofilm Formation among the Clinical Isolates of Staphylococci: An Evaluation of Three Different Screening Methods." *Indian Journal of Medical Microbiology* 24 (1): 25–29. doi:10.1016/S0255-0857(21)02466-X.

Meervenne, Eva Van, Rosemarie De Weirdt, Els Van Coillie, Frank Devlieghere, Lieve Herman, and Nico Boon. 2014. "Biofilm Models for the Food Industry: Hot Spots for Plasmid Transfer?" *Pathogens and Disease* 70 (3): 332–338. doi:10.1111/2049-632X.12134.

Mendoza, Rafael A., Ji-Cheng Hsieh, and Robert D. Galiano. 2019. "The Impact of Biofilm Formation on Wound Healing." *Wound Healing – Current Perspectives*, May. IntechOpen. doi:10.5772/INTECHOPEN.85020.

Mermel, Leonard A. 2011. "What Is the Predominant Source of Intravascular Catheter Infections?" *Clinical Infectious Diseases: An Official Publication of the Infectious Diseases Society of America* 52 (2): 211–212. doi:10.1093/CID/CIQ108.

Miller, J. Michael, Matthew J. Binnicker, Sheldon Campbell, Karen C. Carroll, Kimberle C. Chapin, Peter H. Gilligan, Mark D. Gonzalez, Robert C. Jerris, Sue C. Kehl, Robin Patel, Bobbi S. Pritt, Sandra S. Richter, Barbara Robinson-Dunn, Joseph D. Schwartzman, James W Snyder, Sam Telford, Elitza S Theel, Richard B. Thomson, Melvin P Weinstein, and Joseph D. Yao. 2018. "A Guide to Utilization of the Microbiology Laboratory for Diagnosis of Infectious Diseases: 2018 Update by the Infectious Diseases Society of America and the American Society for Microbiology." *Clinical Infectious Diseases* 67 (6): e1–e94. doi:10.1093/CID/CIY381.

Mohanta, Yugal Kishore, Kunal Biswas, Santosh Kumar Jena, Abeer Hashem, Elsayed Fathi Abd Allah, and Tapan Kumar Mohanta. 2020. "Anti-Biofilm and Antibacterial Activities of Silver Nanoparticles Synthesized by the Reducing Activity of Phytoconstituents Present in the Indian Medicinal Plants." *Frontiers in Microbiology* 11 (June). doi:10.3389/FMICB.2020.01143.

Mu, Dan, Hua Xiang, Haisi Dong, Dacheng Wang, and Tiedong Wang. 2018. "Isovitexin, a Potential Candidate Inhibitor of Sortase A of Staphylococcus Aureus USA300." *Journal of Microbiology and Biotechnology* 28 (9): 1426–1432. doi:10.4014/JMB.1802.02014.

Nafee, Noha, Ayman Husari, Christine K. Maurer, Cenbin Lu, Chiara De Rossi, Anke Steinbach, Rolf W. Hartmann, Claus Michael Lehr, and Marc Schneider. 2014. "Antibiotic-Free Nanotherapeutics: Ultra-Small, Mucus-Penetrating Solid Lipid Nanoparticles Enhance the Pulmonary Delivery and Anti-Virulence Efficacy of Novel Quorum Sensing Inhibitors." *Journal of Controlled Release: Official Journal of the Controlled Release Society* 192 (October): 131–140. doi:10.1016/J.JCONREL.2014.06.055.

Neoh, Koon Gee, Min Li, En Tang Kang, Edmund Chiong, and Paul Anantharajah Tambyah. 2017. "Surface Modification Strategies for Combating Catheter-Related Complications: Recent Advances and Challenges." *Journal of Materials Chemistry B* 5 (11): 2045–2067. doi:10.1039/C6TB03280J.

O'Toole, G., H. B. Kaplan, and R. Kolter. 2000. "Biofilm Formation as Microbial Development." *Annual Review of Microbiology* 54: 49–79. doi:10.1146/ANNUREV.MICRO.54.1.49.

Oechslin, Frank, Philippe Piccardi, Stefano Mancini, Jérôme Gabard, Philippe Moreillon, José M. Entenza, Gregory Resch, and Yok Ai Que. 2017. "Synergistic Interaction Between Phage Therapy and Antibiotics Clears Pseudomonas Aeruginosa Infection in Endocarditis and Reduces Virulence." *The Journal of Infectious Diseases* 215 (5): 703–712. doi:10.1093/INFDIS/JIW632.

Østergaard, Lauge, Nana Valeur, Nikolaj Ihlemann, Henning Bundgaard, Gunnar Gislason, Christian Torp-Pedersen, Niels Eske Bruun, Lars Søndergaard, Lars Køber, and Emil Loldrup Fosbøl. 2019. "Incidence of Infective Endocarditis in Patients Considered at Moderate Risk." *European Heart Journal* 40 (17): 1355–1361. doi:10.1093/EURHEARTJ/EHY629.

Paliwal, Rishi, Shivani Rai Paliwal, Rameshroo Kenwat, Balak Das Kurmi, and Mukesh Kumar Sahu. 2020. "Solid Lipid Nanoparticles: A Review on Recent Perspectives and Patents." *Expert Opinion on Therapeutic Patents* 30 (3): 179–194. doi:10.1080/13543776.2020.1720649.

Parsek, Matthew R., and Pradeep K. Singh. 2003. "Bacterial Biofilms: An Emerging Link to Disease Pathogenesis." *Annual Review of Microbiology* 57: 677–701. doi:10.1146/ANNUREV.MICRO.57.030502.090720.

Paula, Amauri J., Geelsu Hwang, and Hyun Koo. 2020. "Dynamics of Bacterial Population Growth in Biofilms Resemble Spatial and Structural Aspects of Urbanization." *Nature Communications* 11 (1): 1–14. doi:10.1038/s41467-020-15165-4.

Peng, Lu-Yuan, Meng Yuan, Zong-Mei Wu, Ke Song, Chun-Lei Zhang, Qiang An, Fang Xia, Jia-Lin Yu, Peng-Fei Yi, Ben-Dong Fu, and Hai-Qing Shen. 2019. "Anti-Bacterial Activity of Baicalin against APEC through Inhibition of Quorum Sensing and Inflammatory Responses." *Scientific Reports* 9 (1): 1–11. doi:10.1038/s41598-019-40684-6.

Peulen, Thomas Otavio, and Kevin J. Wilkinson. 2011. "Diffusion of Nanoparticles in a Biofilm." *Environmental Science & Technology* 45 (8): 3367–3373. doi:10.1021/ES103450G.

"Phages: Bacterial Eaters from Georgia to Fight Antibiotic Resistance | Science | In-Depth Reporting on Science and Technology | DW | 21.11.2019." 2022. Accessed May 27. https://www.dw.com/en/phages-bacterial-eaters-from-georgia-to-fight-antibiotic-resistance/a-51350421.

Pham, Phuong, Susan Oliver, Edgar H. H. Wong, and Cyrille Boyer. 2021. "Effect of Hydrophilic Groups on the Bioactivity of Antimicrobial Polymers." *Polymer Chemistry* 12 (39): 5689–5703. doi:10.1039/D1PY01075A.

Pires, Diana P., Hugo Oliveira, Luís D. R. Melo, Sanna Sillankorva, and Joana Azeredo. 2016. "Bacteriophage-Encoded Depolymerases: Their Diversity and Biotechnological Applications." *Applied Microbiology and Biotechnology* 100 (5): 2141–2151. doi:10.1007/S00253-015-7247-0.

Pitts, B., A. Willse, G. A. McFeters, M. A. Hamilton, N. Zelver, and P. S. Stewart. 2001. "A Repeatable Laboratory Method for Testing the Efficacy of Biocides against Toilet Bowl Biofilms." *Journal of Applied Microbiology* 91 (1): 110–117. doi:10.1046/J.1365-2672.2001.01342.X.

Ponraj, Diana Salomi, Jeppe Lange, Thomas Falstie-Jensen, Nis Pedersen Jørgensen, Christen Ravn, Anja Poehlein, and Holger Brüggemann. 2022. "Amplicon-Based Next-Generation Sequencing as a Diagnostic Tool for the Detection of Phylotypes of Cutibacterium Acnes in Orthopedic Implant-Associated Infections." *Frontiers in Microbiology* 13 (April). doi:10.3389/FMICB.2022.866893/PDF.

Pouget, Cassandra, Catherine Dunyach-Remy, Alix Pantel, Sophie Schuldiner, Albert Sotto, and Jean Philippe Lavigne. 2021. "New Adapted In Vitro Technology to Evaluate Biofilm Formation and Antibiotic Activity Using Live Imaging under Flow Conditions." *Diagnostics* 11 (10): 1746. doi:10.3390/DIAGNOSTICS11101746.

Rumbaugh, Kendra P., and Karin Sauer. 2020. "Biofilm Dispersion." *Nature Reviews Microbiology* 18 (10): 571–586. doi:10.1038/s41579-020-0385-0.

Sahli, Célia, Sergio E. Moya, John S. Lomas, Christine Gravier-Pelletier, Romain Briandet, and Miryana Hémadi. 2022. "Recent Advances in Nanotechnology for Eradicating Bacterial Biofilm." *Theranostics* 12 (5): 2383. doi:10.7150/THNO.67296.

Saleem, Haleema, and Syed Javaid Zaidi. 2020. "Developments in the Application of Nanomaterials for Water Treatment and Their Impact on the Environment." *Nanomaterials* 10 (9): 1764. doi:10.3390/NANO10091764.

Savage, Victoria J., Ian Chopra, and Alex J. O'Neill. 2013. "Staphylococcus Aureus Biofilms Promote Horizontal Transfer of Antibiotic Resistance." *Antimicrobial Agents and Chemotherapy* 57 (4): 1968–1970. doi:10.1128/AAC.02008-12.

Schooling, Sarah R., and Terry J. Beveridge. 2006. "Membrane Vesicles: An Overlooked Component of the Matrices of Biofilms." *Journal of Bacteriology* 188 (16): 5945–5957. doi:10.1128/JB.00257-06/ASSET/8503AE91-90C2-45CF-AC8C-861664775D3F/ASSETS/GRAPHIC/ZJB016065973007B.JPEG.

Scoffone, Viola Camilla, Gabriele Trespidi, Laurent R. Chiarelli, Giulia Barbieri, and Silvia Buroni. 2019. "Quorum Sensing as Antivirulence Target in Cystic Fibrosis Pathogens." *International Journal of Molecular Sciences* 20 (8): 1838. doi:10.3390/IJMS20081838.

Shao, Jing, Huijuan Cheng, Changzhong Wang, and Yan Wang. 2012. "A Phytoanticipin Derivative, Sodium Houttuyfonate, Induces in Vitro Synergistic Effects with Levofloxacin against Biofilm Formation by Pseudomonas Aeruginosa." *Molecules* 17 (9): 11242–11254. doi:10.3390/MOLECULES170911242.

Shao, Jing, Huijuan Cheng, Daqiang Wu, Changzhong Wang, Lingling Zhu, Zhenxin Sun, Qiangjun Duan, Weifeng Huang, and Jinliang Huang. 2013. "Antimicrobial Effect of Sodium Houttuyfonate on Staphylococcus Epidermidis and Candida Albicans Biofilms." *Journal of Traditional Chinese Medicine* 33 (6): 798–803. doi:10.1016/S0254-6272(14)60015-7.

Silva, N. B. S., L. A. Marques, and D. D. B. Röder. 2021. "Diagnosis of Biofilm Infections: Current Methods Used, Challenges and Perspectives for the Future." *Journal of Applied Microbiology* 131 (5): 2148–2160. doi:10.1111/JAM.15049.

Singh, Pradeep K., Amy L. Schaefer, Matthew R. Parsek, Thomas O. Moninger, Michael J. Welsh, and E. P. Greenberg. 2000. "Quorum-Sensing Signals Indicate That Cystic Fibrosis Lungs Are Infected with Bacterial Biofilms." *Nature* 407 (6805): 762–764. doi:10.1038/35037627.

Singh, Priyanka, Santosh Pandit, Carsten Jers, Abhayraj S. Joshi, Jørgen Garnæs, and Ivan Mijakovic. 2021. "Silver Nanoparticles Produced from Cedecea Sp. Exhibit Antibiofilm Activity and Remarkable Stability." *Scientific Reports* 11 (1). doi:10.1038/S41598-021-92006-4.

Singh, Shriti, Santosh Kumar Singh, Indrajit Chowdhury, and Rajesh Singh. 2017. "Understanding the Mechanism of Bacterial Biofilms Resistance to Antimicrobial Agents." *The Open Microbiology Journal* 11 (1): 53. doi:10.2174/1874285801711010053.

Slachmuylders, Lisa, Heleen Van Acker, Gilles Brackman, Andrea Sass, Filip Van Nieuwerburgh, and Tom Coenye. 2018. "Elucidation of the Mechanism behind the Potentiating Activity of Baicalin against Burkholderia Cenocepacia Biofilms." *PLOS ONE* 13 (1): e0190533. doi:10.1371/JOURNAL.PONE.0190533.

Stepanović, Srdjan, Dragana Vuković, Veronika Hola, Giovanni Di Bonaventura, Slobodanka Djukić, Ivana Ćirković, and Filip Ruzicka. 2007. "Quantification of Biofilm in Microtiter Plates: Overview of Testing Conditions and Practical Recommendations for Assessment of Biofilm Production by Staphylococci." *APMIS* 115 (8): 891–899. doi:10.1111/J.1600-0463.2007.APM_630.X.

Stickler, D. J. 2014. "Clinical Complications of Urinary Catheters Caused by Crystalline Biofilms: Something Needs to Be Done." *Journal of Internal Medicine* 276 (2): 120–129. doi:10.1111/JOIM.12220.

Sun, L. M., K. Liao, S. Liang, P. H. Yu, and D. Y. Wang. 2015. "Synergistic Activity of Magnolol with Azoles and Its Possible Antifungal Mechanism against Candida Albicans." *Journal of Applied Microbiology* 118 (4): 826–838. doi:10.1111/JAM.12737.

Sun, Lingmei, Kai Liao, and Dayong Wang. 2015. "Effects of Magnolol and Honokiol on Adhesion, Yeast-Hyphal Transition, and Formation of Biofilm by Candida Albicans." *PLOS ONE* 10 (2): e0117695. doi:10.1371/JOURNAL.PONE.0117695.

Sutherland, Ian W., Kevin A. Hughes, Lucy C. Skillman, and Karen Tait. 2004. "The Interaction of Phage and Biofilms." *FEMS Microbiology Letters* 232 (1): 1–6. doi:10.1016/S0378-1097(04)00041-2.

Svenson, Sönke, and Donald A. Tomalia. 2005. "Dendrimers in Biomedical Applications--Reflections on the Field." *Advanced Drug Delivery Reviews* 57 (15): 2106–2129. doi:10.1016/J.ADDR.2005.09.018.

Szentmáry, Nóra, Loay Daas, Lei Shi, Kornelia Lenke Laurik, Sabine Lepper, Georgia Milioti, and Berthold Seitz. 2019. "Acanthamoeba Keratitis – Clinical Signs, Differential Diagnosis and Treatment." *Journal of Current Ophthalmology* 31 (1): 16–23. doi:10.1016/J.JOCO.2018.09.008.

Tang, Taishan, Guoqiang Chen, Aizhen Guo, Ye Xu, Linli Zhao, Mengrui Wang, Chengping Lu, Yuan Jiang, and Changyin Zhang. 2020. "Comparative Proteomic and Genomic Analyses of Brucella Abortusbiofilm and Planktonic Cells." *Molecular Medicine Reports* 21 (2): 731–743. doi:10.3892/MMR.2019.10888/HTML.

Thappeta, Kishore Reddy Venkata, Li Na Zhao, Choy Eng Nge, Sharon Crasta, Chung Yan Leong, Veronica Ng, Yoganathan Kanagasundaram, Hao Fan, and Siew Bee Ng. 2020. "In-Silico Identified New Natural Sortase A Inhibitors Disrupt S. Aureus Biofilm Formation." *International Journal of Molecular Sciences* 21 (22): 8601. doi:10.3390/IJMS21228601.

Thi Viet Huong, Do, Phan Minh Giang, Hoang Thi Sim, and Truong Thi To Chinh. 2019. "Triterpenoids and Phytosterols Isolated from Pluchea Indica L. Leaves." *VNU Journal of Science: Natural Sciences and Technology* 35 (2). doi:10.25073/2588-1140/vnunst.4910.

Trampuz, Andrej, Kerryl E. Piper, Melissa J. Jacobson, Arlen D. Hanssen, Krishnan K. Unni, Douglas R. Osmon, Jayawant N. Mandrekar, Franklin R. Cockerill, James M. Steckelberg, James F. Greenleaf, and Robin Patel. 2007. "Sonication of Removed Hip and Knee Prostheses for Diagnosis of Infection." *New England Journal of Medicine* 357 (7): 654–663. doi:10.1056/NEJMOA061588/SUPPL_FILE/NEJM_TRAMPUZ_6 54SA1.PDF.

Trautner, Barbara W., and Rabih O. Darouiche. 2004. "Catheter-Associated Infections: Pathogenesis Affects Prevention." *Archives of Internal Medicine* 164 (8): 842–850. doi:10.1001/ARCHINTE.164.8.842.

Trentin, Danielle Da Silva, Raquel Brandt Giordani, Karine Rigon Zimmer, Alexandre Gomes Da Silva, Márcia Vanusa Da Silva, Maria Tereza Dos Santos Correia, Israel Jacob Rabin Baumvol, and Alexandre José MacEdo. 2011. "Potential of Medicinal Plants from the Brazilian Semi-Arid Region (Caatinga) against Staphylococcus Epidermidis Planktonic and Biofilm Lifestyles." *Journal of Ethnopharmacology* 137 (1): 327–335. doi:10.1016/J.JEP.2011.05.030.

Tseung, Karina Siow Yen Ng How, and Jingjun Zhao. 2016. "Update on the Fungal Biofilm Drug Resistance and Its Alternative Treatment." *Journal of Biosciences and Medicines* 4 (5): 37–47. doi:10.4236/JBM.2016.45004.

Van de Walle, A., J. E. Perez, A. Abou-Hassan, M. Hémadi, N. Luciani, and C. Wilhelm. 2020. "Magnetic Nanoparticles in Regenerative Medicine: What of Their Fate and Impact in Stem Cells?" *Materials Today Nano* 11 (August): 100084. doi:10.1016/J.MTNANO.2020.100084.

van Gennip, Maria, Louise Dahl Christensen, Morten Alhede, Klaus Qvortrup, Peter Østrup Jensen, Niels Høiby, Michael Givskov, and Thomas Bjarnsholt. 2012. "Interactions between Polymorphonuclear Leukocytes and Pseudomonas Aeruginosa Biofilms on Silicone Implants in Vivo." *Infection and Immunity* 80 (8): 2601–2607. doi:10.1128/IAI.06215-11/SUPPL_FILE/ZII999099727SO4.PDF.

Walker, Travis S., Kerry L. Tomlin, G. Scott Worthen, Katie R. Poch, Jonathan G. Lieber, Milene T. Saavedra, Michael B. Fessler, Kenneth C. Malcolm, Michael L. Vasil, and Jerry A. Nick. 2005. "Enhanced Pseudomonas Aeruginosa Biofilm Development Mediated by Human Neutrophils." *Infection and Immunity* 73 (6): 3693–3701. doi:10.1128/IAI.73.6.3693-3701.2005/ASSET/02FDC860-45B6-4012-9375-E9133C10321B/ASSETS/GRAPHIC/ZII0060549310006.JPEG.

Wang, Chaoli, Peng Chen, Youbei Qiao, Yuan Kang, Chaoren Yan, Zhe Yu, Jian Wang, Xin He, and Hong Wu. 2020. "PH Responsive Superporogen Combined with PDT Based on Poly Ce6 Ionic Liquid Grafted on SiO2 for Combating MRSA Biofilm Infection." *Theranostics* 10 (11): 4795. doi:10.7150/THNO.42922.

Wasfi, Reham, Samira M. Hamed, Mai A. Amer, and Lamiaa Ismail Fahmy. 2020. "Proteus Mirabilis Biofilm: Development and Therapeutic Strategies." *Frontiers in Cellular and Infection Microbiology* 10 (August): 414. doi:10.3389/FCIMB.2020.00414/XML/NLM.

Weaver, Abigail A., Nur A. Hasan, Mark Klaassen, Hiren Karathia, Rita R. Colwell, and Joshua D. Shrout. 2019. "Prosthetic Joint Infections Present Diverse and Unique Microbial Communities Using Combined Whole-Genome Shotgun Sequencing and Culturing Methods." *Journal of Medical Microbiology* 68 (10): 1507–1516. doi:10.1099/JMM.0.001068/CITE/REFWORKS.

Werdan, Karl, Sebastian Dietz, Bettina Löffler, Silke Niemann, Hasan Bushnaq, Rolf Edgar Silber, Georg Peters, and Ursula Müller-Werdan. 2013. "Mechanisms of Infective Endocarditis: Pathogen–Host Interaction and Risk States." *Nature Reviews Cardiology* 11 (1): 35–50. doi:10.1038/nrcardio.2013.174.

Willcox, Mark D. P. 2013. "Characterization of the Normal Microbiota of the Ocular Surface." *Experimental Eye Research* 117 (December): 99–105. doi:10.1016/J.EXER.2013.06.003.

Willcox, Mark D. P., Hua Zhu, and Ajay K. Vijay. 2012. "Effect of a Warming Device on Contact Lens Case Contamination." *Eye and Contact Lens* 38 (6): 394–399. doi:10.1097/ICL.0B013E318261AA13.

Wilson, Christina, Rachel Lukowicz, Stefan Merchant, Helena Valquier-Flynn, Jeniffer Caballero, Jasmin Sandoval, Macduff Okuom, Christopher Huber, Tessa Durham Brooks, Erin Wilson, Barbara Clement, Christopher D. Wentworth, and Andrea E. Holmes. 2017. "Quantitative and Qualitative Assessment Methods for Biofilm Growth: A Mini-Review." *Research & Reviews. Journal of Engineering and Technology* 6 (4). NIH Public Access. /pmc/articles/PMC6133255/.

Wongsaroj, Lampet, Kritsakorn Saninjuk, Adisak Romsang, Jintana Duang-nkern, Wachareeporn Trinachartvanit, Paiboon Vattanaviboon, and Skorn Mongkolsuk. 2018. "Pseudomonas Aeruginosa Glutathione Biosynthesis Genes Play Multiple Roles in Stress Protection, Bacterial Virulence and Biofilm Formation." *PLOS ONE* 13 (10): e0205815. doi:10.1371/JOURNAL.PONE.0205815.

Wright, Jesse S., Gholson J. Lyon, Elizabeth A. George, Tom W. Muir, and Richard P. Novick. 2004. "Hydrophobic Interactions Drive Ligand-Receptor Recognition for Activation and Inhibition of Staphylococcal Quorum Sensing." *Proceedings of the National Academy of Sciences of the United States of America* 101 (46): 16168–16173. doi:10.1073/PNAS.0404039101.

Wu, Dan, Xiao Dong Wu, Xue Fu You, Xiao Feng Ma, and Wei Xi Tian. 2010. "Inhibitory Effects on Bacterial Growth and B-Ketoacyl-ACP Reductase by Different Species of Maple Leaf Extracts and Tannic Acid." *Phytotherapy Research* 24 (S1): S35–S41. doi:10.1002/PTR.2873.

Wu, Jiayi, Yu Fan, Xinyue Wang, Xiaoge Jiang, Jing Zou, and Ruijie Huang. 2020. "Effects of the Natural Compound, Oxyresveratrol, on the Growth of Streptococcus Mutans, and on Biofilm Formation, Acid Production, and Virulence Gene Expression." *European Journal of Oral Sciences* 128 (1): 18–26. doi:10.1111/EOS.12667.

Xu, Karen D., Philip S. Stewart, Fuhu Xia, Ching Tsan Huang, and Gordon A. McFeters. 1998. "Spatial Physiological Heterogeneity in Pseudomonas Aeruginosa Biofilm Is Determined by Oxygen Availability." *Applied and Environmental Microbiology* 64 (10): 4035–4039. doi:10.1128/AEM.64.10.4035-4039.1998/ASSET/453595B0-C7D0-4EA3-B72E-912099767FFB/ASSETS/GRAPHIC/AM1080377005.JPEG.

Yang, Longfei, Xin Liu, Lili Zhong, Yujie Sui, Guihua Quan, Ying Huang, Fang Wang, and Tonghui Ma. 2018. "Dioscin Inhibits Virulence Factors of Candida Albicans." *BioMed Research International* 2018. doi:10.1155/2018/4651726.

Yong, Yi Yi, Gary A. Dykes, and Wee Sim Choo. 2019. "Biofilm Formation by Staphylococci in Health-Related Environments and Recent Reports on Their Control Using Natural Compounds." *Critical Reviews in Microbiology* 45 (2): 201–222. doi:10.1080/1040841X.2019.1573802.

Zhao, Min, Shimiao Cheng, Weipin G. Yuan, Jianyong Dong, Kexin Huang, Zhongmin Sun, and Pengcheng Yan. 2015. "Further New Xenicanes from a Chinese Collection of the Brown Alga Dictyota Plectens." *Chemical and Pharmaceutical Bulletin* 63 (12): 1081–1086. doi:10.1248/cpb.c15-00556.

Zhao, Qing, Xiao Ya Chen, and Cathie Martin. 2016. "Scutellaria Baicalensis, the Golden Herb from the Garden of Chinese Medicinal Plants." *Science Bulletin* 61 (18): 1391–1398. doi:10.1007/S11434-016-1136-5.

2 Biofilm Regulation and Quorum Sensing in Bacterial Pathogens

S. Anju, J. Swathi, Y. Aparna, and J. Sarada

2.1 INTRODUCTION

Communities of microbes that are embraced in the matrix of exopolysaccharides have been popularly known as biofilms. The population of microorganisms in a biofilm may be of different species or a single species that aggregate themselves in multilayers. Multiple gradients of matrix in the biofilm structure form microniches of specific species that are optimized in their metabolism with respect to the environment. Microbial cells in biofilm microcolonies develop well-equipped mechanisms to resist harmful chemical compounds, changes in pH, and environmental stress (Gebreyohannes et al., 2019; Flemming et al., 2016).

Biofilms are shaped on biotic surfaces such as connective tissue epithelial layers, endothelium, mucus membrane, intestines, cardiac valves, and bone marrow. These lead to diseases like pharyngitis, pneumonia, bacterial vaginosis, laryngitis, otitis media, endocarditis, mastitis, chronic rhinosinusitis, meningitis, inflammatory bowel diseases, and urinary tract infections. These infections are either chronic or recurrent. Oral cariogenic bacteria that cause tooth decay and gingivitis also are known to form prominent biofilms (Roy et al., 2018).

The biofilm-forming ability seems to be much higher in clinical than in environmental isolates. The ESKAPE group (*Enterococcus* spp., *Staphylococcus aureus, Staphylococcus epidermidis, Klebsiella* spp., *Acinetobacter baumannii, Pseudomonas aeruginosa, Enterobacter* spp.) causes a variety of biofilm-based infections, including wound infections, bacteremia, pneumonia, meningitis, and urinary tract infections. These organisms are known to overcome the action of antibiotics and host defense mechanisms. Most of the bacteria belonging to this group form elaborate biofilms on biotic as well as abiotic surfaces. These bacteria also cause critical infections in the immunocompromised (Sun et al., 2016) (Figure 2.1).

Various microbistatic substances lead to the emergence of antibiotic resistance strains that inhibit the multiplication of the cells and also the low concentration of many microbicidal drugs taken as improper administration. As a result of the antibiotic resistance, it is observed that there is an increased frequency

DOI: 10.1201/9781003297826-2

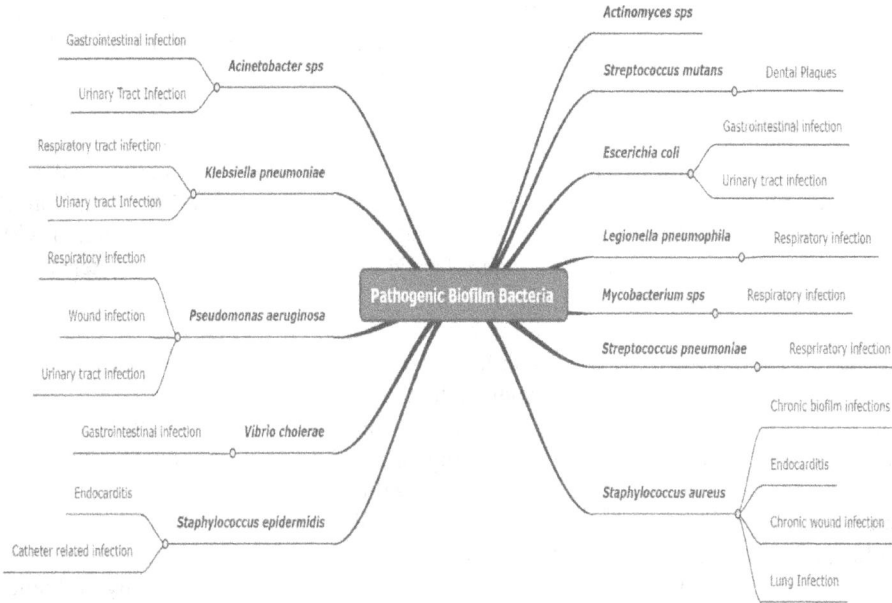

FIGURE 2.1 Pathogenic bacteria forming biofilm.

of disease, emergence of chronic infections, morbidity, and mortality. Many of the medical procedures that require efficient treatment with antibiotics, such as open heart surgery, cancer therapy, organ transplantation, and the use of medical devices, are susceptible to antibiotic-resistant microbial species (Weist and Diaz Hogberg, 2014). Among pathogenic bacteria, certain traits help them to enhance their disease-causing abilities, which mostly involve the production of signal molecules, complex communication systems, and virulence factors that enable a coordinated growth pattern (Stoica et al., 2016).

Regarding infection control related to ESKAPE, the well-known quorum sensing (QS) experimental models, *P. aeruginosa* and *S. aureus*, seem to be the most investigated. The growing frequency of nosocomial infections and acquired resistance mechanisms of the gram-negative species of the ESKAPE group—*Klebsiella* spp., *Enterobacter* spp., and *Acinetobacter* spp.—demand innovative and effective antimicrobial approaches.

2.2 BIOFILM REGULATION IN PATHOGENS

As part of the biofilm lifecycle, bacterial pathogens shift among diverse environments and respond to a number of changes. Instantaneous acclimatization to such changes results in the multiplication and development of biofilm. Most of the bacterial pathogens exhibit multicellular existence required for survival in nature as well as during infections.

The formation of biofilm is induced by different features such as changes in environmental conditions, alterations in nutritional and metabolic properties, oxidative stress, low pH, starvation, heavy metals, toxic compounds, QS signals, subinhibitory concentrations of antimicrobials, and host-derived signals. For example, biofilm formation of *Salmonella typhimurium* is induced by bile salts and acidic stress under oxygen-limiting conditions in the stomach and the small intestine. Various antibiotics at subinhibitory concentrations initiate biofilm formation. Biofilm formation of *Enterococcus faecalis* due to induction of cell wall antibiotics was associated with increased cell lysis, increased extracellular DNA levels, and increased density of bacterial cells (Srivastava et al., 2019).

Posttranscriptional processing for biofilm formation includes the cyclic RNA chemical second messenger molecule cyclic diguanosine monophosphate (c-di-GMP). C-di-GMP controls numerous cellular roles, including motility, virulence, and adhesion, though its main function is to control the shift from a motile planktonic lifestyle to the sessile state resulting in biofilm development. Raised intracellular levels of c-di-GMP encourage the synthesis of EPS, autoaggregation, and surface adhesion leading to the formation of biofilm (Simm et al., 2004). However, reduced intracellular c-di-GMP is associated with decreased biofilm formation. The CsrA, an RNA-binding protein, suppresses biofilm formation by influencing the stability of mRNA transcripts coding polysaccharides that make up the extracellular biofilm matrix. CsrA inhibits or inactivates GGDEF/EAL-encoding proteins that regulate c-di-GMP levels, thereby stimulating motility, instead of biofilm formation. OmrA/B, RprA, GcvB, and McaS regulate biofilm by suppressing csgD, encoding the csgD master regulator responsible for the production of cellulose, curli fimbria, and c-di-GMP. CsrB/CsrC and McaS favor biofilm formation by blocking CsrA activity in pathogens like *E. coli* and *Salmonella* or by positively affecting the production of c-di-GMP (Qrr1-4) and expression of exopolysaccharides (e.g., *Vibrio cholerae*). Degradation of the transcript mqsA of antitoxin by the MqsR toxin leads to inhibition of motility and induction of csgD, favoring curli production.

Environmental factors such as nutrient concentrations of glucose and amino acids, and physiological stresses such as pH, oxidative stress, osmolarity, and antimicrobials are signals facilitating the switch from the planktonic motile to the sessile biofilm state (Figure 2.2).

Pseudomonas aeruginosa RhlA mutants deficient in the synthesis of biosurfactants are found not to show migration-dependent development leading to the development of mushroom-shaped multicellular structures during biofilm formation. The Rhl system controls the expression of pyocyanin and rhamnolipids, which is known to control the deposition of extracellular DNA, a component of the early and late biofilm evolving phases (Muhammad, et al., 2020).

The β-lactam antibiotics result in the release of the extracellular DNA, which is dependent on the autolysin Atl in *Staphylococcus aureus*. The mupirocin-induced biofilm formation of pathogenic *Staphylococcus aureus* was identified due to the upregulation of CidAholin associated with enhanced production of extracellular DNA. Also, similar features were detected in the induction of biofilm formation

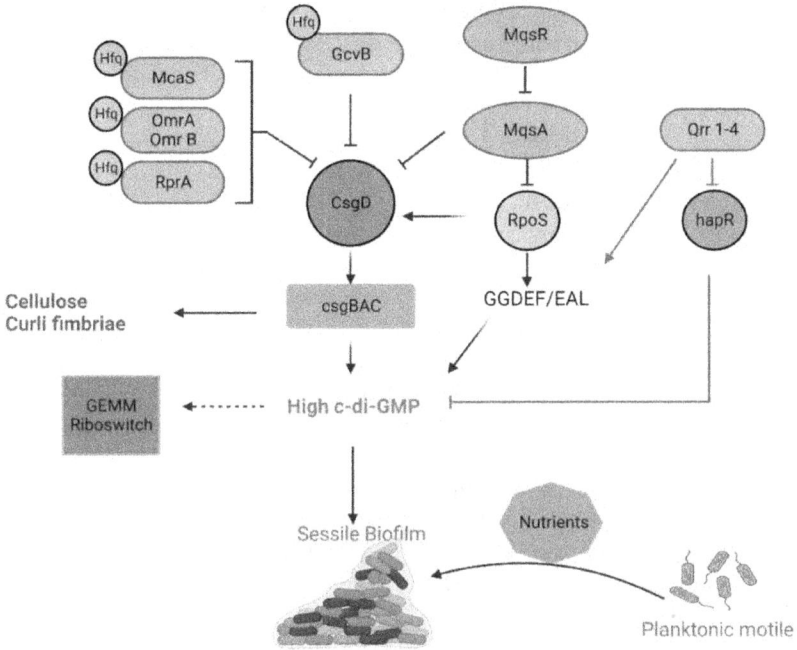

FIGURE 2.2A Biofilm regulation in sessile state.

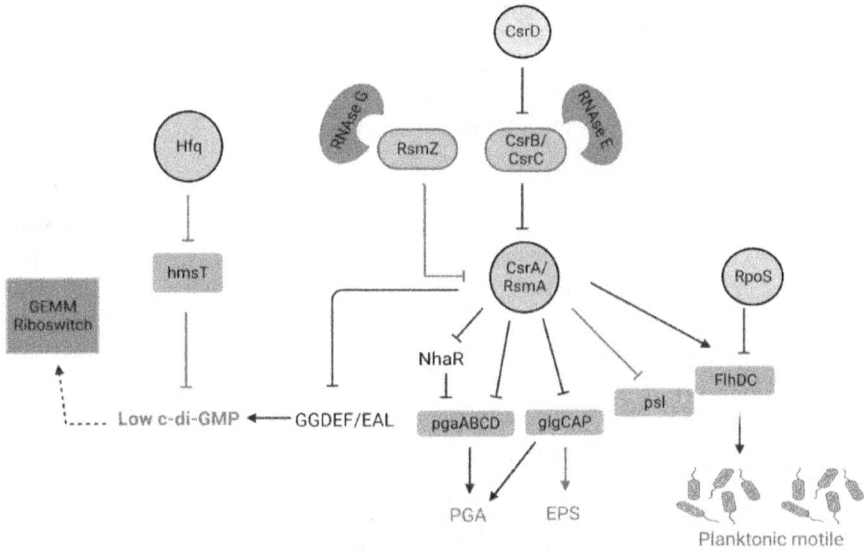

FIGURE 2.2B Biofilm regulation in motile state.

of *Pseudomonas aeruginosa* when aminoglycoside antibiotics regulated the aminoglycoside response regulator (arr). The arr gene encodes inner membrane phosphodiesterase, which targets c-di-GMP, a second messenger regulating cell–surface adhesiveness (Seper et al., 2011).

Induction of the capsular exopolysaccharide in *Acinetobacter baumannii* through a mechanism mediated by the TCS BfmRS in the presence of chloramphenicol and erythromycin has been noticed. Also, azithromycin reduces the biofilm formation of *Pseudomonas aeruginosa* and impedes QS-regulated virulence factors like autoinducer production, swarming, and pyocyanin production (Luna et al., 2019).

Among the biofilm-forming bacteria, *Pseudomonas aeruginosa* is a common infectious agent that leads to most of the infections in the medical setting. Analysis under a microscope shows the *Pseudomonas* biofilm as a mass of cells distinguished into mushroom and stalk-like structures. These are found to be nourished by intervening water channels to allow the flow of nutrients (Passador and Iglewsi, 1995; Hassett et al., 2005).

Pseudomonas aeruginosa has small cationic polyamines like putrescine along with its biosynthetic precursors L-arginine and agmatine that encourage biofilm formation and confer resistance to environmental stimuli of stress. Putrescine and L-arginine upsurge the intracellular c-di-GMP levels. In *Pseudomonas aeruginosa*, SiaDis a diguanylate cyclase that is co-transcribed with siaA/siaB/siaC from the siaABCD operon. The siaABCD encodes a signaling network that is capable of regulating the formation of aggregate cells by modulating the enzymatic activity of SiaD. SiaC combines with SiaD to increase diguanylate cyclase activity, which promotes c-di-GMP synthesis. The communication of SiaC with SiaD is enabled by the inner membrane-associated Ser/Thr SiaA phosphatase, although it is phosphorylated by the SiaB protein kinase. SiaA is triggered by peripheral stress stimuli such as sodium dodecyl sulfate (Diaz-Salazar et al., 2017).

Biofilm formation in *Pseudomonas aeruginosa* is regulated by the two QS systems LasI/LasR and RhlR/RhlI. These are expressed during both early and late biofilm phases. A *LasI* mutant forms flat and indistinguishable biofilms sensitive to sodium dodecyl sulfate.

Furthermore, PqsE thioesterase, part of the 2-alkyl-4-quinolone biosynthesis gene cluster pqsABCDE, is important in the production of rhamnolipids, pyocyanin, and lectin A. *Pseudomonas aeruginosa* intensifies expression Pel and Psl exopolysaccharides upregulating the transcription of two small regulatory RNAs, rsmY and rsmZ. RsmA raises the expression of the type III secretion system (T3SS) and simultaneously represses the type VI secretion system (T6SS).

Other TCSs involved in the biofilm formation of *Pseudomonas aeruginosa* include SagS, BfiRS, BfmRS, and MifRS, which are sequentially phosphorylated during biofilm formation. Deactivation of any one of these limits the formation of biofilm-specific developmental stages. SagS allows the shift from the planktonic state to the sessile by activation of the TCS BfiRS. BfiRS reduces rsmYZ levels, which is necessary for the maturation of *Pseudomonas aeruginosa* biofilm.

BrlR-mediated upregulation of efflux pumps using SagS for resistance to antibiotics is by means of mexAB-oprM and mexEF-oprN. BmfRS regulates biofilm maturation, whereas MifRS modulates microcolony formation. The roc1 locus regulates fimbrial cupB and cupC genes, which encode two response regulators (RocA1 and RocR) and one sensor kinase (RocS1). This cluster, named sadARS, is known to repress type III secretion genes and positively regulate biofilm formation. RocA2 represses the expression of the mexAB-oprM efflux pump, while the RocS1A1R system seems to initiate a signal cascade promoting biofilm formation through Cup fimbriae (Gebreyohannes et al., 2019).

In a similar situation for *Vibrio cholerae* biofilm, the extracellular matrix is composed of *Vibrio* polysaccharides (VPS), and three major matrix proteins—RbmA, RbmC, and Bap1—are responsible for cell–cell and cell–surface adhesion. VpsR and VpsT are identified as principal regulators that positively regulate VPS production. Both VpsR and VpsT are influenced by c-di-GMP promoting transcriptional switch-directing biofilm-regulated genes (Seper et al., 2011).

In *Escherichia coli*, QseBC TCS controlled biofilm formation by upregulating the transcription of bcsA, csgA, fliC, motA, wcaF, and fimA, which are known to be the biofilm-associated genes. The increased transcription of the efflux pump-associated genes marA, acrA, acrB, acrD, emrD, and mdtH conferred antibiotic resistance. BasSR TCS in pathogenic *Escherichia coli* enhances biofilm formation by upregulating the expression of biofilm and the virulence-related genes entC, opgC, gtcE, and fepA. Furthermore, CpxRA TCS senses membrane stress and misfolded proteins, in proper biofilm establishment, motility, adherence, and the formation of type 1 fimbria (Al Safadi et al., 2012).

2.3   QUORUM SENSING IN PATHOGENIC BIOFILM

The bacterial population sends signals about their presence in a place to one another by producing, detecting, and responding to diffusible small signal molecules called autoinducers.

This process of intercellular communication, called quorum sensing, was first described in the marine bioluminescent bacterium *Vibrio fischeri*. *V. fischeri* lives in symbiosis with a number of marine organism hosts. The host uses light formed by *V. fischeri* to attract prey, evade predators, or find a mate. QS controls the regulation of gene expression of numerous endo- and exogenous molecules that are required for the expression of virulence factors, fitness of cells, biofilm formation, exemplifying infection in the host, and escaping host immune responses and antimicrobial substances. The QS mechanism is established with a specific density of signaling molecules referred to as autoinducers. The QS signaling influences the bacterial cells at a distance ranging between 5 and 200 μm (Tamayo et al., 2010; Schulze et al., 2021).

Pathogenic species like *P. aeruginosa*, *E. coli*, *Baumannii*, and *V. cholerae* produce homoserine lactones of different molecular weights and lengths, whereas autoinducing peptides are produced by gram-positive *Staphylococcus aureus* and *Streptococcus* spp.

Acyl homoserine lactones (AHL) are important cellular signaling molecules functioning as part of QS and are used chiefly by gram-negative bacteria. Gram-positive bacteria synthesize oligopeptides as signaling molecules for the development of bio-films. There are three types of QS systems: (i) the acyl homoserine lactone QS system (AHL) in gram-negative bacteria, (ii) the autoinducing peptide (AIP) QS system in gram-positive bacteria, and (iii) the autoinducer-2 (AI-2) system in both gram-negative and gram-positive bacteria. Gram-positive bacteria release AIPs, signaling molecules secreted by membrane transporters. As the surrounding concentration of AIPs increases, these bind to the histidine kinase sensor, which phosphorylates, and as a result, alters target gene expression. In *Staphylococcus* aureus, QS signals are controlled by the *agr*, which is associated with AIP secretion. The production of degradable exoenzymes and toxins as part of virulence are expressed by these genes (Preda and Săndulescu, 2019).

Bacterial cooperation and communication are due to the ability to identify and interpret the signals of AI-2 interspecific signals, which are mediated by LuxS synthase. LuxS activates the methylation cycle and controls the expression of genes associated with the microbial processes of surface adhesion, detachment, toxin production, etc. (Starkey et al., 2014). In gram-negative bacteria signal molecules, AHL synthesis is dependent on a LuxI-like protein. LuxR-like protein is responsible for the recognition of the AHL binding. After that, they activate specific promoter DNA elements and activate the transcription of target genes (Soria-Bustos et al., 2020).

The biochemical mechanism of action of LuxI/LuxR pairs is conserved. The LuxI-like enzymes produce a specific AHL by coupling the acyl side chain of a specific acyl–acyl carrier protein (acyl-ACP) from the fatty acid biosynthetic machinery to the homocysteine moiety of S-adenosylmethionine (SAM).

This intermediate lactonizes to form acyl-HSL, releasing methylthioadenosine. There are hundreds of gram-negative bacteria identified using LuxI/LuxR-type quorum sensing to control a wide range of cellular processes (Utari et al., 2017).

Each species produces a unique AHL or a unique combination of AHL and, as a result, only the members of the same species recognize and respond to their own signal molecule (Richter et al., 2012).

Two types of quorum-sensing systems are identified in gram-positive bacteria. One consists of three components: a signaling peptide (AIP), and a two-component signal transduction system (TCSTS) that specifically detects and responds to an AIP. A signal peptide precursor is produced by gram-positive bacteria that are cleaved as a double-glycine consensus sequence and the activated AIP is then transferred through a peptide-specific ABC transporter into the surrounding environment (Noirot-Gros et al., 2019; Li and Tian, 2012).

The autoinducer (C12-HSL, PQS, IqsR, or C4-HSL) produced by every system interacts with the corresponding receptor (LasR, PqsR, IqsR, or RhlR). The receptors turn on a cascade leading to the expression of a large number of genes. Also, a cross talk of LasR affects PqsR, IqsR, and RhlR. There is also reciprocated communication between PqsR and RhlR. PqsR is responsible for biofilm formation and release of extracellular DNA. Detachment of biofilm cells and maintenance of channels within the matrix are controlled by RhlR (Figure 2.3).

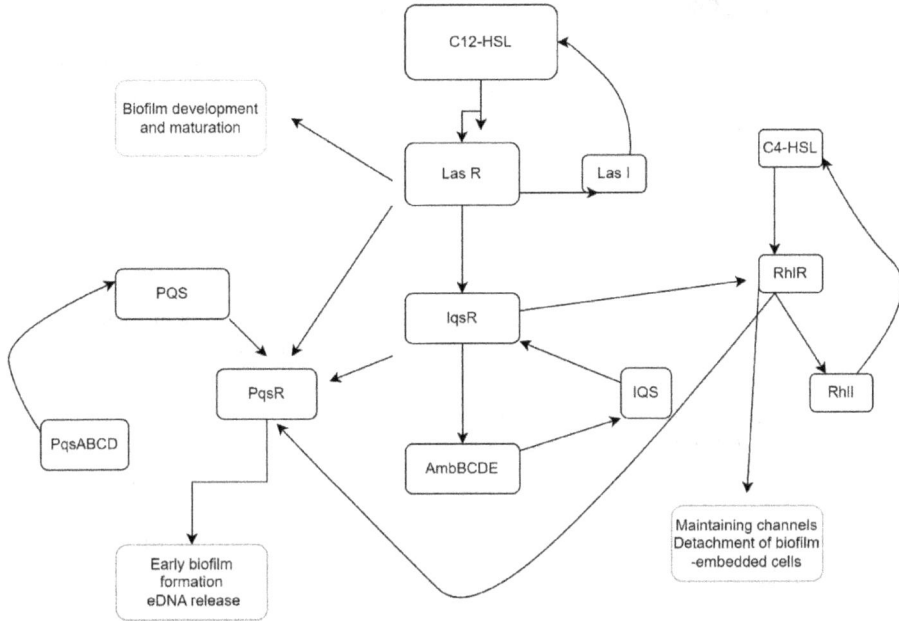

FIGURE 2.3 Cross talk of four QS systems—Las, Rhl, Pqs, and Iqs—*Pseudomonas aeruginosa* for biofilm formation.

Most signaling peptides in gram-positive bacteria consist of 5–25 amino acids and unusual side chains. A membrane-associated histidine kinase protein senses the AIP, and a cytoplasmic response regulator protein enables the cell to respond to the peptide via regulation of gene expression. A second type of quorum-sensing system is recognized in some gram-positive *Streptococci salivarius*, *Streptococci pyogenic*, *Streptococci mutans*, and *Streptococci bovis* groups. This new system is called ComRS, and it has sensors for the small double-tryptophan signal peptide, XIP pheromone. XIP pheromone interacts with a transcriptional regulator to activate competence genes for genetic transformation. *S. mutans* possess ComCDE and ComRS quorum-sensing systems that regulate genetic competence and bacteriocin production. The LuxS-dependent biofilm formation and its molecular mechanism are also identified in clinical isolate of *S. pneumoniae*. Natural biofilms like dental plaque are found to have a LuxS homologue in their genomes (Suntharalingam and Cvitkovitch, 2005).

Quorum sensing in biofilms is complicated, as a range of physical, chemical, and nutritional factors influence signal production, distribution, and efficiency to interact with their receptors in a biofilm. AHL molecules and small peptides diffuse freely in the biofilm matrix; interact with charged molecules; and influence physical, chemical, and biological factors within a biofilm. Since QS activation depends on the diffusion of a signal molecule, QS could be considered diffusion sensing (DS). DS sensing is the direct capability of the individual cells to evolve for autoinducer sensing (Sionov and Steinberg, 2022).

2.4   DRUG RESISTANCE IN PATHOGENIC BIOFILM

The formation of microbial biofilms in diseases causes serious health issues as the biofilms have higher incidences of antimicrobial resistance. When compared to planktonic forms, bacterial cells in biofilm have a thousand times enhanced drug resistance (Olson et al., 2002; Mosaddad et al., 2019).

The physiological barrier of the exopolysaccharide (EPS) matrix along with many regulatory drug-resistant mechanisms prevents the effective diffusion of the majority of antibiotics (Fair and Tor, 2014; Macià et al., 2014). The EPS is found to repel polar-charged molecules of antibiotics and inhibit the entry of detrimental substances that have larger molecular sizes. As time passes, the biofilm environment in its interior becomes anaerobic and is characterized by a lower supply of nutrients and other essential growth factors (Powell et al., 2018).

The pathogenic biofilm causing nosocomial infections are mostly identified to be resistant to multidrug antibiotics. The metabolically active organisms are more susceptible to antibiotics compared to the less active organisms in biofilm (Lewis, 2001).

The anaerobic conditions of biofilm make the antibiotics beta-lactams, aminoglycosides, and fluoroquinolones ineffective due to the absence of oxygen. *P. aeruginosa* biofilm produces a high concentration of alginate in exopolysaccharide, which transforms the disease into a chronic infection. Production of mannuronic acid and glucuronic acid in the EPS protects the biofilm from the action of ceftazidime, ciprofloxacin, and gentamycin.

After horizontal gene transfer and frequent spontaneous mutation among microcolonies in biofilm bacteria, they are found to acclimatize to new hostile environments. *P. aeruginosa* is one of the bacteria that possesses a high level of antibiotic resistance, as it has the capacity for recurrent spontaneous mutation, resulting in the production of β-lactamase that inactivates the β-lactam antibiotics.

eDNA increases biofilm resistance mechanisms by altering the outer membrane conformation of the biofilm and influencing the chelating cations, such as calcium and magnesium, in *P. aeruginosa*, *Acinetobacter baumannii*, *Enterobacter* sp., *S. aureus*, *Enterococcus faecium*, *Klebsiella pneumoniae*, and *Salmonella enterica*. Reduced permeability of the bacterial cell wall for larger molecules of aminoglycosides and the increased expression of low-affinity penicillin-binding proteins have been found to be responsible for antimicrobial resistance in *E. faecium* to β-lactam antibiotics and aminoglycosides (Hedberg and Nord, 1996).

Heterogeneousness in bacterial populations with different QS expression patterns and antibiotic-persisted cells in a biofilm of *S. aureus* has shown cell survival in the presence of antibiotics without development of resistance (Kaplan et al., 2018). Antibiotic-resistant *Staphylococcus aureus* has reduced metabolic activity with less production of ATP in low oxygen and nutrition concentrations, which ultimately elevates tolerance for antibiotics in biofilm. Enzymes, like proteases and nucleases formed by *S. aureus*, diffuse in the biofilm, increasing the viability of the biofilm cells. *Klebsiella pneumoniae* has a thick layer of extracellular formation in the biofilm state along biotic and abiotic surfaces, which increases antibiotic tolerance.

Biofilm organisms such as *P. aeruginosa* develop resistance to antibiotics such as ciprofloxacin and tobramycin due to less oxygen availability in the microenvironment. The heterogeneity also generates a nutritional shortage for certain bacterial populations, favoring enhanced resistance. Biofilm heterogeneity with respect to genotype and phenotype is an important factor in initiating resistance of bacterial communities in biofilms against many antibacterial drugs.

Antibiotic resistance in biofilms can be shifted among the biofilm-forming bacteria through external mechanisms like quorum sensing and EPS. Through metabolic cascades and gene expression, the signal mechanisms can control bacterial behavior (Mirghani et al., 2022).

REFERENCES

Al Safadi, R., Abu-Ali, G. S., Sloup, R. E., Rudrik, J. T., Waters, C. M., Eaton, K. A., and Manning, S. D. (2012). Correlation between in vivo biofilm formation and virulence gene expression in Escherichia coli O104:H4. *PLoS One* 7(7): e41628. https://doi.org/10.1371/journal.pone.0041628

Diaz-Salazar, C., Calero, P., Espinosa-Portero, R., Jimenez-Fernandez, A., Wirebrand, L., Velasco-Dominguez, M. G., et al. (2017). The stringent response promotes biofilm dispersal in Pseudomonas putida. *Scientific Reports* 7: 18055. https://doi.org/10.1038/s41598-017-18518-0

Fair, R. J., and Tor, Y. (2014). Antibiotics and bacterial resistance in the 21st century. *Perspectives in Medicinal Chemistry* 6: 25–64. https://doi.org/10.4137/PMC.S14459

Flemming, H. C., Wingender, J., Szewzyk, U., Steinberg, P., Rice, S. A., and Kjelleberg, S. (2016). Biofilms: An emergent form of bacterial life. *Nature Reviews Microbiology* 14: 563–575. [CrossRef] [PubMed]

Gebreyohannes, G., Nyerere, A., Bii, C., and Sbhatu, D. B. (2019). Challenges of intervention, treatment, and antibiotic resistance of biofilm forming microorganisms. *Heliyon* 5: e02192. [CrossRef] [PubMed]

Hedberg, M., and Nord, C. E. (1996). Beta-lactam resistance in anaerobic bacteria: A review. *Journal of Chemotherapy* 8: 3–16. https://doi.org/10.1179/joc.1996.8.1.3

Kaplan, J. B., Mlynek, K. D., Hettiarachchi, H., et al. (2018). Extracellular polymeric substance (EPS)- degrading enzymes reduce Staphylococcal surface attachment and biocide resistance on pig skin in vivo. *PLoS One* 13: e0205526. https://doi.org/10.1371/journal.pone.0205526

Lewis, K. (2001). Riddle of biofilm resistance. *Antimicrobial Agents and Chemotherapy* 45: 999. https://doi.org/10.1128/AAC.45.4.999-1007.2001

Li, Y. H., and Tian, X. (2012). Quorum sensing and bacterial social interactions in biofilms. *Sensors* 12(3): 2519–2538.

Luna, B. M., Yan, J., Reyna, Z., Moon, E., Nielsen, T. B., Reza, H., et al. (2019). Natural history of Acinetobacter baumannii infection in mice. *PloS One* 14: e0219824. https://doi.org/10.1371/journal.pone.0219824

Macià, M. D., Rojo-Molinero, E., and Oliver, A. (2014). Antimicrobial susceptibility testing in biofilmgrowing bacteria. *Clinical Microbiology and Infection* 20: 981–990. https://doi.org/10.1111/1469-0691.126

Mirghani, R., Saba, T., Khaliq, H., Mitchell, J., Do, L., Chambi, L., ... Rijal, G. (2022). Biofilms: Formation, drug resistance and alternatives to conventional approaches. *AIMS Microbiology* 8(3): 239–277.

Mosaddad, S. A., Tahmasebi, E., Yazdanian, A., et al. (2019). Oral microbial biofilms: An update. *European Journal of Clinical Microbiology & Infectious Diseases* 38: 2005–2019. https://doi.org/10.1007/s10096-019-03641-9-1

Muhammad, M. H., Idris, A. L., Fan, X., Guo, Y., Yu, Y., Jin, X., ... Huang, T. (2020). Beyond risk: Bacterial biofilms and their regulating approaches. *Frontiers in Microbiology* 11: 928.

Noirot-Gros, M. F., Forrester, S., Malato, G., Larsen, P. E., and Noirot, P. (2019). CRISPR interference to interrogate genes that control biofilm formation in Pseudomonas fluorescens. *Scientific Reports* 9: 15954. https://doi.org/10.1038/s41598-019-52400-5

Olson, M. E., Ceri, H., Morck, D. W., et al. (2002). Biofilm bacteria: Formation and comparative susceptibility to antibiotics. *Canadian Journal of Veterinary Research* 66: 86–92.

Passador, L., and Iglewsi, B. (1995). Quorum sensing and virulence gene regulation in Pseudomonas aeruginosa. In *Virulence Mechanisms of Bacterial Pathogens*, Sec. Edn, J. A. Roth, C. A. Bolin, K. A. Brogden, F. C. Minion, and M. J. Wannemuehler, eds. Washington, DC: ASM Press, 65–78.

Powell, L. C., Pritchard, M. F., Ferguson, E. L., et al. (2018). Targeted disruption of the extracellular polymeric network of Pseudomonas aeruginosa biofilms by alginate oligosaccharides. *NPJ Biofilms Microbiomes* 4: 13. https://doi.org/10.1038/s41522-018-0056-3

Preda, V. G., and Săndulescu, O. (2019). Communication is the key: Biofilms, quorum sensing, formation and prevention. *Discoveries* 7(3).

Roy, R., Tiwari, M., Donelli, G., and Tiwari, V. (2018). Strategies for combating bacterial biofilms: A focus on anti-biofilm agents and their mechanisms of action. *Virulence* 9: 522–554. https://doi.org/10.1080/21505594.2017.1313372

Schulze, A., Mitterer, F., Pombo, J. P., and Schild, S. (2021). Biofilms by bacterial human pathogens: Clinical relevance-development, composition and regulation-therapeutical strategies. *Microbial Cell* 8(2): 28.

Seper, A., Fengler, V. H., Roier, S., Wolinski, H., Kohlwein, S. D., Bishop, A. L., Camilli, A., Reidl, J., and Schild, S. (2011). Extracellular nucleases and extracellular DNA play important roles in Vibrio cholerae biofilm formation. *Molecular Microbiology* 82(4): 1015–1037. https://doi.org/10.1111/j.1365-2958.2011.07867

Simm, R., Morr, M., Kader, A., Nimtz, M., and Romling, U. (2004). GGDEF and EAL domains inversely regulate cyclic di-GMP levels and transition from sessility to motility. *Molecular Microbiology* 53: 1123–1134. https://doi.org/10.1111/j.1365-2958.2004.04206.x

Sionov, R. V., and Steinberg, D. (2022). Targeting the holy triangle of quorum sensing, biofilm formation, and antibiotic resistance in pathogenic bacteria. *Microorganisms* 10(6): 1239.

Soria-Bustos, J., Ares, M. A., Gómez-Aldapa, C. A., González-Y-Merchand, J. A., Girón, J. A., and De la Cruz, M. A. (2020). Two Type VI secretion systems of Enterobacter cloacae are required for bacterial competition, cell adherence, and intestinal colonization. *Frontiers in Microbiology* 11: 560488. https://doi.org/10.3389/fmicb.2020.560488

Srivastava, A., Chandra, N., and Kumar, S. (2019). The role of biofilms in medical devices and implants. In *Biofilms in Human Diseases: Treatment and Control*, S. Kumar, N. Chandra, L. Singh, M. Z. Hashmi, and A. Varma (eds). Cham: Springer International Publishing, 151–165. https://doi.org/10.1007/978-3-030-30757-8

Starkey, M., Lepine, F., Maura, D., Bandyopadhaya, A., Lesic, B., He, J., et al. (2014). Identification of Anti-virulence compounds that disrupt quorum sensing regulated acute and persistent pathogenicity. *PLoS Pathogens* 10: e1004321. https://doi.org/10.1371/journal.ppat.1004321

Stoica, P., Chifiriuc, M. C., Rapa, M., and Lazar, V. (2016). Overview of biofilm-related problems in medical devices. In *Biofilms and Implantable Medical Devices*, Y. Deng and W. Lv (eds). Cambridge: Woodhead Publishing, 3–23. https://doi.org/10.1016/b978-0-08-100382-4.00001-0

Sun, S., Zhang, H., Lu, S., Lai, C., Liu, H., Zhu, H., et al. (2016). The metabolic flux regulation of Klebsiella pneumoniae based on quorum sensing system. *Scientific Reports* 6: 38725. https://doi.org/10.1038/srep38725

Suntharalingam, P., and Cvitkovitch, D. G. (2005). Quorum sensing in streptococcal biofilm formation. *Trends in Microbiology* 13(1): 13–6.

Taha, O. A., Connerton, P. L., Connerton, I. F., and El-Shibiny, A. (2018). Bacteriophage ZCKP1: a potential treatment for Klebsiella pneumoniae isolated from diabetic foot patients. *Frontiers in Microbiology* 9: 2127.

Tamayo, R., Patimalla, B., and Camilli, A. (2010). Growth in a biofilm induces a hyperinfectious phenotype in Vibrio cholerae. *Infection and Immunity* 78(8): 3560–3569. https://doi.org/10.1128/IAI.00048-10

Utari, P. D., Vogel, J., and Quax, W. J. (2017). Deciphering physiological functions of AHL quorum quenching acylases. *Frontiers in Microbiology* 8: 1123. https://doi.org/10.3389/fmicb.2017.01123

Vrancianu, C. O., Gheorghe, I., Dobre, E. G., Barbu, I. C., Cristian, R. E., Popa, M., et al. (2020). Emerging strategies to combat β-lactamase producing ESKAPE pathogens. *International Journal of Molecular Sciences* 21: 8527. https://doi.org/10.3390/ijms21228527

Weist, K., and Diaz Högberg, L. (2014). ECDC publishes 2013 surveillance data on antimicrobial resistance and antimicrobial consumption in Europe. *Eurosurveillance* 19: 20962. https://doi.org/10.2807/1560-7917.es2014.19.46.20962

3 Quorum Sensing in Extremophiles

Srinivasan Kameswaran and Bellamkonda Ramesh

3.1 INTRODUCTION

In high cell densities, quorum sensing is a sort of microbial communication that controls gene expression (Bassler, 2002). It is dependent on the cells' generation of signaling molecules that are discharged into the environment. These molecules are continuously produced by every cell, and gene transcription only starts when they reach a specific concentration. The features controlled by quorum sensing are ineffective when carried out by a single cell alone, hence it is believed that the microbial population as a whole can monitor and regulate gene expression and consequently physiology (including metabolism) through this process (Bassler, 2002; Dobretsov et al., 2012; Fuqua et al., 2001).

Bioluminescence, cell competence, horizontal gene transfer, pathogenicity, motility, the development of biofilms, and the synthesis of antibiotics and other secondary metabolites are all known to be regulated by quorum sensing (Rivas et al., 2005; Chaphalkar and Slunkhe, 2010). The regulation of bioluminescence in the marine bacteria *Vibrio harveyi* and *Aliivibrio fischeri* by a number of quorum-sensing mechanisms has been thoroughly defined and reported (Bassler, 2002; Fuqua et al., 1996). Extremophiles are one of the many categories of organisms whose quorum sensing has still to be discovered or characterized in a wide variety of settings and organisms.

A wide range of organisms recognized for their capacity to endure and adapt to "extreme" environmental circumstances are referred to as extremophiles (Pituka and Hoover, 2007). Although this is a manmade definition, the species in this category show the variety of habitats in which life can exist. This includes salinity (high and low), high and low pH levels, extremes of heat and cold, high pressure, nutritional restrictions, or combinations of these conditions. Because microbes need to be able to adapt quickly in order to thrive in a certain niche, short-term oscillations in environmental parameters can also be viewed as harsh conditions. This is especially true in the interesting habitat of microbial mats, which will be discussed later in this chapter. Extremophiles have received a great deal of attention recently because of their potential to shed light on environmental adaptation. The potential use of extremophilic metabolites and extracellular enzymes in business and biotechnology is of great interest to researchers as demand in these fields rises (Van den Burg, 2003). There hasn't been much research done on the use of quorum sensing

DOI: 10.1201/9781003297826-3

in harsh conditions. A small number of individual organisms have been studied to determine the significance of quorum sensing in the adaptation of microorganisms, in general, and extremophiles, in particular, to their environment; however, the function of quorum sensing in the extended microbial biosphere is still largely unknown. A relative richness of knowledge about extremophiles has been made possible by the development of bioinformatic technology and large databases. Although it's not impossible, it might be challenging to cultivate them in the lab because they must endure such extreme circumstances. Therefore, the recent ability to conduct genomic and proteomic investigations on environmental samples has mostly been responsible for allowing significant insight into the capabilities of these bacteria. The goal of this chapter is to evaluate how well we currently understand how quorum sensing might be used in harsh conditions and to give the data supporting this idea.

3.2 QUORUM-SENSING SYSTEMS

The first evidence of quorum sensing was found in the organisms *V. harveyi* and *A. fischeri,* which were observed to create a luminous quality when cell densities reached a certain level. The LuxI–LuxR, or AI-1, quorum-sensing system was discovered to be a genetic mechanism shared by this and other gram-negative bacteria. These first observations led to the discovery of a second, more universal sensing system, albeit it is debatable whether this system is a true signaling system. The autoinducer-2 (AI-2) system is described by Bassler (2002), Fuqua et al. (2001), and Fuqua et al. (1996).

Acylated homoserine lactones (AHLs) are used as autoinducers in the LuxI–LuxR system as seen in *Vibrio* spp. In this quorum-sensing mechanism, it is these molecules that are released and received. More than 70 different microbial species have now been found to use AHL-based signaling (Dobretsov et al., 2012; Fuqua et al., 2001). It is interesting to note that although this system was initially noticed in the proteobacterial phylum, it has most recently been discovered in archaea (Zhang et al., 2012) and cyanobacteria (Sharif et al., 2008). The LuxI synthase or a homologue produces AHLs. AHLs all have a consistent central ring structure, but their side-chain composition varies greatly. These can have oxo or hydroxyl groups and come in different lengths, which enable the signaling molecules to be species-specific (Dobretsov et al., 2012). Depending on the size of the molecule and the surrounding environment, the molecules either actively travel out of or reenter the cells by passive diffusion.

The effectiveness of signaling is significantly influenced by the chemical characteristics of the AHL side chain, such as the number of carbon atoms in the alkyl side chain. Long-chain alkyl groups (such as C10–C14) are significantly more stable than short-chain alkyl groups at high pH levels (>8.2). This shows that cells may be able to identify this physicochemical value by adjusting the ratios of short- and long-chain sides, which are affected by the pH of the surroundings. The AHLs bind to the *lux* box, a promoter region, which causes transcription of the linked genes when extracellular concentrations of the signals reach a crucial level (Miller and Bassler, 2001). It's interesting to note that AHLs have been demonstrated to quickly deteriorate at high temperatures and alkaline pH levels, with the lactone ring being attacked by nucleophiles. If the pH is significantly dropped to a pH of 2.0, this lactone ring has the capacity to rebuild (Yates et al., 2002). Longer-chain AHLs might be used by microorganisms that thrive in harsher environments since they seem to be more resistant to chemical deterioration (Yates et al., 2002; Decho et al., 2009). For the microbial mats that are mentioned in a later section, this mechanism has been postulated.

The autoinducer molecules used in the AI-2 quorum-sensing system are all similar, in contrast to the signaling molecules present in the LuxI–LuxR system (Xavier and Bassler, 2005). As a result, it has been suggested that the AI-2 quorum-sensing system is a global system that enables communication between different species. The S-ribosylhomocysteine lyase gene, which is encoded by the *luxS* gene, controls the AI-2 system by cleaving bonds in S-ribosylhomocysteine (SRH) to produce the precursors of AI-2 signals. The linked genes determine the function of the AI-2 signal, which varies (Chaphalkar and Salunkhe, 2010). Due to the widespread nature of *luxS*, the protein that synthesizes the diesters, the autoinducer 2 or AI-2 system, which uses furanosyl borate diesters as a messenger molecule, was initially described as a bacterial Esperanto or universal language (Chen et al., 2002). This hypothesis, however, has come under fire because it is not certain if diesters always function as signaling molecules. Given that the *luxS* gene is a component of a metabolic system that recycles S-adenosyl-L-methionine, it is plausible that the AI-2 molecule is only a by-product and not a real signal (Diggle et al., 2006).

Gram-positive bacteria use peptide-based signaling systems, whereas gram-negative bacteria use AHLs as autoinducers. The latter is made up of formed, processed peptides that are typically shorter than 40 amino acids long and are moved to the extracellular space via active transport. The interaction between the signal molecules and the exterior regions of membrane-bound sensor proteins causes an intracellular reaction (Bassler, 2002). It has been discovered that the production of these chemicals is cell-density dependent, and as a result, this is now understood to be a type of quorum sensing. The excellent thermostability of the molecules in peptide-based signaling is a huge advantage (Johnson et al., 2005). A peptide-based signaling system may be useful in a hyperthermal environment, for example, as AHLs are susceptible to thermal destruction.

Pseudomonas aeruginosa is one example of a bacterium that can produce and react to a variety of quorum-sensing signals, including species-specific systems that use the quinolone molecule (Diggle et al., 2006). Some people have been seen to use multiple quorum-sensing systems. For instance, *V. harveyi* regulates bioluminescence and the development of biofilms using a highly integrated network made up of three separate quorum-sensing systems (Dobretsov et al., 2012). Although this may be more common, these multicomponent systems seem to be restricted to the *Vibrio* spp. (Miller and Bassler, 2001).

Although studies first concentrated on microbes that could send quorum-sensing signals, it has been shown that a number of bacteria can nevertheless receive and react to signals even when they cannot give them. For instance, *Salmonella* sp. lacks a LuxI–LuxR homologue but does possess the SdiA receptor, which is similar to

LuxR and enables the response to stimuli supplied by other organisms (Smith et al., 2001). This has come to be recognized as the concept of eavesdropping, and it raises more concerns when quorum sensing is thought of as a communal activity, especially in mixed-species cultures (Dobretsov et al., 2012).

3.3 QUORUM SENSING DETECTION USING BIOSENSORS

Biosensors are frequently used to detect the presence of quorum-sensing molecules such as AHLs or furanosyl borate diesters. Biosensors are strains of organisms designed to respond to a quorum-sensing molecule by producing a measurable phenotype, such as luminescence or pigment synthesis (Steindler and Venturi, 2007). It is significant to note that biosensor strains depend on foreign sources to activate rather than producing their own quorum-sensing molecules. Biosensors have limitations that must be taken into account even if they are useful tools for the study of quorum-sensing behavior, especially when investigating severe conditions where little is known. There are numerous biosensors available for AHLs and furanosyl borate diester systems (Steindler and Venturi, 2007; Rajamani et al., 2007). The sensitivity of these biosensors can vary; for example, certain biosensors are more suited to detecting short-chain AHLs than longer-chain variants (Steindler and Venturi, 2007). To verify any potential findings, it is possible to search for these molecules using analytical chemical techniques. Non-quorum-sensing molecules can also activate and inhibit biosensors.

The environment that the organism being investigated is from should also be taken into account before choosing a biosensor. AHL stimulation, for instance, causes the AHL biosensor *Chromobacterium violaceum* CV026 to create a purple pigment (McClean et al., 1997). Because *C. violaceum* CV026 has a reputation for being particularly sensitive to salinity, adjustments to biosensor methods may be taken into account while studying halophilic organisms (Llamas et al., 2005). Extreme environmental circumstances can also make it difficult to extract quorum-sensing molecules; for instance, *Natronococcus occultus* thrives in alkaline saline environments, and this alkalinity would also shorten the half-life of AHL molecules. The molecules can be re-formed through acidification procedures to remove AHLs from alkaline settings (Yates et al., 2002; Paggi et al., 2003).

3.4 QUORUM SENSING IN PARTICULAR GROUPS OF EXTREMOPHILES

3.4.1 Halophiles

Organisms known as halophiles flourish in settings with high salt concentrations. The two states of salinity and alkalinity are frequently observed together (Visscher et al., 2010) because of the dynamics of alkaliphilic (high pH) environments. Microbes from the three kingdoms of life—Bacteria, Archaea, and Eukarya—represent the halophiles. The halophiles prefer settings with salt concentrations of around 2.5 M and need these salts for growth, whereas the non-halophiles can grow in the absence of salt and in low quantities (Margesin and Schinner, 2001). Alkaliphiles are those that need a pH of greater than 9 to survive, but some halophiles can also withstand high temperatures (Pituka and Hoover, 2007; Penesyan et al., 2010).

Investigation into the synthesis of AHLs in *Halomonas* isolates from various sites revealed that all four species under consideration had the capacity to do so (Llamas et al., 2005). AHL synthesis in culture has been successfully identified, but the function of the signaling molecules in these microbial species are yet unknown. The creation of exopolysaccharide (EPS), which is known to protect cells from desiccation and improve communication by forming specialized channels, was mentioned by the authors as having a function in the formation of biofilms (Decho, 1990, 2000). The finding that the bacteria could all create identical AHLs, with the exception of *Halomonas ventosae*, and that they could each make many types of AHLs is of special relevance in these studies.

A salt marsh on the German coast yielded gram-positive, moderately halophilic *Halobacillus halophilus* bacteria. Due to its severe Cl⁻ dependence, it has established itself as a model organism for the study of salt adaptation. The presence of chloride ions is necessary for *H. halophilus* to develop and divide its cells, with optimal growth taking place at 0.8–1.0 M Cl⁻. Numerous other physiological processes, including the development of flagella and motility, have also been demonstrated to be influenced by anion concentration (Averhoff and Muller, 2010). Several molecules involved in the creation of putative AI-2 signals are encoded by the luxS operon in the bacterium *H. halophilus*. The presence of Cl⁻ ions is crucial for the operon's expression, which is growth-phase dependent (Averhoff and Muller, 2010). In 2.0 M NaCl, the peak of expression was seen during the mid-exponential period. This is LuxS's first known instance of a chloride-dependent system. Although more research is required to establish, there has been some speculation that the LuxS signaling pathway and cell motility are related (Sewald et al., 2007).

Also demonstrated to participate in quorum sensing in saline conditions are eukaryotic algae. In hypersaline salterns, the eukaryote *Dunaliella salina* is a microalgae that has been observed to create quorum-quenching molecules that block the activity of quorum-sensing signals (DasSarma et al., 2006; Natrah et al., 2011).

3.4.2 Heavy-Metal-Resistant Microbes and Acidophiles

Due to the significant industrial applications, severe acidophiles are a group that is extensively researched for their capacity to survive high concentrations of heavy metals. This group includes the acidophilic archaeon *Ferroplasma acidarmanus* Fer1, which was discovered in the Iron Mountain mine in California. Although it frequently dominates these biofilm forms by up to 85% of its cellular mass, it is typically seen in mixed-species biofilms. The ability of the bacteria to remain protected from acidic conditions is thought to give the biofilm mode of life a competitive advantage in these situations (Baker-Austin et al., 2010). Although a direct functional connection still has to be established, it was discovered that the *F. acidarmanus* genome contains many genes relevant to biofilm production and motility. No LuxR or LuxS homologues were found. Unique morphological alterations in biofilm formations point to a specific cellular response mechanism. These alterations were noticed in single-species cultures, which clearly implies that intra- but not interspecies cell signaling played a role (Baker-Austin et al., 2010).

The divergently oriented genes *afeI* and *afeR*, which are coupled and are predicted to create proteins that are comparable to the LuxI–LuxR proteins, are present in the genome of the very acidophilic bacterium *Acidithiobacillus ferrooxidans*. This bacterium is frequently connected to bioleaching processes and likes settings with a pH range of 1–2. Due to their strong resemblance to the Lux proteins, these genes were first discovered by bioinformatics (Rivas et al., 2005) and have subsequently undergone extensive research. *A. ferrooxidans* is very tolerant to heavy metals in addition to acidic conditions. Cu^{2+} is a trace element that is necessary for life, although large amounts of it can be hazardous (Wenbin et al., 2011).

Studies have looked into how these genes' expression and the products they produce are affected by high Cu^{2+} concentrations as well as synthetic furanones. It is known that furanones can prevent quorum sensing (Penesyan et al., 2010). Results showed a substantial decrease in Cu^{2+} ion tolerance in the presence of furanone compounds, indicating that quorum sensing is important for heavy-metal resistance (Wenbin et al., 2011). This study additionally evaluated *A. ferrooxidans'* generation of AHLs to support these conclusions. The ability of *A. ferrooxidans* to produce a wide variety of AHLs had been demonstrated in earlier research, and in this case, a number of long-chain AHLs that are known to be stable in acidic environments were found (Decho et al., 2009). The amount of these AHLs that the bacterium produced was dramatically decreased by the presence of furanones (Wenbin et al., 2011). Now, genomic study has demonstrated that *A. ferrooxidans* has a second potential quorum-sensing system. Act is the name of the AHL synthase-encoding orthologue of hdtS found in *Pseudomonas fluorescens*. Its resemblance to well-known genes suggests that it contributes to the fluidity and production of membranes. It has been proposed that the two distinct quorum-sensing systems control how well the bacteria can use various energy sources (Rivas et al., 2007).

Acidophilic microorganisms employed in biomining include *Acidithiobacillus thiooxidans* and *Leptospirillum ferrooxidans*. Due to these organisms' strong evolutionary and functional link to *A. ferrooxidans*, studies have tried to find quorum-sensing mechanisms in them. It was discovered that while *L. ferrooxidans* does not make AHLs, *A. thiooxidans* does. However, a LuxI–LuxR homologue made up of the divergent genes lttI and lttR was discovered in *L. ferrooxidans* after genomic research. The putative proteins generated by these genes resemble known quorum-sensing molecules found in the bacteria *Geobacter uraniireducens* very closely (Ruiz et al., 2008). *Escherichia coli* genes implicated in cell growth, biofilm formation, and motility, including chemotaxis and flagellum generation, have also been compared (Moreno-Paz et al., 2010).

The human body presents a variety of acidic, oxic, and anoxic environments, making it a potentially harsh environment that presents several difficulties for bacteria. The bacterium that causes the disease cholera, which is prevalent in many areas, particularly in the poor world, is called *Vibrio cholerae*. It is extremely virulent, and the toxins it produces are what give the sickness its characteristics.

The pathogenicity of *V. cholerae* is due to its highly evolved quorum-sensing system, which also enables its survival in the human host. Quorum sensing is a key component of the genetic traits of *V. cholerae* that enable it to successfully live in the human host, and these traits have been well-documented. Many of these genes have an impact on biofilm development and *Vibrio* polysaccharide (VPS) synthesis. VPS is an extracellular substance that is essential for bacterial adhesion to a surface and the development of biofilms. Depending on the environment, *V. cholerae* biofilms exhibit significant variations, and numerous distinct genes have been linked to these variations (Hammer and Bassler, 2003). It is *V. cholerae*'s capacity to alter the structure of its biofilm in response to environmental modifications that enables it to successfully colonize and infect the human body. The stomach's extremely acidic environment (pH 1) is one of the obstacles that germs trying to enter the human body through the alimentary canal must overcome. When *V. cholerae* enters the stomach, they produce too much VPS, which causes them to form thick, sticky biofilms. This is made possible by the absence of Hap, a quorum-sensing regulator that prevents the VPS operon from being expressed. CqsA then functions as an autoinducer synthase to achieve this. Production of HapR continues, leading to a conformational change in the biofilm when the cells have exited the stomach and the biofilm's protection is no longer needed (Hammer and Bassler, 2003; March and Bentley, 2004).

Helicobacter pylorus is another bacterium that is known to live in the human stomach. It is an opportunistic pathogen. Due to the challenges in duplicating these conditions, this bacterium has only recently been able to be cultured in a lab. This is because it is well evolved to this niche environment. The synthesis of AI-2 has been linked to the regulation of flagella gene transcription in *H. pylori*, which results in immotility (Rader et al., 2007).

3.4.3 THERMOPHILES

Due to the AHL lactone ring's heat lability, quorum sensing was at first believed to be difficult in even a somewhat thermophilic environment (Schopf et al., 2008). Despite this original result, it has now been proposed that quorum sensing plays a crucial function in these situations.

AHL signaling has been shown to be important in the thermophilic bacteria *Thermus* sp. GH5's reaction to cold shock. Although this is a situation when AHLs would be most stable, quorum-sensing signals have only been picked up in the early stages of the cold shock response. The chemical AHL precursors were overexpressed, and the AHL production cycle was stimulated. These AHL precursors' synthesis under cold shock was connected to the development of biofilms. *Thermotoga maritima*'s genome had a gene that codes for a short-chain amino acid, which was expressed at a much higher rate in denser cell populations and was thought to be a potential quorum-sensing molecule (Johnson et al., 2005).

As it has been observed to create symbiotic connections with sessile microorganisms, indicating some type of cellular communication, the hyperthermophilic archaeon *Pyrococcus furiosus* has been researched for its potential quorum-sensing abilities. It was proposed that quorum sensing was involved in this process, but the notion was immediately rejected since the LuxI/R- or LuxS-type proteins are not encoded by the genome, making it unlikely to find classic models of quorum sensing (Nichols et al., 2009). Contrary to early speculation, it was shown that *P. furiosus* and *T. maritima*, when cultured together, were capable of producing an AI-2-type signal through a number of biotic and abiotic stages. Additionally, the genome of *T. maritima* lacks a homologue that codes for LuxS. Despite the signal being present, there was no discernible phenotypic change in response to this compound (Nichols et al., 2009).

Additional research on *T. maritima* has shown an EPS synthesis pathway that points to the possibility of peptide-based quorum sensing. *T. maritima* and *Methanocaldococcus jannaschii*, both of which lack the luxS gene and have no AHLs in the culture media, were cultivated in co-culture together. However, it was discovered that EPS synthesis was significantly increased in larger cell densities, leading researchers to speculate that quorum sensing may be involved despite the absence of any recognized genetic criteria (Johnson et al., 2005). It has been suggested that these putative quorum-sensing signals contribute to the heat shock response because it has been noted that *T. maritima* exhibits a transcriptome-based stress response resembling that seen in AI-2 signaling (Nichols et al., 2009).

3.4.4 PSYCHROPHILES

There is a specific shortage of knowledge about the psychrophiles' possible quorum-sensing capabilities. Even though the ecological significance of cold-adapted microorganisms is being intensively examined, quorum sensing function in these conditions has received very little attention. In this field, the development of bioinformatics has revealed some of the capabilities of microbes, but it is still unclear how these organisms work and interact with their surroundings.

Although it was discovered that the psychrophile *Pseudoalteromonas haloplanktis* contains the mtnN gene, which is thought to be involved in the creation of putative AI-2 signals, no LuxS homologue was found (Medigue et al., 2005). Several different genes are encoded in the genome that may be signs of a different, less well-known quorum-sensing system. This includes the putative multidomain aconitate hydratase gene PSHAa0159, which can serve as a signal during the stationary growth phase. Additionally, it has genes that are known to be necessary for the gammaproteobacteria to produce diffusible signaling molecules (Medigue et al., 2005).

Numerous alternative regulatory mechanisms have been discovered through examination of the *Psychromonas ingrahamii* genome. Although much information is not known, a LuxR orthologue has been reported. The resilience of this creature in the sea ice where it is found may be significantly influenced by biofilms, according to the authors, but this has not yet been fully explored. According to one theory, the microorganisms' ability to produce EPS enables them to reduce the freezing point of the environment, which increases the amount of water available for growth (Riley et al., 2008).

3.4.5 PIEZOPHILES

The piezophiles, formerly known as barophiles, are a class of microorganisms distinguished by their predilection for high-pressure environments. Several microorganisms have now been isolated effectively from high-pressure settings, especially deep ocean depths.

A bacterium called *Photobacterium profundum* SS9, which was discovered at a water depth of 3600 m, has been used as a model organism for research on piezophiles. *P. profundum* is closely related to *V. harveyi* and *A. fischeri*, two organisms in the family Vibrionaceae that were the first to exhibit quorum sensing. In an effort to identify AI-2 signaling networks in *P. profundum*, comparative genomic investigations have discovered that, despite the presence of a LuxS homologue, it appears to serve only a metabolic purpose (Rezzonico and Duffy, 2008). Additionally, a novel, as-yet-unidentified quorum-sensing system is said to be present in *P. profundum*. This putative quorum-sensing system shares 35% of its sequence with the LuxMN and AinSR systems in *V. harveyi* and *A. fischeri*, supporting the notion that quorum sensing may be crucial in high-pressure environments (Reen et al., 2006) and highlighting the need to reevaluate other genomes when new quorum-sensing systems are found.

The deep sea is also home to the piezophilic bacteria *Shewanella benthica* and *Shewanella violacea*. The luxS gene is present in all *Shewanella* species, according to documentation (Bodor et al., 2008), although its role in these piezophiles has not yet been studied. Numerous *Shewanella* species have shown that they can disrupt quorum sensing in other species and degrade AHLs. By preventing zoospore establishment, several of these microorganisms were able to severely impact cross-domain signaling (Tait et al., 2009). Studies that looked at the potential for LuxS-type signaling by analyzing the genomes of *Shewanella* spp. concluded that this was more closely related to phylogenetic affiliation than it was to the environment of a microbe. As a result, there is a good chance that the piezophilic *Shewanella* spp. performs quorum quenching as well as quorum sensing (Bodor et al., 2008).

We still have a lot to learn and understand about this particular class of microbes. Our knowledge of this unusual habitat is limited because it can be challenging to cultivate microorganisms in high-pressure environments. While cutting-edge molecular genetic tools have given us some understanding of their physiology, there is still much to learn about how they interact with their surroundings.

3.4.6 RADIATION-RESISTANT MICROORGANISMS

Due to special DNA repair processes, the bacteria *Deinococcus radiodurans* is one of many that can withstand high doses of radiation. It is known that *D. radiodurans* can survive inside nuclear reactors, and its genes have been extracted and studied for potential industrial use. Although the entire genome of *D. radiodurans* has been annotated and presented, not much is known about its multicellular activities. It has a *luxS* homologue that participates in the recycling of S-adenosylhomocysteine (SAH), which generates AI-2 signals. Although the purposes of this system and its by-products have not been explored, it has been discovered to contain a two-step Pfs/ LuxS pathway for the creation of AI-2 signals (Sun et al., 2004).

Deinococcus gobiensis, a different radioresistant bacteria, has displayed a number of chemical reactions after being exposed to ultraviolet (UV) radiation (Yuan et al., 2012). The gidA gene, which encodes the glucose-inhibited cell division protein A and regulates the posttranscriptional regulation of quorum-sensing genes in *Pseudomonas aeruginosa,* has yet to be studied. The RhlR-dependent and RhlR-independent routes used by *P. aeruginosa* for this function are similar to those seen in many quorum-sensing soil symbionts. Though its strong resemblance to these well-known quorum-sensing systems suggests a role for quorum sensing in UV-resistant bacteria, the precise function of this gene in *D. gobiensis* is still unknown (Yuan et al., 2012).

3.4.7 ARCHAEA

Although the archaea are sometimes referred to as extremophiles and may be found in the majority of the conditions listed earlier, there has never been any proof of quorum sensing in the archaeal domain. Traditional LuxI–LuxR and AI-2 quorum sensing systems were first attempted to be identified in archaea, but this research failed (Miller and Bassler, 2001; Decho et al., 2009). However, recent research has produced some intriguing findings. Through the enzymatic (lactonase) breakdown of this signal, sulfur-reducing archaea of the Crenarchaeota phylum have been demonstrated to directly interact with AHL-based signaling systems, such as those now present in bacteria (Ng et al., 2011). It is still unknown how this lactonase affects the surrounding microbial population and the environment. AHLs may be used as messenger molecules for archaeal quorum-sensing systems, according to recent research. The haloalkaliphile *Natronococcus occultus* provided the first clue that archaea might have an AHL-based quorum-sensing system.

A haloalkaliphilic archaeon called *N. occultus* has been discovered to produce an extracellular protease both during famine and the late exponential and stationary growth phases (Paggi et al., 2003). As this protease was seen in the stages of growth allowing for ideal cell density, it was believed that synthesis of this enzyme was quorum-sensing dependent (Paggi et al., 2003). Additionally, *N. occultus* extracts at these specific times were able to trigger an AHL biosensor. Although not convincing, this AHL biosensor activation raises the possibility that AHLs play a role in mediating the production of extracellular enzymes, which are frequently quorum-regulated in bacteria.

The Kenyan saline waterbody Lake Magadi is the source of the haloalkaliphile *Natrialba magadii* archaeon. Nep, a protease similar to halolysin that is stable in high salt concentrations, is known to be produced by *N. magadii* (Penesyan et al., 2010). Nep is created during the stationary period of growth and is thought to be a reaction to the lack of available nutrients. It has not yet been proven that AHLs and quorum sensing are responsible for the upregulation of Nep synthesis. Unable to be isolated, a possible quorum-sensing molecule was discovered (Penesyan et al., 2010), and a bioinformatic examination of the *N. magadii* genome produced no genes that resembled conventional quorum-sensing genes.

The methanogenic archaeon *Methanothrix* (*Methanosaeta*) *harundinacea* produces carboxylated AHLs, and filament production is triggered by these signals, according to a recent study (Zhang et al., 2012). N-carboxyl-decanoyl-homoserine lactone (carboxylated C10 HSL), N-carboxyl-dodecanoyl-homoserine lactone (carboxylated C12 HSL), and N-carboxyl-tetradecanoyl-homoserine lactone were the three substances specifically found (Zhang et al., 2012). This is the first instance of quorum sensing in archaea in the direct sense. Analytical chemistry methods were used to identify these carboxyl AHLs, and this particular class of AHL has not yet been found in bacteria. The homoserine lactone (HSL) ring's carboxyl group appears to be joined to the amino group (Zhang et al., 2012). It is still unknown how carboxylation affects chemical stability and, thus, the potential environmental signal. Bacterial AHLs were not able to trigger filament synthesis in *M. harundinacea*, even though carboxyl AHLs from this archaeon were able to activate bacterial biosensors (Zhang et al., 2012), suggesting the possibility of one-way cross talk. As a result, the possibility of interspecies and even interdomain signaling is highly important and warrants more research.

Since both *N. occultus* and *N. magadii* are found in highly alkaliphilic habitats, alterations to conventional quorum-sensing molecules would be required for them to work in these harsh situations (Decho et al., 2009). Short-chain AHLs are also unstable in alkaline environments. An increase in chain length, which can help AHLs endure alkaline environments for a longer period of time, is one such change (Yates et al., 2002; Decho et al., 2009). Other chemical changes, such as the carboxylation mentioned earlier in *M. harundinacea* (Zhang et al., 2012), might also be important.

Finally, given that other compounds, including diketopiperazines, have been shown to activate biosensors (Holden et al., 1999) and are found in haloarchaea (Tommonaro et al., 2012), it is possible that they are acting as quorum-sensing molecules.

3.5 MICROBIAL MATS: QUORUM SENSING IN AN EXTREME ENVIRONMENT

Although the majority of this review has been on quorum sensing in individual organisms, this discussion will now utilize microbial mats as an example to show this phenomenon in a specific environmental situation. An excellent example of an extreme habitat is microbial mats, where resident microorganisms are exposed to a variety of varying conditions (Braissant et al., 2009; Decho, 2010). Numerous EPS molecules are present in these organo-sedimentary systems (Braissant et al., 2009), which may be crucial in influencing cell signaling (Decho, 2000). They undergo substantial variations in O_2, H_2S, and pH in response to diel cycles because they are made up of a diversified community of microbial functional groups. Large changes in geochemical and physicochemical conditions are caused by the activities of photosynthesis and aerobic respiration dominating the microbial mat's metabolism during the day and fermentation and anaerobic respiration (sulfate reduction) doing so during the night (Visscher et al., 2010). For instance, this causes a significant fluctuation in the pH levels within the mat, which can range from >11 during the peak of photosynthesis to 5.5 at night (Decho et al., 2009). This quorum necessitates that sensing be effective, efficient, and well adaptive to these varying environments.

Early research has indicated that AHLs are susceptible to high pH, therefore it is likely that the diel fluctuations typical of microbial mats lead to AHL breakdown, particularly in the afternoon, which disrupts cell signaling. When compared to the overnight setting, it was demonstrated that the shorter-chain (7) AHLs were present at much lower amounts during the day (Decho et al., 2009). Because the short-chain AHLs are less effective at night, samples from natural mats and organisms isolated from mats frequently have acyl side chains with lengths between C12 and C14. In microbial mats, a wide variety of AHLs have been found, and a pattern has been proposed in which longer-chain AHLs are created during the day and shorter chains are formed at night. As a result, the bacteria within the biofilm would be able to time their gene expression to be most advantageous or appropriate (Decho et al., 2009).

In the higher levels of the microbial mats, in particular, confocal imaging has shown dense clusters of microorganisms (Decho et al., 2010). When taking into account the requirement for change and dissemination of these signals throughout the microbial mat, the complexity of the microbial communication system becomes apparent. Larger molecules can't travel as far as smaller ones, and quorum-sensing systems in microbial mats face some unusual difficulties since they must communicate with cells of the same species across long distances despite the immediate high cell density (Decho et al., 2010). Quorum sensing may be used to monitor the diversity (and metabolism) of species in the environment rather than individuals of the same species in mixed-species habitats, such as the microbial mats that feature a high diversity of AHLs. The idea that the LuxR–LuxI-type proteins could mediate interspecies communication under these circumstances is still present (Fuqua et al., 1996).

Additionally, it has been demonstrated in numerous investigations that oxygen-sensitive sulfate reduction occurs during the peak of oxygenic photosynthesis, necessitating physiologic adjustments (Visscher et al., 1992). The ability of both physiological groups to coexist in an environment with supersaturated O_2 concentrations was predicted to be enabled by interspecies communication between sulfate-reducing bacteria (SRB) and sulfide-oxidizing bacteria (SOB). Early experiments have demonstrated that a mixture of long-chain AHLs, like those produced by SRB, stimulate sulfide oxidation by SOB in mats. The latter metabolism would eliminate the harmful sulfur dioxide that SRB and oxygenic photosynthesis create as well as O_2. Exopolymeric components are a crucial component of the microbial mat because they serve as the matrix for a 3D design and permit the existence of dense cell clusters. In these systems, communication may depend on certain EPS characteristics, such as nanochannels (Decho et al., 2010). The EPS matrix may also play a crucial role in the mat's operation by shielding quorum-sensing chemicals from desiccation, excessive UV radiation, H_2O_2, OH radicals, and singlet O_2.

3.6   APPLICATIONS OF BIOTECHNOLOGY

Extremophiles and the products they produce have as many biotechnological uses as there are types of organisms. Many times, as with the acidophiles, it seems that research on bacteria has started with an eye on potential industrial applications. The possibilities offered by extremophiles are wide ranging and include industrial operations, aquaculture, bioremediation, medical interventions, and usage in the food business.

By altering environmental factors, quorum-sensing devices are frequently used to promote advantageous microbial interactions. The agriculture sector has exploited this idea to encourage healthy soil growth, and operations in aquaculture have done the same. Due to their production of quorum-sensing inhibitors, halophilic organisms such as the microalga *Dunaliella salina* may have the ability to support aquaculture (Natrah et al., 2011).

As was already noted, *Acidithiobacillus ferrooxidans* is frequently utilized in bioleaching procedures (Rivas et al., 2005) as well as in the biohydrometallurgy method (Wenbin et al., 2011) for recovering metals like copper, gold, and uranium from metal ores. Similar to this, *Ferroplasma acidarmanus* is employed in biomining, which uses the microorganisms' metal sulfide oxidation to liberate metals from sulfide rocks (Baker-Austin et al., 2010). It is possible to optimize these processes, for which they have previously been highly chosen, employing the quorum-sensing systems of both of these organisms, as is done in the agriculture sector.

Due to their capacity to catalyze processes and potential commercial applications in harsh environments, extremophiles have recently attracted a lot of attention (Gupta et al., 2014; Dumorné et al., 2017; Geng et al., 2018). Even though extremozymes were discovered several decades ago, scientists are still primarily focused on genetically modifying existing enzymes to increase their activity and screening novel enzymes from various sources to identify those with the necessary properties for use in biotechnological and industrial applications. Extremophiles' enzymes and other biomolecules are already widely used in industry. These are all obtained from the acidophiles alone and include amylases, ligases, plasmids, and maltose-binding proteins (Sharma et al., 2012). Table 3.1 lists some of the biological products produced by extremophiles that are already being used or have the potential to be exploited in industrial settings. The use of quorum sensing has tremendous potential for optimizing the synthesis of these substances. The biotechnological industry may find some extracellular enzymes isolated from these harsh settings useful, and some of these extracellular enzymes may be quorum-controlled (Paggi et al., 2003).

Since quorum sensing and the synthesis of antibiotics are closely related, the medical industry has potential for quorum-sensing applications (Penesyan et al., 2010). In-depth research is being done on AHLs and their derivatives in order to utilize them as antibacterial platforms in the medical industry. As they prevent bacterial colonization without eliminating all natural microbes or causing antibiotic resistance factors, they represent an appealing substitute for conventional antibiotics (Dobretsov et al., 2012). The employment of extremophiles in this situation would permit the usage of acid-stable compounds, which would be necessary, for instance, in the digestive system.

TABLE 3.1

Extremophiles and their bioproducts with industrial applications

Microorganism	Bioproduct	Application	Reference
Alteromonas sp. ML117	β-Galactosidase	Food	Yao et al., 2019
Erwinia sp. E602	Cold-adapted β-Galactosidase	Dairy industry	Xia et al., 2018
Anoxybacillus flavithermus *Bacillus licheniformis*	β-Galactosidase	Bioremediation, food, biosensor	Rani et al., 2019
Thermophilic *Anoxybacillus* sp. GXS-BL	α-Amylase	Pharmaceutics, food, detergent, textile and bioenergy industries	Liao et al., 2019
Anoxybacillus thermarum FRM-RBK02	α-Amylase	Food, biorefinery, detergent	Mantiri et al., 2019
Bacillus mojavensis SO-10	α-Amylase	Food, detergent, biorefinery	Ozdemir et al., 2018
Paenicibacillus barengoltzii	Chitinase	Cellulose-to-ethanol conversion	Yang et al., 2016
Thermophilic *Anoxybacillus* sp. HBB16	Alkaline lipase	Detergent synthesis, wastewater treatment, and biodiesel production	Burcu Bakir and Metin, 2017
Bacillus cereus FT 1	Alkaline protease	Food, leather, pharmaceuticals, detergents, and bioremediation	Asha and Palaniswamy, 2018
Bacillus subtilis Lucky9	Alkali-tolerant xylanase	Food and biofuel	Chang et al., 2017
Cellulomonas fimi ATCC484	Thermostable endoglucanase	Biorefinery	Saxena et al., 2018

Quorum sensing has been extensively studied for the field of food microbiology. Numerous food products include quorum-sensing signals, and since microbial infection frequently leads to food spoiling, it might be possible to use quorum-sensing inhibitors to stop microbial development. For instance, milk spoiling has been linked to the bacteria *Serratia proteamaculans*. The milk did not degrade as quickly when a mutant strain was put into milk cultures that did not produce AHLs (Bai and Rai, 2011). Alternative food processing sterilizing techniques like high pressure are advantageous because they maintain the product's color and flavor. This procedure comprises a brief increase in pressure that renders microorganisms inactive or lethal. While generally advantageous, this also destroys the microorganisms that are exploited in the food industry for their ability to impart flavor and other desired qualities. While piezophiles do not currently have any applications in the food industry, it has been proposed that using their metabolites in these high-pressure techniques may be very advantageous (Abe and Horikoshi, 2001), albeit it is unknown whether these metabolites are quorum-regulated.

The manufacturing of consumables has also been linked to quorum-sensing applications. For instance, the production of specific aromas in wine is strongly dependent on the activities of yeast and bacteria. The final output can be significantly impacted by how yeast–yeast interactions balance out against yeast–bacterial interactions. It has been proposed that evaluating quorum sensing as a technique of keeping a balance in this connection may be a new way of getting the desired outcomes of specific product features (Fleet, 2003).

3.7 CONCLUSIONS

Although the extremophiles are a large, diversified, and well-studied population, we know very little about their capacity to generate and receive quorum-sensing signals. The identification of quorum-sensing genes in bacteria and speculation about how they might use these to interact with their environment has been made possible by the development of genomic sequencing and bioinformatic databases. Traditional quorum-sensing models have been shown in numerous studies to be inadequate because, although organisms can make AHLs and other quorum-sensing molecules, we frequently still do not fully understand the genetic basis for their synthesis or regulation. There is a substantial knowledge gap regarding the quorum-sensing capabilities of extremophiles.

A variety of phenotypes that aid in survival in diverse conditions are regulated by quorum-sensing systems, which are still being discovered in new situations. Due to the challenges associated with cultivating extremophiles, quorum sensing in these species has not yet been thoroughly studied. Quorum sensing has had significant ecological effects throughout evolutionary time, notably concerning interspecies or even interdomain signaling. It's conceivable that there are new chemicals and receptors out there just waiting to be found. It is important for us to comprehend how the environment affects quorum-sensing signals as well as the degree to which such changed molecules might still influence phenotypes. We are starting to unravel the mysteries of quorum sensing in harsh conditions with the use of bioinformatics, genome sequencing, and emerging technologies like plasmid-based biosensors.

REFERENCES

Abe, F. and Horikoshi, K. 2001. The biotechnological potential of piezophiles. *Trends in Biotechnology* 19:102–108.

Asha, B. and Palaniswamy, M. 2018. Optimization of alkaline protease production by *Bacillus cereus* FT1 isolated from soil. *Journal of Applied Pharmaceutical Science* 8:119–127.

Averhoff, B. and Muller, V. 2010. Exploring research frontiers in microbiology- recent advances in halophilic and thermophilic extremophiles. *Research in Microbiology* 161:506–514.

Bai, A.J. and Rai, V.R. 2011. Bacterial quorum sensing and food industry. *Comprehensive Reviews in Food Science and Food Safety* 10(3):183–193.

Baker-Austin, C., Potrykus, J., Wexler, M., Bond, P.L. and Dopson, M. 2010. Biofilm development in the extremely acidophilic archaeon 'Ferroplasma acidarmanus' Fer1. *Extremophiles* 14(6):485–491.

Bassler, B.L. 2002. Small talk: Cell-to-cell communication in bacteria. *Cell* 109(4):421–424.

Bodor, A., Elxnat, B., Thiel, V., Schulz, S. and Wagner-Döbler, I. 2008. Potential for luxS related signalling in marine bacteria and production of autoinducer-2 in the genus *Shewanella*. *BMC Microbiology* 8(1):1–9.

Braissant, O., Decho, A.W., Przekop, K.M., Gallagher, K.L., Glunk, C., Dupraz, C. and Visscher, P.T. 2009. Characteristics and turnover of exopolymeric substances in a hypersaline microbial mat. *FEMS Microbiology Ecology* 67(2):293–307.

Burcu Bakir, Z. and Metin, K. 2017. Production and characterization of an alkaline lipase from thermophilic *Anoxybacillus* sp. HBB16. *Chemical and Biochemical Engineering Quarterly* 31(3):303–312.

Chang, S., Guo, Y., Wu, B. and He, B. 2017. Extracellular expression of alkali tolerant xylanase from *Bacillus subtilis* Lucky9 in E. coli and application for xylooligosaccharides production from agro-industrial waste. *International Journal of Biological Macromolecules* 96:249–256.

Chaphalkar, A. and Salunkhe, N. 2010. Phylogenetic analysis of nitrogen-fixing and quorum sensing bacteria. *International Journal of Bioinformatics Research* 2:17–32.

Chen, X., Schauder, S., Potier, N., Van Dorsselaer, A., Pelczer, I., Bassler, B.L. and Hughson, F.M. 2002. Structural identification of a bacterial quorum-sensing signal containing boron. *Nature* 415(6871):545–549.

DasSarma, S. and DasSarma, P. 2006. Halophiles. In *Encyclopedia of Life Sciences (General and Introductory Life Sciences)*. London, UK: Wiley.

Decho, A.W. 1990. Microbial exopolymer secretions in ocean environments: Their role (s) in food webs and marine processes. *Oceanography and Marine Biology: An Annual Review* 28(7):73–153.

Decho, A.W. 2000. Microbial biofilms in intertidal systems: An overview. *Continental Shelf Research* 20(10–11):1257–1273.

Decho, A.W., Visscher, P.T., Ferry, J., Kawaguchi, T., He, L., Przekop, K.M., Norman, R.S. and Reid, R.P. 2009. Autoinducers extracted from microbial mats reveal a surprising diversity of N-acylhomoserine lactones (AHLs) and abundance changes that may relate to diel pH. *Environmental Microbiology* 11(2):409–420.

Decho, A.W., Norman, R.S. and Visscher, P.T. 2010. Quorum sensing in natural environments: Emerging views from microbial mats. *Trends in Microbiology* 18(2):73–80.

Diggle, S.P., Cornelis, P., Williams, P. and Cámara, M. 2006. 4-quinolone signalling in *Pseudomonas aeruginosa*: Old molecules, new perspectives. *International Journal of Medical Microbiology* 296(2–3):83–91.

Dobretsov, S., Teplitski, M. and Paul, V. 2012. Mini-review: Quorum sensing in the marine environment and its relationship to biofouling. *Biofouling* 25:413–427.

Dumorné, K., Camacho Córdova, D., Astorga-Eló, M. and Renganathan, P. 2017. Extremozymes: A potential source for industrial applications. *Journal of Microbiology and Biotechnology* 27:649–659.

Fleet, G.H. 2003. Yeast interactions and wine flavour. *International Journal of Food Microbiology* 86(1–2):11–22.

Fuqua, C., Winans, S.C. and Greenberg, E.P. 1996. Census and consensus in bacterial ecosystems: The LuxR-LuxI family of quorum-sensing transcriptional regulators. *Annual Review of Microbiology* 50:727–752.

Fuqua, C., Parsek, M.R. and Greenberg, E.P. 2001. Regulation of gene expression by cell-to-cell communication: Acyl-homoserine lactone quorum sensing. *Annual Review of Genetics* 35:439.

Geng, A., Cheng, Y., Wang, Y., Zhu, D., Le, Y., Wu, J., Xie, R., Yuan, J.S. and Sun, J. 2018. Transcriptome analysis of the digestive system of a wood-feeding termite (Coptotermes formosanus) revealed a unique mechanism for effective biomass degradation. *Biotechnology for biofuels* 11(1):1–14.

Gupta, G.N., Srivastava, S., Khare, S.K. and Prakash, V. 2014. Extremophiles: An overview of microorganism from extreme environment. *International Journal of Agriculture, Environment and Biotechnology* 7(2):371.

Hammer, B.K. and Bassler, B.L. 2003. Quorum sensing controls biofilm formation in *Vibrio cholerae*. *Molecular Microbiology* 50(1):101–104.

Holden, M.T., Ram Chhabra, S., De Nys, R., Stead, P., Bainton, N.J., Hill, P.J., Manefield, M., Kumar, N., Labatte, M., England, D. and Rice, S. 1999. Quorum-sensing cross talk: isolation and chemical characterization of cyclic dipeptides from Pseudomonas aeruginosa and other gram-negative bacteria. *Molecular microbiology* 33(6):1254–1266.

Johnson, M.R., Montero, C.I., Conners, S.B., Shockley, K.R., Bridger, S.L. and Kelly, R.M. 2005. Population density-dependent regulation of exopolysaccharide formation in the hyperthermophilic bacterium *Thermotoga maritima*. *Molecular Microbiology* 55(3):664–674.

Liao, S.M., Liang, G.E., Zhu, J., Lu, B.O., Peng, L.X., Wang, Q.Y., Wei, Y.T., Zhou, G.P. and Huang, R.B. 2019. Influence of calcium ions on the thermal characteristics of α-amylase from thermophilic *Anoxybacillus* sp. GXS-BL. *Protein and Peptide Letters* 26(2):148–157.

Llamas, I., Quesada, E., Martínez-Cánovas, M.J., Gronquist, M., Eberhard, A. and Gonzalez, J.E. 2005. Quorum sensing in halophilic bacteria: Detection of N-acyl-homoserine lactones in the exopolysaccharide-producing species of *Halomonas*. *Extremophiles* 9(4):333–341.

Mantiri, F.R., Rumende, R.R.H. and Sudewi, S. 2019. Identification of α-amylase gene by PCR and activity of thermostable α-amylase from thermophilic *Anoxybacillus thermarum* isolated from Remboken hot spring in Minahasa, Indonesia. *IOP Conference Series: Earth and Environmental Science* 217(1):012045. IOP Publishing.

March, J.C. and Bentley, W.E. 2004. Quorum sensing and bacterial cross-talk in biotechnology. *Current Opinion in Biotechnology* 15(5):495–502.

Margesin, R. and Schinner, F. 2001. Potential of halotolerant and halophilic microorganisms for biotechnology. *Extremophiles* 5(2):73–83.

McClean, K.H., Winson, M.K., Fish, L., Taylor, A., Chhabra, S.R., Camara, M., Daykin, M., Lamb, J.H., Swift, S., Bycroft, B.W. and Stewart, G.S. 1997. Quorum sensing and *Chromobacterium violaceum*: Exploitation of violacein production and inhibition for the detection of N-acylhomoserine lactones. *Microbiology* 143(12):3703–3711.

Médigue, C., Krin, E., Pascal, G., Barbe, V., Bernsel, A., Bertin, P.N., Cheung, F., Cruveiller, S., D'Amico, S., Duilio, A. and Fang, G. 2005. Coping with cold: The genome of the versatile marine Antarctica bacterium *Pseudoalteromonas haloplanktis* TAC125. *Genome Research* 15(10):1325–1335.

Miller, M.B. and Bassler, B.L. 2001. Quorum sensing in bacteria. *Annual Review of Microbiology* 55(1):165–199.

Moreno-Paz, M., Gómez, M.J., Arcas, A. and Parro, V. 2010. Environmental transcriptome analysis reveals physiological differences between biofilm and planktonic modes of life of the iron oxidizing bacteria *Leptospirillum* spp. in their natural microbial community. *BMC Genomics* 11(1):1–14.

Natrah, F.M.I., Kenmegne, M.M., Wiyoto, W., Sorgeloos, P., Bossier, P. and Defoirdt, T. 2011. Effects of micro-algae commonly used in aquaculture on acyl-homoserine lactone quorum sensing. *Aquaculture* 317(1–4):53–57.

Ng, F.S., Wright, D.M. and Seah, S.Y. 2011. Characterization of a phosphotriesterase-like lactonase from *Sulfolobus solfataricus* and its immobilization for disruption of quorum sensing. *Applied and Environmental Microbiology* 77(4):1181–1186.

Nichols, J.D., Johnson, M.R., Chou, C.J. and Kelly, R.M. 2009. Temperature, not LuxS, mediates AI-2 formation in hydrothermal habitats. *FEMS Microbiology Ecology* 68(2):173–181.

Ozdemir, S., Fincan, S.A., Karakaya, A. and Enez, B. 2018. A novel raw starch hydrolyzing thermostable α-amylase produced by newly isolated *Bacillus mojavensis* SO-10: Purification, characterization and usage in starch industries. *Brazilian Archives of Biology and Technology* 61:399.

Paggi, R.A., Martone, C.B., Fuqua, C. and De Castro, R.E. 2003. Detection of quorum sensing signals in the haloalkaliphilic archaeon *Natronococcus occultus*. *FEMS Microbiology Letters* 221(1):49–52.

Penesyan, A., Kjelleberg, S. and Egan, S. 2010. Development of novel drugs from marine surface associated microorganisms. *Marine Drugs* 8(3):438–459.

Pituka, E.V. and Hoover, R.B. 2007. Microbial extremophiles at the limits of life. *Crit. Rev. Microbiol* 33:183–209.

Rader, B.A., Campagna, S.R., Semmelhack, M.F., Bassler, B.L. and Guillemin, K. 2007. The quorum-sensing molecule autoinducer 2 regulates motility and flagellar morphogenesis in *Helicobacter pylori*. *Journal of Bacteriology* 189(17):6109–6117.

Rajamani, S., Zhu, J., Pei, D. and Sayre, R. 2007. A LuxP-FRET-based reporter for the detection and quantification of AI-2 bacterial quorum-sensing signal compounds. *Biochemistry* 46(13):3990–3997.

Rani, V., Sharma, P. and Dev, K. 2019. Characterization of thermally stable β galactosidase from *Anoxybacillus flavithermus* and *Bacillus licheniformis* isolated from Tattapani hotspring of North Western Himalayas, India. *International Journal of Current Microbiology and Applied Sciences* 8(1):2517–2542.

Reen, F.J., Almagro-Moreno, S., Ussery, D. and Boyd, E.F. 2006. The genomic code: Inferring Vibrionaceae niche specialization. *Nature Reviews Microbiology* 4(9):697–704.

Rezzonico, F. and Duffy, B. 2008. Lack of genomic evidence of AI-2 receptors suggests a non-quorum sensing role for luxS in most bacteria. *BMC Microbiology* 8(1):1–19.

Riley, M., Staley, J.T., Danchin, A., Wang, T.Z., Brettin, T.S., Hauser, L.J., Land, M.L. and Thompson, L.S. 2008. Genomics of an extreme psychrophile, *Psychromonas ingrahamii*. *BMC Genomics* 9(1):1–19.

Rivas, M., Seeger, M., Holmes, D.S. and Jedlicki, E. 2005. A Lux-like quorum sensing system in the extreme acidophile *Acidithiobacillus ferrooxidans*. *Biological Research* 38(2–3):283–297.

Rivas, M., Seeger, M., Jedlicki, E. and Holmes, D.S. 2007. Second acyl homoserine lactone production system in the extreme acidophile *Acidithiobacillus ferrooxidans*. *Applied and Environmental Microbiology* 73(10):3225–3231.

Ruiz, L.M., Valenzuela, S., Castro, M., Gonzalez, A., Frezza, M., Soulere, L., Rohwerder, T., Queneau, Y., Doutheau, A., Sand, W., Jerez, C. and Guiliani, N. 2008. AHL communication is a widespread phenomenon in biomining bacteria and seems to be involved in mineral-adhesion efficiency. *Hydrometallurgy* 94:133–137.

Saxena, H., Hsu, B., de Asis, M., Zierke, M., Sim, L., Withers, S.G. and Wakarchuk, W. 2018. Characterization of a thermostable endoglucanase from *Cellulomonas fimi* ATCC484. *Biochemistry and Cell Biology* 96(1):68–76.

Schopf, S., Wanner, G., Rachel, R. and Wirth, R. 2008. An archaeal bi-species biofilm formed by *Pyrococcus furiosus* and *Methanopyrus kandleri*. *Archives of Microbiology* 190(3):371–377.

Sewald, X., Saum, S.H., Palm, P., Pfeiffer, F., Oesterhelt, D. and Müller, V. 2007. Autoinducer-2-producing protein LuxS, a novel salt-and chloride-induced protein in the moderately halophilic bacterium *Halobacillus halophilus*. *Applied and Environmental Microbiology* 73(2):371–379.

Sharif, D.I., Gallon, J., Smith, C.J. and Dudley, E.D. 2008. Quorum sensing in Cyanobacteria: N-octanoyl-homoserine lactone release and response, by the epilithic colonial cyanobacterium *Gloeothece* PCC6909. *The ISME Journal* 2(12):1171–1182.

Sharma, A., Kawarabayasi, Y. and Satyanarayana, T. 2012. Acidophilic bacteria and archaea: Acid stable biocatalysts and their potential applications. *Extremophiles* 16(1):1–19.

Smith, M.B., Smith, J.N., Swift, S., Heffron, F. and Ahmer, B.M. 2001. SdiA of *Salmonella enterica* is a LuxR homolog that detects mixed microbial communities. *Journal of Bacteriology* 183(19):5733–5742.

Steindler, L. and Venturi, V. 2007. Detection of quorum-sensing N-acyl homoserine lactone signal molecules by bacterial biosensors. *FEMS Microbiology Letters* 266(1):1–9.

Sun, J., Daniel, R., Wagner-Döbler, I. and Zeng, A.P. 2004. Is autoinducer-2 a universal signal for interspecies communication: A comparative genomic and phylogenetic analysis of the synthesis and signal transduction pathways. *BMC Evolutionary Biology* 4(1):1–11.

Tait, K., Williamson, H., Atkinson, S., Williams, P., Cámara, M. and Joint, I. 2009. Turnover of quorum sensing signal molecules modulates cross-kingdom signalling. *Environmental Microbiology* 11(7):1792–1802.

Tommonaro, G., Abbamondi, G.R., Iodice, C., Tait, K. and De Rosa, S. 2012. Diketopiperazines produced by the halophilic archaeon, *Haloterrigena hispanica*, activate AHL biore-porters. *Microbial Ecology* 63(3):490–495.

Van Den Burg, B. 2003. Extremophiles as a source for novel enzymes. *Current Opinion in Microbiology* 6(3):213–218.

Visscher, P.T., Prins, R.A. and van Gemerden, H. 1992. Rates of sulfate reduction and thiosulfate consumption in a marine microbial mat. *FEMS Microbiology Letters* 86(4):283–293.

Visscher, P.T., Dupraz, C., Braissant, O., Gallagher, K.L., Glunk, C., Casillas, L. and Reed, R.E. 2010. Biogeochemistry of carbon cycling in hypersaline mats: Linking the present to the past through biosignatures. In *Microbial Mats* 14:443–468. Dordrecht: Springer.

Wenbin, N., Dejuan, Z., Feifan, L., Lei, Y., Peng, C., Xiaoxuan, Y. and Hongyu, L. 2011. Quorum-sensing system in *Acidithiobacillus ferrooxidans* involved in its resistance to Cu2+. *Letters in Applied Microbiology* 53(1):84–91.

Xavier, K.B. and Bassler, B.L. 2005. Interference with AI-2-mediated bacterial cell–cell communication. *Nature* 437(7059):750–753.

Xia, Y., He, L., Mao, J., Fang, P., Ma, X. and Wang, Z. 2018. Purification, characterization, and gene cloning of a new cold-adapted β -galactosidase from *Erwinia* sp. E602 isolated in northeast China. *Journal of Dairy Science* 101:6946–6954.

Yang, S., Fu, X., Yan, Q., Guo, Y., Liu, Z. and Jiang, Z. 2016. Cloning, expression, purification and application of a novel chitinase from a thermophilic marine bacterium *Paenibacillus barengoltzii*. *Food Chemistry* 192:1041–1048.

Yao, C., Sun, J., Wang, W., Zhuang, Z., Liu, J. and Hao, J. 2019. A novel cold-adapted β-galactosidase from *Alteromonas* sp. ML117 cleaves milk lactose effectively at low temperature. *Process Biochemistry* 82:94–101.

Yates, E.A., Philipp, B., Buckley, C., Atkinson, S., Chhabra, S.R., Sockett, R.E., Goldner, M., Dessaux, Y., Cámara, M., Smith, H. and Williams, P. 2002. N-acylhomoserine lactones undergo lactonolysis in a pH-, temperature-, and acyl chain length-dependent manner during growth of *Yersinia pseudotuberculosis* and *Pseudomonas aeruginosa*. *Infection and Immunity* 70(10):5635–5646.

Yuan, M., Chen, M., Zhang, W., Lu, W., Wang, J., Yang, M., Zhao, P., Tang, R., Li, X., Hao, Y. and Zhou, Z. 2012. Genome sequence and transcriptome analysis of the radioresistant bacterium *Deinococcus gobiensis*: Insights into the extreme environmental adaptations. *PloS One* 7(3):e34458.

Zhang, G., Zhang, F., Ding, G., Li, J., Guo, X., Zhu, J., Zhou, L., Cai, S., Liu, X., Luo, Y. and Zhang, G. 2012. Acyl homoserine lactone-based quorum sensing in a methanogenic archaeon. *The ISME Journal* 6(7):1336–1344.

4 Single- and Dual- Species Biofilms of Human Pathogenic Bacteria and Application of Bacteriophages on Biofilms

Pallavali Roja Rani, Guda Dinneswara Reddy, Degati Vijayalakshmi, Durbaka Vijaya Raghava Prasad, and Jeongdong Choi

4.1 INTRODUCTION

Biofilm formation is a self-protecting mechanism by a self-produced extracellular matrix of pathogenic bacteria. In biofilms, bacteria are embedded in a matrix, i.e., extracellular polymeric substances (EPS; consisting of carbohydrates, proteins, lipids, and endogenous DNA) attached to a solid support. EPS acts as a safeguard against stresses such as starvation, desiccation, disinfectants, UV radiation, and antimicrobial agents (1).

Biofilms may be composed of one or more species in a single or multilayered form. These layers can generate microniches; microorganisms constrict the optimal metabolic reactions in that environment. Generally, biofilms need a solid support; a biotic or abiotic surface can initiate the attachment process (2).

According to the National Institutes of Health (NIH), 60% to 80% of pathogenic microorganisms associated with infections can form biofilms. Biofilms are associated with medical devices such as contact lenses, catheters, prostheses, heart stunts; and a variety of biotic surfaces including skin, mucosal-associated tissues, and the respiratory and digestive systems. Bacteria embedded within the biofilms showed increased resistance to most antibiotics compared to planktonic bacteria. This may be due to decreased penetration of antibiotics or inactivation of antibiotics within the extracellular matrix. Microorganisms have escaped from the immune system by preventing phagocytosis, immune cell modulation, releasing toxins, and altering the physiological status (3–5).

DOI: 10.1201/9781003297826-4

Biofilms are densely packed communities of microorganisms growing on biotic and abiotic surfaces or surround themselves by secreting extracellular polymers (6, 7). Within a biofilm, the bacteria communicate with each other by producing chemotactic factors or pheromones. This phenomenon is called quorum sensing (8). If the availability of major nutrients, chemotaxis of bacteria, surface adhesions, and the presence of surfactants are responsible for forming biofilms, then this is one of the important survival strategies of pathogens (9, 10). The formation of biofilms is thought to begin when the bacteria scene environmental conditions are not suitable, which triggers the transition to stay on those surfaces or solid support. The structural and physiological complexity of biofilms has led to an idea enforced on coordinated and cooperated groups, which are analogues to multicellular organisms (11). In humans, biofilms are responsible for the development of many diseases, most of which are associated with the use of medical devices (12). Major problems of biofilms are their inherent tolerance of defense mechanisms and antibiotic therapy. Therefore, there is an urgent need to manifest alternative ways to prevent and control biofilm-associated infections (13–17).

The microorganisms growing in biofilms are intrinsically more resistant to antimicrobial agents than planktonic cells. A high dose of antimicrobial agents is required to inactivate the biofilm growth. According to NIH reports, more than 80% of infections, such as dental plaques, urogenital tract infections, peritonitis, and urogenital infections, are associated with biofilms (18, 19). Both gram-positive and gram-negative bacteria are capable of forming biofilms, which include *Staphylococcus aureus*, *Streptococcus*, *Escherichia coli*, *Klebsiella pneumoniae*, *Pseudomonas aeruginosa*, and *Proteus* species (20–22). Pathogenic bacterial biofilms have been thought of as a source of infection and often they are very difficult to treat with available antibiotics because they develop resistance to current antimicrobial treatment mechanisms and often act as a source of a high number of bacterial communities. The bacteria encased in the biofilm showed an elevated drug-resistant nature and was even difficult for the host immune system to clear (23–25).

Presently, several strategies are used to eradicate biofilm formation and minimize the microbial load on the infectious sites. One of the widely employed methods for the treatment of biofilms is bacteriophage therapy. Bacteriophages have been used for the treatment of bacterial diseases in plants, animals, and humans. Approved by the US Food and Drug Administration, phages are used to remove bacterial food contaminants in stored food items and to eradicate *Listeria monocytogenes* (26, 27). The use of bacteriophages to control biofilms is one of the best methods. Phages can replicate at the site of infection, thereby increasing the number of progenies, where the bacterial load is predominant, and where the biofilm is formed. Moreover, a single virion will produce hundreds of progeny phages and bacteriophages will produce degrading enzymes for the extracellular polysaccharide of the bacteria (28).

Bacterial communities in the extracellular matrix showed special features that deviated from the planktonic bacterial cells such as (a) intercellular signals between the community (quorum sensing), which regulates the maturation and detachment of the biofilms to objects; (b) activation of secondary messengers, which plays a role in the formation of biofilms, in flagellar movements, and production of extracellular polysaccharides; and (c) bap protein 12 plays a role in the formation of the matrix with the help of matrix scaffold proteins and creates the suitable environment for the bacteria to live in the biofilm (24, 29, 30). The formation of biofilms depends on many internal and external factors such as moist surfaces, energy sources on the site of the wound, type of bacterial association, availability of receptors for bacterial attachment, temperature, and pH. There are various methods available to detect biofilms, these include the tissue culture plate, tube method (31), and Congo red agar method (32).

Biofilms are thought to underlie much of the resistance reported to antibiotics. As an outline of the life cycles of bacterial biofilms, it is exemplified that *P. aeruginosa* is a motile bacterium that has the capacity to produce more biofilm than the non-motile, except *S. aureus*, which forms extensive biofilm. The lytic bacteriophages replicate inside the host and release progeny particles that can infect a greater number of bacteria. It has also been assumed that biofilms confer resistance to bacteriophages due to the impermeability of the biofilm matrix. However, although they are larger than antibiotics, bacteriophages are still much smaller than their bacterial host. Since many of the bacteriophages can infect the bacteria within biofilm selectively, one can make an argument that the phages have convoluted with biofilms and infection of biofilms would be expected. There are four mechanisms to destroy the biofilms by phages: (1) destruction of cells producing the biofilm matrix, (2) progeny bacteriophages diffuse through biofilms, (3) the biofilm matrix is attacked by enzymes induced by bacteriophages from their host, and (4) persistent cells are infected by bacteriophages that remain dormant until their reactive and died (10, 33–35).

It is very important to note that different bacterial species produce different exopolysaccharides, thus depolymerase active against polysaccharides by one species may not digest that produced by others. The complexity (viability) in the exopolysaccharides is lower than that of the host where the bacteriophages have the broad activity to target the exopolysaccharides (36), which is evidenced by the young biofilms. However, it blocks the activity of antibiotics, where amikacin showed 100× the minimum inhibitory concentration (MIC) activity enhancing bacterial growth. Even though it has been shown to be sensitive at the MIC by disc susceptibility while growing planktonically.

Sharma et al. (9) reported the onset of antibiotic resistance developed in the early stage of biofilms, thus the bacteriophages can kill bacteria in situations where conventional antibiotics cannot do so (16, 37, 38). As a result, massive and often readily available and diversified bacteriophages isolated from the natural environment target the bacteria including biofilms. It is further possible to optimize bacteriophages for their intended application either through initial selection, serial passage, or other standard techniques. Hence, bacteriophage possesses unique properties and shows considerable promise in the control of biofilms. However, such applications are still evolving and large-scale productions are still under development. Thus, identification is the most effective approach or a speculative nature is needed to reach the best practices for appropriate use.

4.2   BIOFILM FORMATION STAGES

Biofilm usually forms by the following four steps: (1) bacterial attachment to suitable objects, (2) microcolony formation by the association of different bacterial cells in the vicinity of the site of infection, (3) maturation of the bacterial biofilms by using nutrients available at the site of infection, and (4) bacterial dispersion or detachment of the biofilm mostly by external enzymes such as proteases and nucleases, which degrades the external matrix of the biofilm (39–42) (Figure 4.1).

BIOFILM FORMATION

1. Attachment
2. Maturation
3. Detachment

BIOFILM INTEGRITY AND COMPOSITION

Carbohydrates
Proteins
Lipids
Extracellular DNA

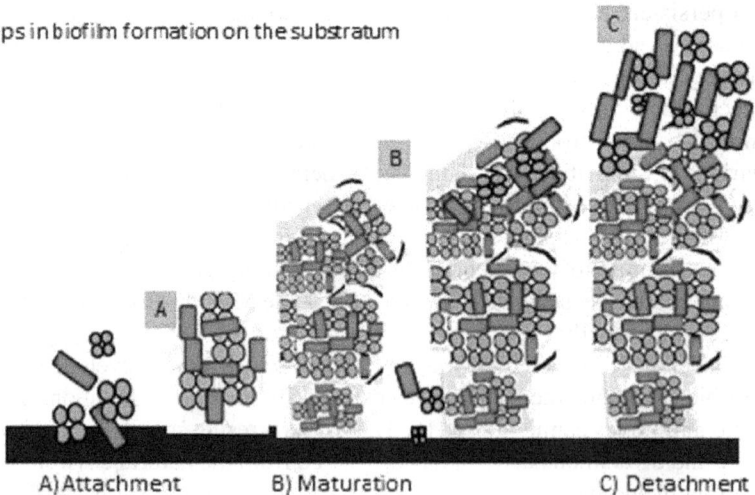

Steps in biofilm formation on the substratum

A) Attachment   B) Maturation   C) Detachment

FIGURE 4.1 Stages involved in the formation of biofilm on the solid substratum. (A) Attachment of bacteria onto the solid support, (B) maturation of the attached bacteria, and (C) detachment of biofilm forming a bacterial group and attaching to another solid surface.

4.3 QUALITATIVE AND QUANTITATIVE DETERMINATION OF BIOFILM-FORMING BACTERIA

Biofilm formation is a process whereby microorganisms irreversibly attach to and grow on a surface and produce an extracellular polymer that facilitates attachment and matrix formation. The most prevalent bacterial species of septic wound patients were the prominent biofilm producers which were screened by using the tube adherence method, Congo red agar method, microtiter plate method, and electron microscopic method.

4.3.1 TUBE ADHERENCE METHOD

Biofilm formation was investigated by the tube adherence test with slight modifications. Whereby using 10 mL of brain heart infusion broth (HiMedia, Mumbai) inoculated with selected bacterial strains of *P. aeruginosa*, *S. aureus*, *E. coli*, and *K. pneumoniae* (100 µL) and incubated for 24 hours at 37°C, using a shaker at 130 rpm. After incubation, the culture medium was removed and washed twice with phosphate buffer saline (PBS pH 7.4). Then the tubes were stained with 0.1% crystal violet, then washed and air dried for 24 hours. The presence of a layer of stained material adhered to the inner wall of the tube indicates biofilm formation (Figure 4.2).

4.3.2 CONGO RED AGAR METHOD

Biofilm formation was also demonstrated by the Congo red agar method (43). Bacteria species *P. aeruginosa*, *S. aureus*, *E. coli*, and *K. pneumoniae* isolated from septic wounds were suspended in brain heart infusion (BHI) broth (HiMedia, Mumbai) by mixing 0.08% Congo red (Kmphasol, Mumbai) supplemented with 1% glucose and incubated at 37°C for 24 to 48 hours. After incubation, the Congo red agar media plates were observed for the phenotypic characteristics of the colonies raised. Biofilm formers appear with black color, whereas non-biofilm producers form red color colonies (Figure 4.3).

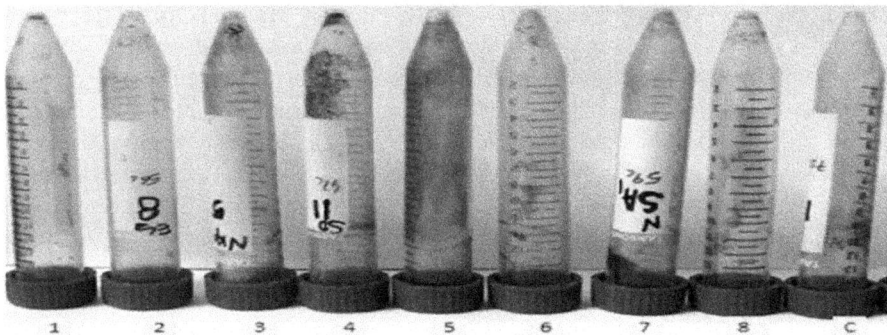

FIGURE 4.2 Tube adhesion test of biofilm formers.

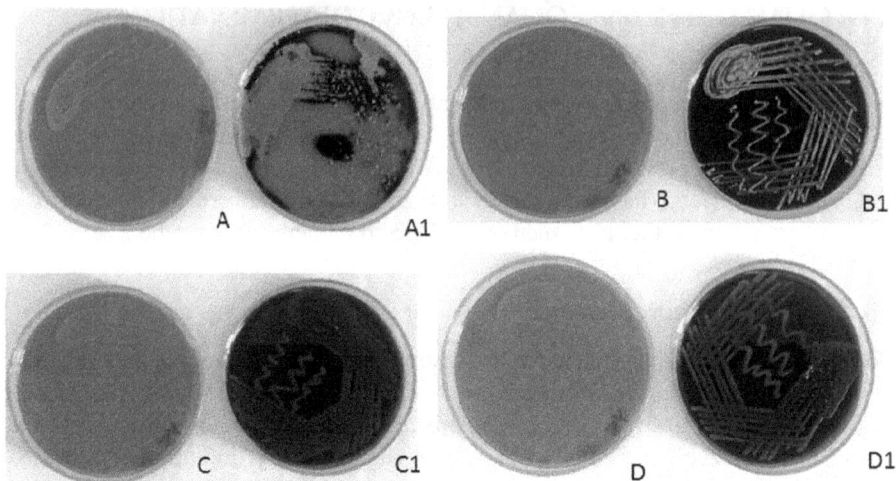

FIGURE 4.3 Detection of biofilm formers by Congo red agar. A, B, C, and D are the non-biofilm formers of *S. aureus*, *P. aeruginosa*, *K. pneumoniae*, and *E. coli* strains, respectively. A1, B1, C1, and D1 are the biofilm formers of *S. aureus*, *P. aeruginosa*, *K. pneumoniae*, and *E. coli* strains, respectively.

4.3.3 MICROTITER PLATE METHOD

The biofilm formation phenomenon was also investigated by using 96-well flat-bottom tissue culture plates. It is a semiquantitative method for the determination of the biofilms. Precisely, 24-hour-old bacterial suspensions were prepared in BHI broth with 1% glucose and maintained up to the mid-log phase (A 600 = 0.1 (~10^7 CFU/mL) for microtiter plate method. Then, 100 µL of bacterial suspension of each bacterium was inoculated into individual wells of a microtiter plate and then incubated overnight at 37°C, extending up to 48 hours. Further, the plates were gently aspirated and washed with 1X phosphate buffer saline (PBS pH 7.4), followed by staining with 100 µL of 0.1% crystal violet (Qualigens, Mumbai) for 30 minutes at room temperature. Excess crystal violet stain was decanted and washed with distilled water. Crystal violet bound to the biofilms and then dissolved in 95% ethanol. Then, the biofilm was quantified by measuring the absorbance of the supernatant read at 570 nm. For all the selected bacterial strains biofilm assay was performed in triplicate and then the mean absorbance value was calculated. Bacterial strains that showed twice that of negative control, i.e., BHI broth with non-biofilm formers (2X ≥ OD 570), were positive for biofilms, whereas those strains with values less than the negative control were considered as non-biofilm-forming strains (Table 4.1 and Figures 4.4 and 4.5).

TABLE 4.1
Standard OD values of strong, moderate, and weak biofilm formers

Biofilm formation	OD value
Zero	Less than 0.05
Weak	0.05 to 0.12
Moderate	0.12 to 0.24
Strong	Greater than 0.24

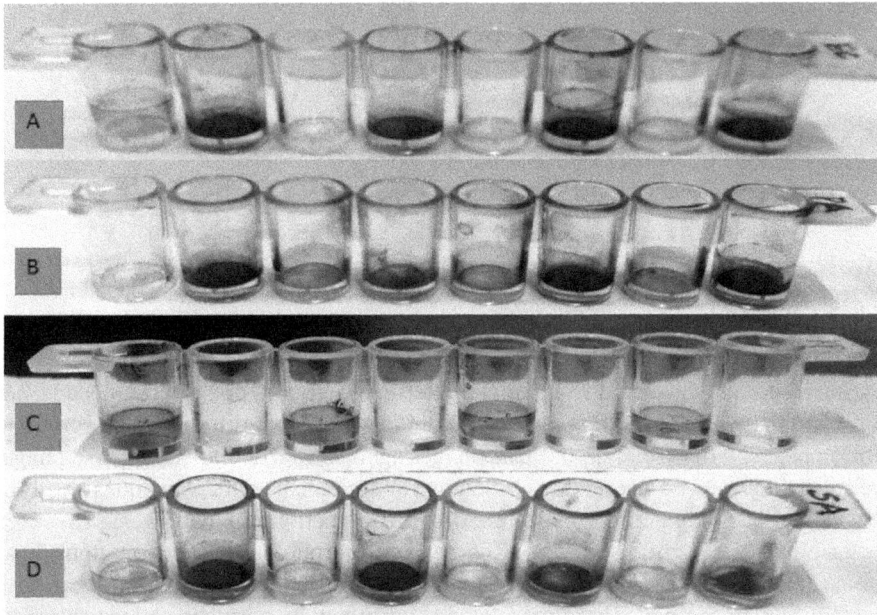

FIGURE 4.4 Biofilm formation of *S. aureus*, *P. aeruginosa*, *K. pneumoniae*, and *E. coli* in microtiter plates.

4.4 BACTERIOPHAGES AS BIOFILM DISRUPTORS

4.4.1 INTRODUCTION TO BACTERIOPHAGES

Bacteriophages are naturally occurring viruses that infect bacteria, are ubiquitous, have a huge influence on the environment where bacteria exist, and they are one of the important biomass producers on Earth. So far, more than 5000 classified bacteriophages are known and are easily identified in water sources, sewage, soil, and even ocean depths (44).

Bacteriophages are eaters of harmful and useful bacteria. Bacteriophages are a class of viruses that require a host like bacteria with specific receptors on the surface

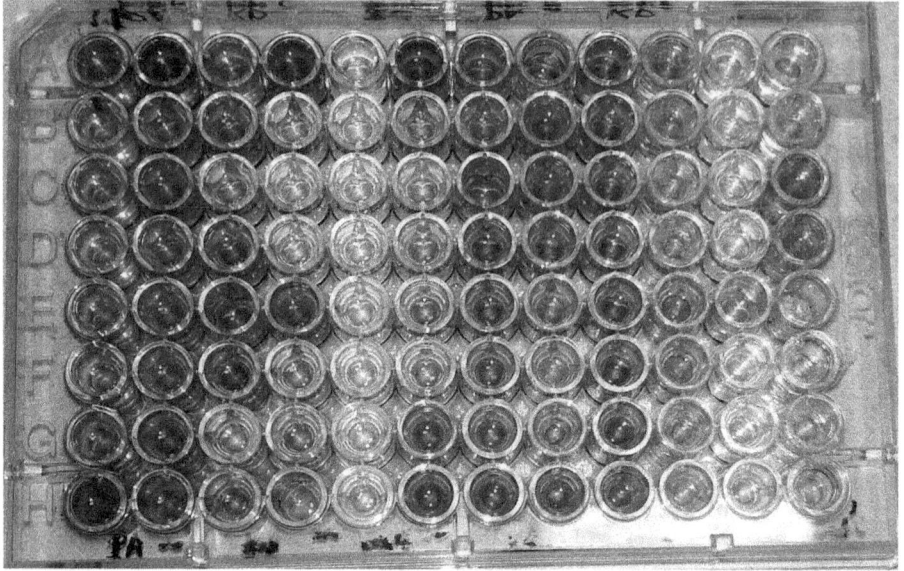

FIGURE 4.5 Crystal violet staining of biofilms. Eight- and 96-well microtiter plates show the biofilm formation of predominant isolates of septic wound infections.

of cell walls because they are intracellular obligate parasites. The phages for selective bacteria can be isolated from fecal matters, sewage soil, hot springs, oceans, etc. For example, water from the Ganga in India has been found to be a rich source of vibrio phages. After isolation of these phages against a particular stain, these phages are most likely to be useful for clinicians for treatment, which includes the lytic phages that have high efficacy and broad-spectrum activity on pathogens. However, bacteriophages can be classified on the basis of morphology, genetic content, host, habitat, or life cycle. Usually, phages exhibit different life cycles within their host-virulent and temperate. Therefore, during the infection, virulent phages associate with metabolic activity, directing the bacterial molecular machinery into the synthesis of the new phage particles. The host cell lyses and the viral progeny is released. Hence, they may be termed virulent phages. Similarly, temperate phages, those initiating the lysogeny by integrating their host, maintain the quiescent stage (prophage), and it is vertically transferred with the bacterial genome as the host cell reproduces until the lytic cycle is induced (45).

The genome size varies between 100 kb and 300 kb. Most of the examples show that bacterial species have sensitivity toward one or more phages. Almost all phages have DNA as the genetic material and few phages have RNA as genetic material, in single-stranded form. Electron microscopic studies with negative staining revealed that 97% of phages are tailed and the remaining 3% of phages are tailless like filamentous, polyhedral, and pleomorphic phages (46). Tailed phages have an advantage with a tail, for the adsorption of the virion to receptors of the bacteria. Except for the filamentous phages, all the phage groups have a polyhedral capsid plus genome. This capsid is usually joined to a tail, which is a helical protein structure required for the adsorption of the virion to the bacterial cell. Felix de Herelle was the first scientist to use the term "bacteriophages," a biological principle that has the potential capacity to attack and kill bacteria. Phage therapy is an ancient bactericidal method for specific bacteria. Phage therapy was first introduced by de Herelle in 1919 for the treatment of shigella dysentery in rabbits and humans in Paris. The early strong interest in phage therapy is reflected in some 800 papers published on the topic between 1917 and 1956. During 1920–1940, bacteriophage therapy became the major method for the treatment of different microbial diseases. During the 1920s–1930s, bacteriophage therapy began to become more widespread, as the United States pharmaceutical company Eli Lilly produced phages for staphylococcus infections. Along with Eli Lilly, Bristol-Meyers and Abbott laboratories were also producing phages for therapy. But in 1940, Alexander Fleming accidentally discovered the antibiotic penicillin from *Penicillium notatum* from mold culture. This discovery became the most advantageous method for killing bacteria. Eventually, phage therapy was confined to Eastern Europe and the former Soviet Union. The industrialization of antibiotics in the 1940s, however, changed the focus of anti-infective research and development in the best away from phage treatments and toward natural products and their semi-synthetic derivatives with antibacterial effects. From 1940 onward, a series of discoveries on antibiotic development like penicillin, streptomycin, kanamycin, and neomycin were produced as secondary metabolites, and purified products were used for antibiotic therapy. After their initial discovery in the early 1900s, they were shown to be effective at treating bacterial infections, even though their mechanism of action was not known. Research in this area was stopped in the Western world upon the discovery of antibiotics. However, now that the era of antibiotics is becoming challenging with the rise of a resistance pattern in microorganisms' phages, again being turned to as a possible weapon in the fight against multidrug-resistant bacterial infections (47–50).

Nowadays, due to the evolution of multidrug-resistant bacteria, the entire world is looking for alternatives to antibiotics, that is, bacteriophages. Bacteriophages that undergo the lytic cycle are suitable and applied candidates for phage therapy. In addition, bacteriophages do not cause human allergies nor do they change the structure, odor, or flavor of food products. Despite the huge amount of research on phage therapy, there are few reports available on the pharmacokinetics of therapeutic phage preparation. The therapeutic phages are assumed to lyse the selective target bacteria by replicating inside.

4.4.2 BACTERIOPHAGE THERAPY AND ITS APPLICATION

Now, over 60 years later, interest again is turning to phages, as adjunct therapies in the control of bacterial pathogens that emerged as resistant to antibiotics because of the increase of antibiotic resistance. Researchers are showing interest in phages as therapeutic agents in medical, veterinary, poultry, agriculture, and aquaculture applications. Antibiotic resistance is now observed in the following organisms: *Staphylococcus aureus, Salmonella, Mycobacterium tuberculosis, Acinetobacter,*

Escherichia coli, Streptococcus pneumonia, Campylobacter jejuni, Helicobacter pylori, Pseudomonas aeruginosa, Haemophilus influenza, and *Clostridium difficile* (51–54). There is evidence that phage particles do not disturb the normal intestinal flora and there have been no side effects reported. It is also suggested that they can be used prophylactically and in established infections because of their cell-perpetuating nature. In the presence of susceptible bacterial infection, multiple administrations were not required. Despite unlimited advantages, some disadvantages have also been observed (55). Bacteriophages are not recommended for patients in critical condition. The phage preparations are not recommended to apply through intraperitoneal and intravenous injections routes. Usually, phage preparations contain live bacteria. Rapid clearance of phages is completed by the spleen, liver, and other filtering organs. Development of the lysogeny state would be a big problem. Antiphage antibodies are another problem because they won't be able to interfere with acute treatment lasting a week. Because of these reasons, reoccurrence of the same bacterial infection progressed. Bacteriophages injected in diseased patients suffering from cutaneous boils caused by staphylococcus, saw improvement (reduced pain and fever) within 48 hours. Mershivalli and colleagues (2009) proved that the phage cocktail consists of all the lytic phages exclusively used for burn wound patients infected by *Staphylococcus aureus* and *P. aeruginosa*. There is remarkable control of otitis media caused by drug-resistant *Pseudomonas aeruginosa* for which a clinical trial of the therapeutic phage preparations has been employed. So far, phages have been reported effectively in treating bacterial diseases such as cerebrospinal meningitis; skin infections caused by *P. aeruginosa, S. aureus, K. pneumoniae,* and *E. coli*; and cystic fibrosis, eye infections, neonatal sepsis, urinary tract diseases, and cancers. In an important report by Markoishivi et al. (2003) the phages impregnated polymers used to treat venous stasis skin ulcers. Similarly, using the same principle, combinational therapy has been implemented by using biodegradable polymers embedded with ciprofloxacin and bacteriophages. The phages can also be applied to treat various infections of the urogenital system by direct infection or topical applications. As per phage therapy, MRSA is simply another stain treated by phages that can be accomplished by local application. There is a need to provide the phage preparation for the systemic application to treat patients suffering from an immune-compromised state. With the increasing worldwide prevalence of antibiotic resistance, bacteriophage endolysins represent a very promising novel alternative therapeutic against infections. Phage endolysins or lysins are enzymes that damage cellular integrity by hydrolyzing peptidoglycan components. There is also evidence that phage lysins have been employed for the reduction of nasopharyngeal carriage of *K. pneumoniae*. Phage therapy has been successfully tested for protecting fish from experimentally induced bacterial infections in aquaculture and has been approved in the USA. While several research groups continue to develop whole phage as alternative treatments, the isolation and optimization of purified phage components as antibacterial opens new opportunities in the fight against viral infections. According to the scientific classification, a combination of three bacteriophage cocktails was more effective against *Enterobacter cloaca* than the single bacteriophage. The combined treatment of bacteriophage cocktail and polysaccharide depolymerase were the best tools for the control of bacteriophages. Findings suggest that the combinational treatment of bacteriophages and chlorine is a promising method to control and remove bacterial biofilms from various surfaces. In contrast, bacteriophages seem to have an abundant ability to target the bacteria growth, but a high number of bacteria present within biofilms facilitates the action of bacteriophages by developing an efficient and rapid infection in the host and consequent amplification of bacteriophages. In general, these phages have the intrinsic property to make the biofilm susceptible to their action, i.e., they are known to induce enzymes that degrade the extracellular matrix. Some cultured biofilms are better examples to support the replication of bacterio-phages than other planktonic systems. It is perhaps surprising that bacteriophages as the natural predators of the bacteria can target the common form of bacterial life. Biofilms are thought to underlie much of the resistance reported to antibiotics. As an outline of the life cycles of bacterial biofilms, it is exemplified that *P. aeruginosa* is a motile bacterium that has the capacity to produce a vast amount of biofilms com-pared to non-motile bacteria, except *S. aureus*, which forms extensive biofilms. The lytic bacteriophages replicate inside the host and release progeny particles can infect a greater number of bacteria. It has also been assumed that biofilms confer resis-tance to bacteriophages due to the impermeability of the biofilm matrix. However, although they are larger than antibiotics, bacteriophages are still much smaller than their bacterial host. Since many bacteriophages can infect the bacteria within bio-film selectively, one can make an argument that the phages have convoluted with biofilms and that infection of biofilms would be expected. There are four mecha-nisms to destroy the biofilms by phages: (1) destruction of cells producing the biofilm matrix, (2) progeny bacteriophages diffuse through biofilms, (3) the biofilm matrix is attacked by enzymes induced by bacteriophages from their host, and (4) persistent cells are infected by bacteriophages that remain dormant until they become active. (10, 33–35). It is very important to note that different bacterial species produce dif-ferent exopolysaccharides, thus depolymerase active against polysaccharides by one species may not digest that produced by others. The complexity (viability) in the exopolysaccharides is lower than that of the host where the bacteriophages have the broad activity to target the exopolysaccharides (36), which is evidenced by the young biofilms. However, it blocks the activity of antibiotics, where amikacin showed 100× the MIC activity enhancing bacterial growth. Even though it has been shown to be sensitive at the MIC by disc susceptibility while growing planktonically (37, 38).

4.5 DETERMINATION OF PHAGE ACTION ON BIOFILMS BY EMPLOYING ELECTRON MICROSCOPIC METHODS

4.5.1 SCANNING ELECTRON MICROSCOPIC METHODS

Biofilms grown on borosilicate glass coverslips previously placed into the wells of a 24-well microtiter plate were used. All the biofilms formed were incubated with 100 μL of individual selective bacteriophage for both single- and dual-species bio-film in the wells for 4 hours. After treatment, the coverslips were washed twice with PBS and dried for 20 hours at 37°C. The biofilms coated on glass slides were fixed with glutaraldehyde (2.5%) and dehydrated through a series of graded ethanol

(30%–100%) for 5 minutes. Further, the glass slides were sputtered with gold after critical point drying and the aggregated biofilms were examined using scanning electron microscopy (FEI, Tecnai G-2S Twin). The scanning electron microscopic images of various conditions are reported in the following.

4.5.1.1 Dynamic Conditions of Single-Species Biofilm
See Figure 4.6.

4.5.1.2 Dynamic Conditions of Single-Species Biofilm
See Figure 4.7.

4.5.1.3 Dual-Species Biofilm
Dual-species biofilm studies show multidrug-resistant bacteria grown in three different combinations, i.e., *S. aureus*, which is a gram-positive bacteria, with a gram-negative bacterium, *P. aeruginosa*, *K. pneumoniae*, and *E. coli*. Under static conditions, there was appreciable growth of mixed bacterial growth on coverslips when challenged with respective phage cocktails. There was a drastic complete eradication observed with dual-species biofilms (Figure 4.8).

4.5.2 Confocal Scanning Electron Microscopic Method

Staining with the FilmTracer™ LIVE/DEAD® Biofilm viability kit (Molecular Probes, Life Technologies Ltd.) was performed according to the instructions provided by the manufacturer. The working solution of fluorescent stains was prepared

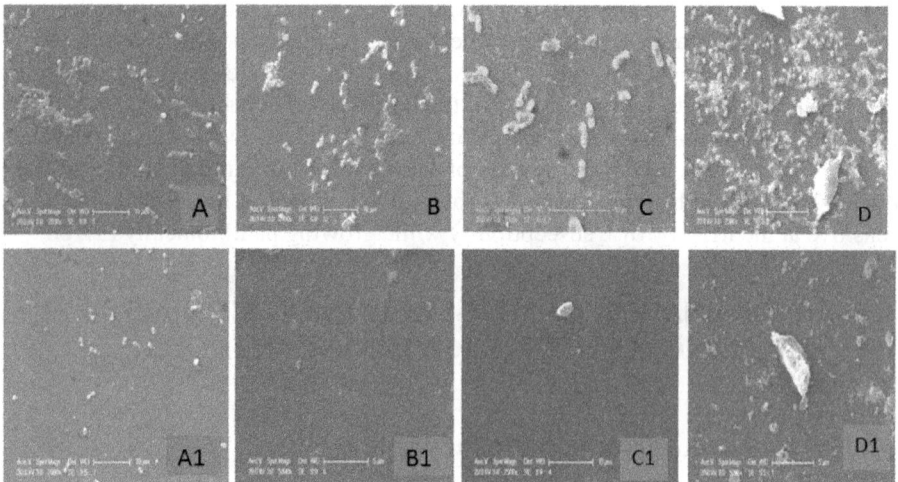

FIGURE 4.6 Scanning electron microscopic images of *P. aeruginosa*, *E. coli*, *K. pneumoniae*, and *S. aureus* (A, B, C, and D) with respective bacteriophages (A1, B1, C1, and D1) biofilm growing on the glass coverslip under dynamic conditions at 37°C for 12 hours (under dynamic conditions).

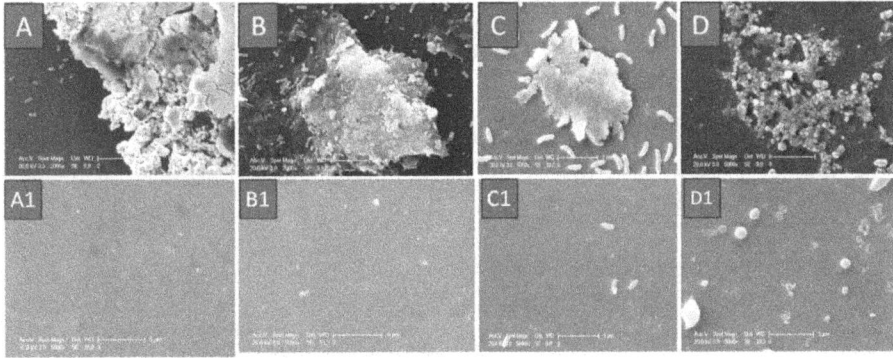

FIGURE 4.7 Scanning Electron microscopic images of *P. aeruginosa, E. coli, K. pneumoniae,* and *S. aureus* (A, B, C, and D) with respective bacteriophages (A1, B1, C1, and D1) biofilm growing on the glass coverslip under static conditions at 37°C for 12 hours (under static conditions).

by adding 3 μL of SYTO® 9 stains and 3 μL of propidium iodide (PI) stain to 1 mL of filter-sterilized water. Also, 200 μL of staining solution was deposited on the glass coverslip surface coated with biofilms of selected multidrug-resistant bacterial isolates treated with selective phages. After 15 minutes of incubation in the dark at room temperature, the samples were washed with sterile saline to remove excess dye and rinsed with water from the base of the support material. Stained biofilms were examined with a confocal laser microscope (Leica model TCS SP5; Leica Microsystems CMS GmbH) using a 20X dry objective (HC PL FLUOTAR 20.0 X 0.50 DRY) plus a 2× electronic zoom. To minimize the air contact and maintain a constant sample moisture condition, a coverslip was reversely placed on the specimen (Figure 4.9).

A 488 nm laser line was used to excite SYTO 9, while the fluorescent emission was detected from 500 to 540 nm. PI was excited with a 561 nm laser line and its fluorescent emission was detected from 600 to 695 nm. Images from at least four randomly selected areas were acquired for each disk. For each of them, sequential optical sections of 2 μM were collected along the z-axis over the complete thickness of the sample to be subsequently analyzed biofilm, i.e., SYTO 9 for live cells and PI applied for dead cell markers.

4.6   CONCLUSION

The drug-resistant nature of bacterial pathogens to antibiotics has become a great burden to human healthcare. Drug resistance is a common and natural mechanism in microorganisms. Since the 1930s, antibiotics have been used for the treatment of various diseases, but this has led to the emergence of multidrug-resistant bacterial strains. The World Health Organization reported that 60% of pathogens have attained resistance to major available antibiotics. It is anticipated that all pathogens will acquire 100% drug resistance. One of the reasons for better adaptation of microorganisms to antibiotics may be self-medication along with continual usage.

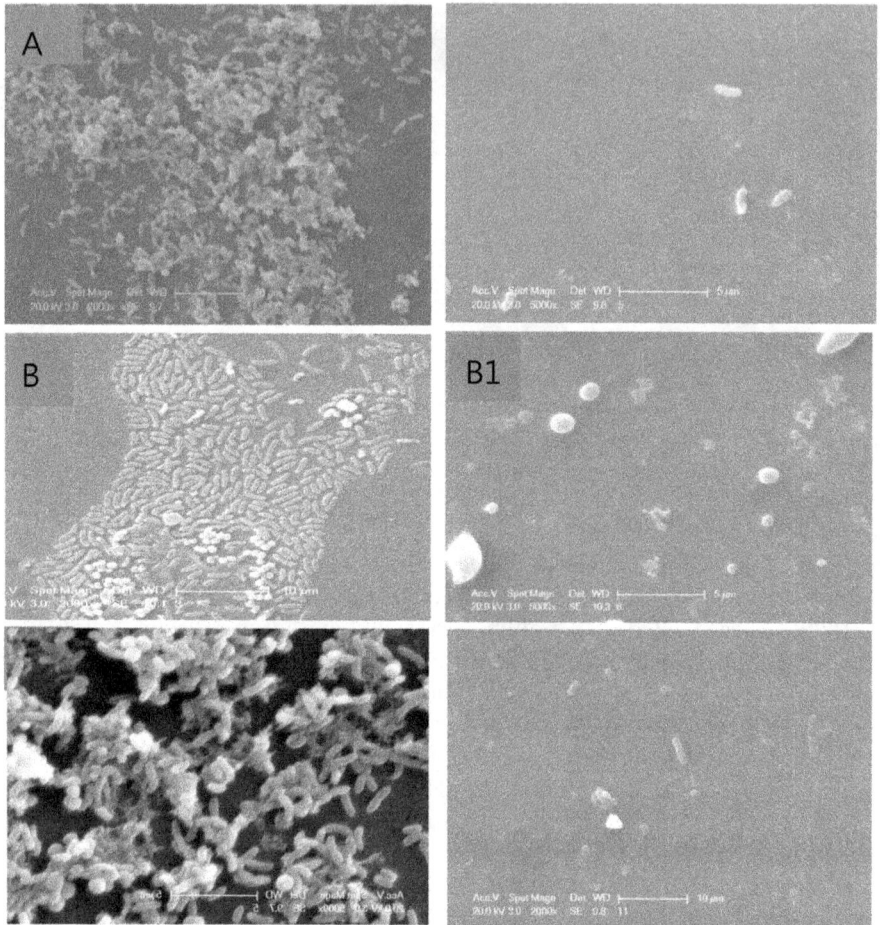

FIGURE 4.8 Dual species biofilms treated with respective phage cocktails. Scanning electron microscopic images of a 4-hour phage cocktail treated dual-species biofilms of multidrug-resistant bacterial isolates on the coverslip at 12 hours of incubation. (A) *S. aureus* with *P. aeruginosa*, (A1) treated with phage cocktail (phage vB_SAnS_SADP1 + vB_PAnP_PADP4). (B) *S. aureus* with *K. pneumoniae*, (B1) treated with phage cocktail (phage vB_SAnS_SADP1 + vB_KPnM_KPDP1. (C) *S. aureus* with *E. coli*, (C1) treated with phage cocktail (phage vB_SAnS_SADP1 + vB_ECnM_ECDP3. Drastic reductions of biofilms were observed after phage cocktail treatment when compared with test samples (only biofilms without phage cocktails).

Multidrug-resistant organisms emerge not only by accumulation but also by absorbing antibiotics from outside the environment. But, crucially, the response to an antibiotic attack on the bacteria by adaptation and the pinnacle of evolution, "survival of the fittest," is the broad consequence of the immense genetic plasticity of pathogens, which triggers the responses resulting in adaptive mutations, acquisition

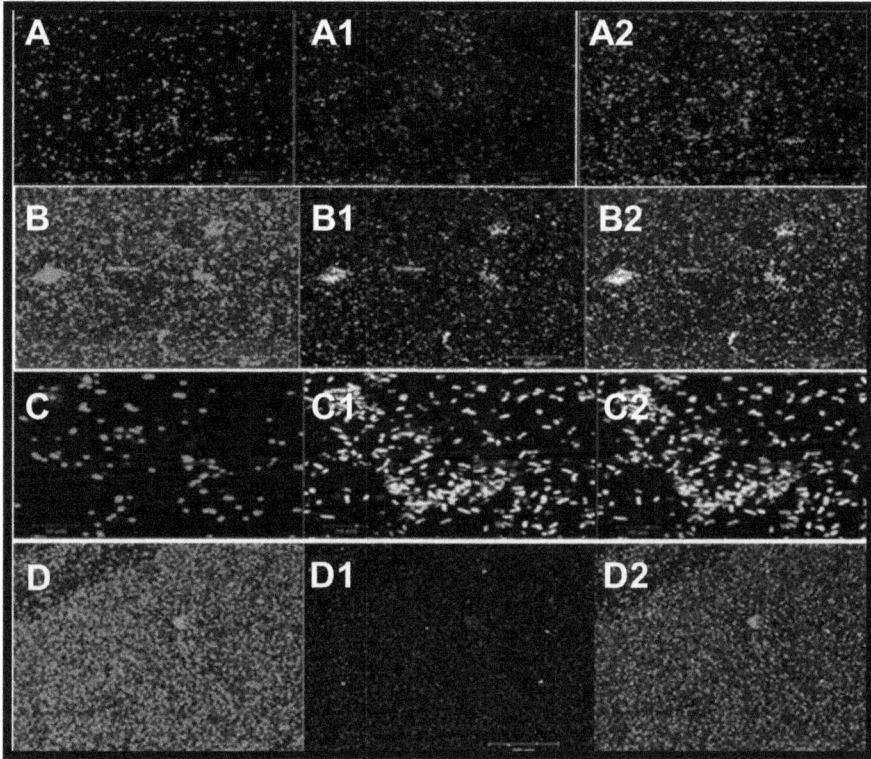

FIGURE 4.9 Bacteriophage lytic activity on 48-hour-old biofilms after 2 and 4 hours of incubation as analyzed by confocal laser scanning microscope. Biofilm of multidrug-resistant *P. aeruginosa*, *K. pneumoniae*, *E. coli*, and *S. aureus* incubated for 48 hours. A, B, C, and D biofilms were treated with respective phages for 4 hours. A1, B1, C1, and D1 were treated with SM buffer (control). A2, B2, C2, and D2 were treated with 2 hours incubation with respective phages.

of genetic elements, or altering the gene expression that alternatively produces resistance to virtually all antibiotics currently available.

Microorganisms growing in biofilms are intrinsically more resistant to antimicrobial agents than planktonic cells. A high dose of antimicrobial agents is required to inactivate the biofilm growth. According to the National Institutes of Health (NIH), more than 80% of infections are associated with biofilms, including dental plaques, urogenital tract infections, and peritonitis. Both gram-positive and gram-negative bacteria can form biofilms, including *Staphylococcus aureus*, *Streptococcus*, *Escherichia coli*, *Klebsiella pneumoniae*, and *Proteus* species.

The formation of biofilms depends on many internal and external factors such as moist surfaces, energy sources on the site of the wound, type of bacterial association, availability of receptors for bacterial attachment, temperature, and pH.

The following four stages support biofilm formation: (1) bacterial attachment to the suitable objects, (2) microcolony formation by the association of different bacterial cells in the vicinity of the site of infection, (3) maturation of the bacterial biofilms by using nutrients available at the site of infection, and (4) bacterial dispersion or detachment of the biofilm, mostly by external enzymes such as proteases and nucleases, which degrades the external matrix of the biofilm.

Bacteriophages are obligate parasites of host bacterium and ubiquitous in nature. Selection of bacteriophages has been thoroughly emphasized by scientists, particularly in Ganga water in India. It is the basic research to pave the way to detect the bacteriophages. After isolation of these types of phages against a particular stain, these selected phages are more likely to be useful for clinicians for appropriate treatment, which includes the lytic phages that have high efficacy and a broad-spectrum activity on pathogens. As a result, massive and often readily available diversified bacteriophages are isolated from the natural environment. Almost all of them target the bacteria including biofilms. It is further possible to optimize bacteriophages for their intended application of initial selection or serial passage or other standard techniques. Hence, bacteriophages pose unique properties and show considerable promise in the control of biofilms. However, such applications are still evolving and large-scale production is still under development. Thus, identification is the most effective approach or a speculative nature is required to reach the best practices for appropriate use.

REFERENCES

1. Harper DR, Parracho HMRT, Walker J, Sharp R, Hughes G, Werthén M, et al. Bacteriophages and biofilms. *Antibiotics*. 2014;3(3):270–84.
2. Muhammad MH, Idris AL, Fan X, Guo Y, Yu Y, Jin X, et al. Beyond risk: Bacterial biofilms and their regulating approaches. *Front Microbiol*. 2020;11(May):1–20.
3. Barzegari A, Kheyrolahzadeh K, Mahdi S, Khatibi H, Sharifi S, Memar MY, et al. The battle of probiotics and their derivatives against biofilms. *Infect Drug Resist*. 2020;13:659–72.
4. Gutiérrez D, Rodríguez-Rubio L, Martínez B, Rodríguez A, García P. Bacteriophages as weapons against bacterial biofilms in the food industry. *Front Microbiol*. 2016;7(Jun):1–15.
5. Khan F, Bamunuarachchi NI, Pham DTN, Tabassum N, Khan MSA, Kim YM. Mixed biofilms of pathogenic Candida-bacteria: Regulation mechanisms and treatment strategies. *Crit Rev Microbiol* [Internet]. 2021;47(6):699–727. Available from: https://doi.org/10.1080/1040841X.2021.1921696
6. Tait K, Skillman LC, Sutherland IW. The efficacy of bacteriophage as a method of biofilm eradication. *Biofouling*. 2002;18(4):305–11.
7. Milho C, Silva MD, Alves D, Oliveira H, Sousa C, Pastrana LM, et al. Escherichia coli and Salmonella Enteritidis dual-species biofilms: Interspecies interactions and antibiofilm efficacy of phages. *Sci Rep*. 2019;9(1):1–15.
8. Kaistha, S.D. Bacteriophages in biofilm control. *EC Microbiology*. 2017;10:47–52.
9. Sharma G, Sharma S, Sharma P, Chandola D, Dang S, Gupta S, et al. Escherichia coli biofilm: Development and therapeutic strategies. *Journal of Applied Microbiology*. 2016;121(2):309–19.
10. Zhu J, Miller MB, Vance RE, Dziejman M, Bassler BL, Mekalanos JJ. Quorum-sensing regulators control virulence gene expression in Vibrio cholerae. *Proceedings of the National Academy of Sciences*. 2002;99(5):3129–34.

11. Fernández L, González S, Campelo AB, Martínez B, Rodríguez A, García P. Low-level predation by lytic phage phiIPLA-RODI promotes biofilm formation and triggers the stringent response in Staphylococcus aureus. *Sci Rep.* 2017;7:40965.

12. Brandão GA, Pereira A, Brandão AM, de Almeida H, Motta RH. Does the bracket composition material influence initial biofilm formation? *Indian Journal of Dental Research.* 2015;26(2):148–51.

13. Pirnay JP, De Vos D, Verbeken G, Merabishvili M, Chanishvili N, Vaneechoutte M, et al. The phage therapy paradigm: Prêt-à-porter or sur-mesure? *Pharmaceutical Research.* 2011;28(4):934–7.

14. Santos SB, Carvalho CM, Sillankorva S, Nicolau A, Ferreira EC, Azeredo J. The use of antibiotics to improve phage detection and enumeration by the double-layer agar technique. *BMC Microbiol.* 2009;9:148.

15. Pires D, Sillankorva S, Faustino A, Azeredo J. Use of newly isolated phages for control of Pseudomonas aeruginosa PAO1 and ATCC 10145 biofilms. *Res Microbiol.* 2011;162(8):798–806.

16. Sillankorva S, Neubauer P, Azeredo J. Isolation and characterization of a T7-like lytic phage for Pseudomonas fluorescens. *BMC Biotechnol.* 2008;8:80.

17. Steier L, Oliveira SD De. Bacteriophages in dentistry – State of the art and perspectives. *Dent J.* 2019;7(1):6.

18. Cornelissen A, Ceyssens PJ, T'Syen J, van Praet H, Noben JP, Shaburova OV, et al. The t7-related pseudomonas putida phage φ15 displays virion-associated biofilm degradation properties. *PLoS One.* 2011;6(4):e18597.

19. Burrowes B, Harper DR, Anderson J, McConville M, Enright MC. Bacteriophage therapy: Potential uses in the control of antibiotic-resistant pathogens. *Expert Review of Anti-Infective Therapy.* 2011;9(9):775–85.

20. Mahgoub EM, Elfatih M, Omer A. Aerobic bacteria isolated from diabetic septic wounds. 2015;3:91–99.

21. Omole IA, Stephen E. Antibiogram profile of bacteria isolated from wound infection of patients in three hospitals in Anyigba, Kogi state, Nigeria. *FUTA Journal of Research in Sciences.* 2014;10:258–266.

22. Elkadi OA. Phage therapy: The new old antibacterial therapy. Vol. 2014. *El Mednifico Journal.* 2014;2:311–312.

23. Leiman PG, Chipman PR, Kostyuchenko VA, Mesyanzhinov VV, Rossmann MG. Three-dimensional rearrangement of proteins in the tail of bacteriophage T4 on infection of its host. *Cell.* 2004;118(4):419–29.

24. Yuan Y, Qu K, Tan D, Li X, Wang L, Cong C, et al. Microbial Pathogenesis Isolation and characterization of a bacteriophage and its potential to disrupt multi-drug resistant Pseudomonas aeruginosa bio films. *Microbial Pathogenesis.* 2019;128(July 2018):329–36.

25. Gutiérrez D, Fernández L, Rodríguez A, García P. Role of bacteriophages in the implementation of a sustainable dairy chain. *Front. Microbiol.,* 2019;10(January):1–14.

26. Marsh EJ, Luo H, Wang H. A three-tiered approach to differentiate Listeria monocytogenes biofilm-forming abilities. *FEMS Microbiol Lett.* 2003;228(2):203–10.

27. Abbatiello A, Agarwal D, Bersin J, Lahiri G, Schartz J, Volini E. Well-being: A strategy and a responsibility. 2018; Deloitte Global Human Capital Trends. 2018;62:65–70.

28. Vieira A, Silva YJ, Cunha Â, Gomes NCM, Ackermann HW, Almeida A. Phage therapy to control multidrug-resistant Pseudomonas aeruginosa skin infections: In vitro and ex vivo experiments. *European Journal of Clinical Microbiology and Infectious Diseases.* 2012;31(11):3241–9.

29. Yazdi M, Bouzari M, Ghaemi EA. Isolation and characterization of a lytic bacteriophage (vB-PmiS-TH) and its application in combination with ampicillin against planktonic and biofilm forms of proteus mirabilis isolated from urinary tract infection. *J Mol Microbiol Biotechnol.* 2018;28(1):37–46.

30. Sanchez CJ, Mende K, Beckius ML, Akers KS, Romano DR, Wenke JC, et al. Biofilm formation by clinical isolates and the implications in chronic infections. *BMC Infect Dis.* 2013;13(43).
31. Christensen GD, Simpson WA, Younger JJ, Baddour LM, Barrett FF, Melton DM, et al. Adherence of coagulase-negative staphylococci to plastic tissue culture plates: a quantitative model for the adherence of staphylococci to medical devices. *Journal of Clinical Microbiology.* 1985;22:996–1006.
32. Hassan A, Usman J, Kaleem F, Omair M, Khalid A, Iqbal M. Evaluation of different detection methods of biofilm formation in the clinical isolates. *Brazilian Journal of Infectious Diseases.* 2011;15(4):305–11.
33. Ryan EM, Gorman SP, Donnelly RF, Gilmore BF. Recent advances in bacteriophage therapy: How delivery routes, formulation, concentration and timing influence the success of phage therapy. *Journal of Pharmacy and Pharmacology.* 2011;63(10):1253–64.
34. Dalmasso M, Strain R, Neve H, Franz CMAP, Cousin FJ, Ross RP, et al. Three new Escherichia coli phages from the human gut show promising potential for phage therapy. *PLoS One.* 2016;11(6):e0156773.
35. Zameer F, Rukmangada MS, Chauhan JB, Khanum SA, Kumar P, Devi AT, et al. Evaluation of adhesive and anti-adhesive properties of Pseudomonas aeruginosa biofilms and their inhibition by herbal plants. *Iran J Microbiol.* 2016;8(2):108–119.
36. Zhang G, Zhao Y, Paramasivan S, Richter K, Morales S, Wormald PJ, et al. Bacteriophage effectively kills multidrug resistant Staphylococcus aureus clinical isolates from chronic rhinosinusitis patients. *Int Forum Allergy Rhinol.* 2018;8(3):406–414.
37. Santos SB, Carvalho CM, Sillankorva S, Nicolau A, Ferreira EC, Azeredo J. The use of antibiotics to improve phage detection and enumeration by the double-layer agar technique. *BMC Microbiol.* 2009;9:148.
38. Oliveira A, Ribeiro HG, Silva AC, Silva MD, Sousa JC, Rodrigues CF, et al. Synergistic antimicrobial interaction between honey and phage against Escherichia coli biofilms. *Front Microbiol.* 2017;8:2407.
39. Zhvania P, Hoyle NS, Nadareishvili L, Nizharadze D, Kutateladze M. Phage therapy in a 16-year-old boy with Netherton Syndrome. *Front Med (Lausanne).* 2017;4:94.
40. Kumari S, Harjai K, Chhibber S. Isolation and characterization of Klebsiella pneumoniae specific bacteriophages from sewage samples. *Folia Microbiol (Praha).* 2010;55(3):221–7.
41. Sanmukh SG, Khairnar K, Khairnar S, Narayan Paunikar W. Novel applications of bacterial and algal viruses in advancement of molecular biology and for enhancement of bio-fuel production. In *Emerging Technologies of the 21st Century* (pp. 199–212). New India Publishing Agency, New Delhi.
42. Kwiatek M, Mizak L, Parasion S, Gryko R, Olender A, Niemcewicz M. Characterization of five newly isolated bacteriophages active against Pseudomonas aeruginosa clinical strains. *Folia Microbiol (Praha).* 2015.
43. Freeman DJ, Falkiner FR, Keane CT. New method for detecting slime production by coagulase negative staphylococci. *Journal of Clinical Pathology.* 1989;42(8):872–874.
44. Maganha de Almeida Kumlien AC, Borrego CM, Balcázar JL. Antimicrobial resistance and bacteriophages: An overlooked intersection in water disinfection. *Trends Microbiol* [Internet]. 2021;29(6):517–27. Available from: https://doi.org/10.1016/j.tim.2020.12.011
45. Gandham P. Bacteriophages: Their use in the treatment of infections in the future. *Int J Curr Microbiol Appl Sci* [Internet]. 2015;4(2):867–79. Available from: http://www.ijcmas.com/vol-4-2/Pavani Gandham.pdf
46. Ackermann HW. Frequency of morphological phage descriptions in the year 2000. *Arch Virol.* 2001;146(5):843–57.

47. Dias RS, Eller MR, Duarte VS, Pereira ÂL, Silva CC, Mantovani HC, Oliveira LL, Silva EDAM, De Paula SO. Use of phages against antibiotic-resistant Staphylococcus aureus isolated from bovine mastitis. *J Anim Sci*. 2013;91:3930–3939.

48. Roja P, Degati R, Lakshmi V, Vijaya D, Prasad R. Lytic bacteriophages and phage cocktails seems to be a future alternatives against multi-drug resistant bacterial infections. 2019;(June). Available from: www.preprints.org

49. Roja RP, Vijaya LD, Narala VRR, Vijaya RPD. Isolation and characterization of a lytic bacteriophage (VB_PAnP_PADP4) against MDR- Pseudomonas aeruginosa isolated from septic wound infections. *Afr J Biotechnol*. 2019;18(15):325–33.

50. Pallavali RR, Degati VL, Lomada D, Reddy MC, Durbaka VRP. Isolation and in vitro evaluation of bacteriophages against MDR-bacterial isolates from septic wound infections. Das G, editor. *PLoS One* [Internet]. 2017 Jul 18 [cited 2022 Mar 24];12(7):e0179245. Available from: https://dx.plos.org/10.1371/journal.pone.0179245

51. Abedon ST. Phage-antibiotic combination treatments: Antagonistic impacts of antibiotics on the pharmacodynamics of phage therapy? *Antibiotics*. 2019;8(4):182.

52. Chanishvili N. Phage therapy-history from Twort and d'Herelle through soviet experience to current approaches. Vol. 83, *Advances in Virus Research*. 2012:3–40.

53. Abedon ST, Danis-Wlodarczyk KM, Alves DR. Phage therapy in the 21st century: Is there modern, clinical evidence of phage-mediated efficacy? *Pharmaceuticals*. 2021;14(11):1157.

54. Essa N, Rossitto M, Fiscarelli EV. Phages and phage therapy: Past, present and future. *Microbiologia Medica*. 2020;35(1).

55. Nilsson AS. Phage therapy-constraints and possibilities. *Ups J Med Sci*. 2014;119(2):192–8.

5 Biofilm-Associated Drug Resistance and Progress of Antibiofilm Therapy Strategies by Perspective Microcrystals and Nanocrystals

*J. Ramkumar, K. SenthilKannan,
N. Balamurugapandian, K.S. Radha, and R. Divya*

5.1 INTRODUCTION

The assortment and occurrence of transmittable ailments have increased year over year in exemplary elevation over the past nearly three decades. However, advancements in the medical field and medicinal/pharma sectors considerably reduced fatalities (Smith et al. 2014). Many scientists and technocrats are researching and focusing on studies on recognizing the complicated perseverance and extent of contagious illness (Jones et al. 2008) to find an apparent approach to the phenomenon. The cause is mainly by the bacteria and fungi that stick onto the exteriors forming multifarious biofilms (BFs) that defend from impending destructive or traumatic surroundings (Aparna and Yadav 2008). BFs are complicated structure configurations that are repeatedly correlated using the materialization of an assortment of confronts such as leveled genetic material transport, antimicrobial resistance, and persistent or frequent diseases. They consist of a diverse neighborhood of microorganisms to facilitate permanently sticking to abiotic otherwise biotic faces throughout the assembly of additional polymer specimens (Sadekuzzaman et al. 2015). Cell features of bacteria and fungi that were properly entrenched and enclosed by a bi-film have been experiential to be ten- to thousand-fold supplementary resistant to healing using antimicrobial sequencing (Davies 2003) than the counteract partners. The fundamentally multifarious antimicrobes confrontation exhibited by BFs and the inadequate overabundance of novel antimicrobial medicines (Pierce et al. 2015) point toward the necessity for substituting curatives that may perhaps fight contagions coupled using

DOI: 10.1201/9781003297826-5

biofilms. Date and sequence coupled with BFs displayed that their concerto and systems were necessary for forming the defense displayed by the essential microorganisms (Dos Santos Ramos et al. 2018). Numerous efforts by researchers have used microtechnology and nanotechnology to fight biofilms. Microtechnology and nanotechnology display exclusive features, for instance, medicine transporters and potential anti-BF contenders. This chapter's discussion is related to the expected standards essentially and clinically vital to microbial BF construction through extraordinary prominence on fungi BFs and BF and anti-BF stratagems.

5.2 BF AND ITS RESISTIVE FUNCTION

Biofilm progress is a convoluted procedure to facilitate numerous chronological levels. Bacteria and yeast contribute to comparable biofilm configuration procedures, while filamentous fungi necessitate many further levels, including the construction of established filaments and terminal biofilm morphological status to ascertain BFs (Costa-Orlandi et al. 2017). In general, biofilm configuration engages the connectivity of cells, pursued by the configuration of the microcolony, maturation, and dispersion. The preliminary accessory to exteriors is reversing nature as those cells were tranquil and prone toward healing by antibiotics. BFs were inherent, lively configurations to add to the expansion of the resistive process in microorganisms and participate as a functional part in the materialization of AMR (Yin et al. 2019). Microorganisms extend AMR as an advancement reaction toward staying alive in intimidating surroundings (Briones et al. 2008). Biofilm correlated to the effect of resistance is needed on numerous supplementary aspects, including physiological stipulation, the density of cells, quorum sensing (QS), extracellular matrixes, and forbearance.

5.3 BFS IN HEALTHCARE

According to the Centers for Disease Control (CDC 2020), 1 in 30 patients get a healthcare-related infection on any day. Roughly 60%–70% of healthcare is ascribed to biofilm configuration on medical appliances (Bryers 2008; Francolini and Donelli 2010). The permanent presence of devices is the ultimate exterior for biofilm arrangement as fewer microorganisms are necessary for migration to human tissues (Zimmerli et al. 2004; Vergidis and Patel 2012; Nowakowska et al. 2014; Khatoon et al. 2018). *E. faecium*, *S. aureus*, *K. pneumoniae*, *A. baumannii*, *P. aeruginosa*, and *Enterobacter* species (EF-SA-KP-AB-PA-EB) are several familiar drug-resistant bacteria allied with healthcare (Santajit et al. 2016). In the interim, *Candida* spp. is the main familiar fungi variety examined (Percival et al. 2015), with rising cases originating from non-*Candida albicans* types (Deorukhkar et al. 2014; Khan et al. 2017). BF-connected infectivities were not only intricate to spot and care for but could also enhance transience paces while dropping the effectiveness of medicinal applications. The current methodologies to attend to BF-correlated healthcare accentuate the consequence of avoiding diseases throughout life through techniques and restrict the customs except obligatory or erratically (Römling and Balsalobre 2012; Septimus and Moody 2014). Modern approaches investigate the prospect of incorporating the antimicrobial and permanent presence of medicinal appliances in the course of covering or impregnation next to regular injury-covering procedures to avoid the development of BF on those exteriors (Septimus and Moody 2014; Percival 2017; Baillie and Douglas 1998). This new modus operandi to avoid or take care of BF shows potential as it could decrease the occurrence and the pace of contagions coupled with means of permanent medicinal stratagems, eventually dropping the death rate.

5.4 CHARACTERISTICS OF BFS

The features and concerto of BF have a circumlocutory effect on the receptiveness en route for antimicrobials.

5.4.1 PHYSIOLOGICAL CONDITION AND EXTRACELLULAR MATRIX

The physiological affirmative of microorganisms surrounded by BF can be subjective by ecological features, which could influence their requirements and supply to AMR (Dumitru et al. 2004; Walters et al. 2003; Ramage et al. 2012; Scorzoni et al. 2017). The extracellular matrix is a significant feature of BF that shields from aggressive surroundings, for instance, antimicrobes mediators and host-resistant arrangement (Taraszkiewicz et al. 2012). It serves as the standard mechanical and elucidates the structural constancy, avoids the attack of antimicrobial mediators, and aids in the association of nutrients and energy in BF (Ross et al. 1991; Cramton et al. 1999; Steinberg et al. 2015; Al-Fattani and Douglas 2006).

5.5 FACTORS CAUSATIVE TO DRUG RESISTANCE

BF interconnected resistance relies on numerous aspects together with cell density, quorum sensing, and overexpression of targeted drugs.

5.5.1 CELL DENSITY AND QUORUM SENSING

Fungi BFs are compactly colonized with yeasts, hyphae, and pseudo-hyphae set in a systematic array for significant purposes such as nutrition perfusions, waste eviction, and water controls (Dominguez et al. 2019; Silva et al. 2009; Martinez and Casadevall 2007; Beauvais et al. 2007; Ramage et al. 2011; Rajendran et al. 2013; Martins et al. 2009; Raghupathi et al. 2018; Perumal et al. 2007; Kirby et al. 2012). Cell density is illustrated as an imperative aspect formerly surveyed, as BF of *C. albicans* had abridged receptiveness enrooted for azole-type drugs. In contrast, cell densities were improved from one thousand to one lakh thousand cells/mL (Kirby et al. 2012; Dong et al. 2001). QS is distinctively portrayed as the capability of microorganisms to correspond and harmonize the actions throughout the discharge of signal particles branded as QS molecules or QS particles in a populace-reliant approach (Turan et al. 2017; Albuquerque and Casadevall 2012; Papenfort and Bassler 2016; Sturme et al. 2002; Deep et al. 2011; Pereira et al. 2013; Cao et al. 2005; Dou et al. 2017; Li et al. 2018).

5.5.2 Presence of Persister Cells

Persister cells are the inactive cells contained by BF to proficiently bear antifungal mediators and source recurring diseases. Persister cells are established in the mutual planktonic type of cells and BF in bacterial cases, while they have only been experiential in BF for fungi classes. There were phenotypic variations of the undomesticated type matching parts through indistinguishable inherent summary as an antimicrobial predisposed cell (Scorzoni et al. 2017; Taraszkiewicz et al. 2012; LaFleur et al. 2006) and, thus, short of an inherited resistive system. The persister cell pattern is self-regulating of BF configuration, as it was formerly perceived in a reliable altitude still in altered twists to identify imperfection in BF creation (Miyaue et al. 2018). A topical revision on *E. coli* has been signified to facilitate persister cells that might display a long upholding outcome after being concealed from BF (Al-Dhaheri et al. 2010). The incidence of persister cells is simply experiential when microbicidal mediators were utilized and effectively accounted for, decreasing the propensity to antimicrobial negotiators and enhancing endurance. By conversing effect, AMR signifies with the purpose of cells so as to staying alive of antifungal were not resistant (Miyaue et al. 2018; Al-Dhaheri et al. 2010; Bink et al. 2011; Wuyts et al. 2018; Vincent et al. 2013; Cohen et al. 2013). The specific classification at the back of these phenotypes is uncertain; conversely, using fungus-conjectured reaction leads to progression and resistance (Delarze et al. 2015).

5.5.3 Antimicrobial Tolerance and Substitute Rehabilitation for BF Alleviation

Antimicrobial forbearance is the capability of microorganisms to stay alive when exposed to a higher level of concentrated antibiotics that surpass the minimum inhibition level of concentration (Vincent et al. 2013; Cohen et al. 2013; Delarze et al. 2015; Brauner et al. 2016; Held et al. 2018), which might lead to healing malfunctioning. Several studies have interpreted that poor development situations also show the way to forbearance (Held et al. 2018; Lederberg et al. 1948; Caza et al. 2019; Akins et al. 2005; Liu et al. 2020; Uppuluri et al. 2008; Lin et al. 2018). Similarly, *E. coli* is appropriately secluded and carries on penicillin revelation in the nonexistence of an amino acid. Though antibiotics and antifungal medicines were the strongholds for taking care of microbe contagions, optional or allied remedial advanced methodologies were adopted for their efficiency in fighting BF-associated medicinal resistance. The subsequent segments portray the assortment of replacement counteractive/curative are being studied for justifying BF resistance (Li et al. 2015; Robbins et al. 2011; Donnelly et al. 2007).

5.5.4 Antimicrobial Photodynamic Therapy (APDT) and Antimicrobial Lock Therapy (ALT)

Antimicrobial photodynamic therapy (APDT) exchange, also known as photodynamic initiation or photodynamic antimicrobial chemotherapy, is an alternative treatment strategy for biofilm infections confined to small areas. Nontoxic photosensitizer, molecular oxygen, and visible light work synergistically to create APDT (De Melo et al. 2013; Rosa et al. 2014; Walraven et al. 2012). Antimicrobial lock therapy (ALT) is a complementary healing employed to cure contagions caused by BF connected to medical devices. The idea behind ALT is that injecting antimicrobials that were 100 to 1000 times more potent than the planktonic types into an intravascular catheter lumen will cause it to remain "locked" for a predetermined period and result in the uninterrupted discharge of antimicrobials (Justo et al. 2014; Schinabeck et al. 2004). The results of several clinical studies show that ALT is a successful way to get rid of microbial infections without having to take out catheters. Additionally, it was agreed that ALT showed superior therapeutic results when combined with already effective antimicrobials (Schinabeck et al. 2004; Lazzell et al. 2009; Ghannoum et al. 2011; Delattin et al. 2016).

5.5.5 Antimicrobial Peptides (AMPs)

Short (less than a hundred amino acids), positively charged, and amphiphilic peptides known as antimicrobial peptides (AMPs) can interact with biological membranes. The wide range of characteristics exhibited by AMPs includes anti-BF, anticancer, antimicrobial, and immunomodulatory characteristics. Peptide, a synthetic short cationic AMP with about nine types of amino acids, showed anti-BF outcomes and properly kept pace with BF-related genetic specimens (Galdiero et al. 2019; Raheem et al. 2019; De La Fuente-Núñez et al. 2012; Martinez et al. 2006; Ruiz-Ruigomez et al. 2016).

5.5.6 Electrical Methods and Antimicrobial Coatings

Direct current (DC) application is a potential anti-BF therapeutic used in electrical methods to lessen or stop the growth of BF. Upon attraction or repulsion, BF begins to form. The application of DC will increase the electrostatical forces that repel microorganisms, interrupt their adhesion, and change the pH and temperature of the environment to further prevent the formation of BF. Antimicrobial coatings offer a promising alternative to electrical methods for treating infections caused by BF. Anti-BF layers were applied to medical devices with BF formations to stop microorganisms from adhering to surfaces. De Prijck et al. (2010) found that polydimethylsiloxane (PDMS) materials with immobilized quaternized polyDMAEMA (dimethyl aminoethyl methacrylate) and polyethyleneimine prevented the growth of *C. albicans* BF (Nowakowska et al. 2014; Boda et al. 2016; Sandvik et al. 2013; Zander and Becker 2018; Carlson et al. 2008; CDC 2021).

5.6 NANOTECHNOLOGY AND MICROTECHNOLOGY IN THE PREVENTION OF MICROBIAL RESISTANCE; NANOTECHNOLOGY AND ITS METHODS FOR REDUCING BIOFILMS

With more reports of multidrug resistance in various microorganisms, the emergence of new resistance mechanisms is steadily increasing. According to the CDC, 35,000 of the nearly 2,8 million cases of antibiotic-resistant contagions that happen each year in the U.S. alone result in death. There were insufficient alternative thera-peutics to treat infections brought on by these microorganisms due to the restricted availability. The platforms for reducing biofilm-associated resistance based on microtechnology and nanotechnology were depicted in supplementary details in the subsequent segments. Surface charges and solubility, two distinctive nanomaterial physiochemical characteristics, help regulate biodistribution and aid in intracellular uptake and clearance (Eleraky et al. 2020; Armstead and Li 2011; Kuan et al. 2012; Paul and Sharma 2010; Martin-Serrano et al. 2019; Yadav and Raizaday 2016; Keane et al. 2013; Davey 2008). Their tiny size plays a vital part in many applications.

5.6.1 Types of Nanomaterials

Organic and inorganic nanomaterials are distinguished by their composition and physical characteristics. Biocompatible, hydrophilic, nontoxic, and more stable than organic materials were inorganic nanomaterials like gold or magnetic nanoparticles. However, organic nanomaterials with high levels of biocompatibility and biode-gradability, like polymeric nanoparticles and liposomes, were the best choices for clinically specified relevance. Both types of nanomaterials have recompense and drawbacks, but if used properly, both can be advantageous. The primary categories of novel nanomaterials with anti-BF properties were depicted (Eleraky et al. 2020; Armstead and Li 2011; Kuan et al. 2012; Paul and Sharma 2010; Martin-Serrano et al. 2019; Yadav and Raizaday 2016; Keane et al. 2013; Davey 2008).

5.6.1.1 Quantum Dots (QDs)

In honor of the "quantum confinement" effect, quantum dots (QDs) were lumines-cent colloidal semiconductor crystals that range in size from 2 to 20 nm and in some cases 2 to 10 nm. They display unique, tunable broad absorption properties with narrow, continuous, and size-dependent emission spectra (Eleraky et al. 2020; Armstead and Li 2011; Kuan et al. 2012; Paul and Sharma 2010; Martin-Serrano et al. 2019; Yadav and Raizaday 2016; Keane et al. 2013; Davey 2008). Due to quantum size effects, QDs can concurrently emanate distinct colors of different wavelengths when exposed to extensive uninterrupted excitation.[101] According to reports, QDs emit nearly a hundred times brighter light than the majority of organic dyes or pro-teins. They have intermittently been used as substitutes for conventional luminous pigments or indicators because they were highly stable against photobleaching.[103] They have been suggested as the perfect tool for several biomedical uses, including due to their capacity for surface functionalization and photoluminescence. Although recent studies have demonstrated the potential of QDs as an antibiofilm, they have also been used frequently for identifying and visualizing structures. These activities were linked to their combined capacity to produce, through contact inhibition, gra-phene oxide (GO) QDs covalently functionalized with polyvinylidene fluoride mem-brane stopped the growth of *E. coli* and the development of BF. According to recent research, QDs were a good candidate for various biomedical applications because of their distinctive properties. However, because of the expensive precursors and low reproducibility, QDs have yet to be widely used (Acharya et al. 2017; Morrow et al.

2010; Li et al. 2015; Zeng et al. 2016; Garcia et al. 2018; Garcia et al. 2020; Shaikh et al. 2019; Bhattacharya et al. 2016). Most of the studies were still in the in vitro phase, demonstrating the necessity for in vivo case studies to ascertain whether the results were comparable.

5.6.1.2   Nanoparticles Made of Carbon: Nanodiamonds and Dendrimers

The attractive properties of carbon nanomaterials like carbon nanotubes (CNTs) are used for clinically persuading uses like drug deliverance, drug and organism imaging, and analysis. They demonstrated each carbon family member's particular electrical, optical, and mechanical characteristics. Nanodiamonds (NDs) were a typical class of nanoparticles of carbon using a curtailed octahedral class of structural design to facilitate the measurement among 1 to 4 nm in radius. They have consisted of an extremely structured diamond interior encircled by a cover of sets to provide the steadiness of the particles. They were a capable drug deliverance medium for an extensive variety of healings appropriate to the physical as well as the chemical characterizations and inferences, for instance, the diminutive size of the particles, transparency, high biocompatible nature, photoluminescence, and lucrative type of synthesis. In comparison to quantum dots, NDs were measured as the uncontaminated substitute for imaging intentions. NDs demonstrate exterior studies pertaining to the zone properties and nontoxicity temperament to progress the efficacy of their deliverance attributes, for illustration, the intracellular discharge of the materials, which separates them from supplementary carbon-type materials. They were extremely steady in acidic and chemical mediums such as the small appetite value of the pH put side by side with the metal as well as the metal oxide type of nanoparticles. Numerous types of research on NDs examined the prospective type of improved dental resins. Properly purposeful NDs were experiential to put forth action against the microbes and the characteristics comparable to the one reported by means of CNTs, which might enlarge the hydrophilic nature of the surfaces to avoid microorganisms from sticking onto these exteriors, therefore thwarting the BF pattern. Trithiomannoside clustering paired to NDs displays effective reticence of *E. coli* linkage to yeasts as well as the BF cells, with successive inhibition of BF creation and was accounted to be more than 90 times proficient to unpaired NDs, and the anti-BF action was augmented nearly 135 times measure up to their unpaired counteracting components. The actions of NDs included against polymethylmethacrylate (PMMA) nanocombinations have been accounted to display enhanced mechanoefficiency and resistance to fungi. In addition, the insertion of NDs was observed to boost the mechanobehavioral potency of composites such as dentistry resin to facilitate them to withstand more laborious impacts. Dendrimers are small-sized, molecules of more valence typically of the order of nanometer scale, with divisional nonlinear structures. They were the ultimate carriers for biomedicinal relevances, as their dendrite level of structural design was able to manipulate to outfit the intention. The toxic property linked using dendrimers was endorsed to the elevated cationic accusations on their margin, which may show the way to membrane disruption. Proposals to reduce the toxic property comprise choosing the proper level of neutralist or type of anionic dendrimers that were of biocompatibility by the chemically modified ones. The dendrimers showed anti-BF and antimicrobial action in opposition to cells of the BF (Zhang et al. 2009; Chen et al. 2016; Chang et al. 2008; Szunerit et al. 2016; Khanal et al. 2015; Cao et al. 2018; Mangal et al. 2019; Nimesh et al. 2013; Tsai and Imae 2011; Johansson et al. 2008; Ge et al. 2017; Han et al. 2019; Gao et al. 2020; Lee et al. 2017).

5.6.2 MICROTECHNOLOGY AND BF

Microtechnology involves the operation, surveillance, and fabrication or assembling of structural parameters at the micrometer level of measurement. Microfluidics is an imperative division of microtechnology to expand the attention to the perceptiveness of BF. Microfluidics engage the operation and organize the small quantity of microfluidics in sectors or in the proper routes to the locale to the growing of BF. Earlier investigation pertaining to the utilization of microfluidics scheduled BF comprises the work on BF pattern and linkage and other usage and studies (Gao et al. 2020; Lee et al. 2017; Zhang et al. 2016; Lee et al. 2008; Bahar et al. 2010; Kim et al. 2010; Kim et al. 2015; Hong et al. 2012; Shumi et al. 2013; Molina et al. 2015). The microsensors, for instance, microelectrodes, are a special division of microtechnology used in BF. The microelectrodes were micrometer electrodes used to scrutinize alterations in the chemically and physiologically relevant restrictions in BF (Moya et al. 2014; Becerro et al. 2014; Hou et al. 2017; Lin et al. 2219; Waghule 2000; Singh et al. 2010; Khalid et al. 2020; Teughels et al. 2006; Sima et al. 2016; Xu et al. 2017).

5.6.2.1 Microparticles for Deliverance of Antimicrobials

Microparticles are the majority universal form of microtechnology used for drug deliverance. They were defined as particles with a radius of 1 to 1000 micrometers, not including the walling and central part structural elucidation or composition. They were appropriate applicants for treatment by medicinal deliverance as they were alleviated dynamic mediators and showed changeable drug-discharge outlines together with the proscribed discharge of medicines. Subordinate classes of microparticles include microspheres (microparticles shaped like spheres) and microcapsules (microparticles by way of special walls and core specimens). Microparticle medium specimens were collected of each with an inorganic or organic class of nature of the materials. The inorganic class of materials, for example, gold, was used for the distinctive assets including enhanced permanence and magnetic impactness. Supplementary work collected hybrid microparticles of a combination of inorganic and organic constituents persuaded for enhanced and enlarged work (Moya et al. 2014; Becerro et al. 2014; Hou et al. 2017; Lin et al. 2219; Waghule 2000; Singh et al. 2010; Khalid et al. 2020; Teughels et al. 2006; Sima et al. 2016; Xu et al. 2017).

5.6.2.2 New Microtechnology Mythological Way for Anti-BF Effectiveness and Coatings with Microparticles

The opportunity to integrate antimicrobes mediators amid microparticles, for instance, microspheres and microcapsules, to contest BFS has gained popularity. Numerous microtechnology methods through anti-BF portfolios comprise microrods, microswimmers, and microneedles. Additional topical techniques, for instance, microtextured and micropatterned exteriors, were studied for their capability to stop BF patterns throughout the peripheral geography (Moya et al. 2014; Becerro et al. 2014; Hou et al. 2017; Lin et al. 2219; Waghule 2000; Singh et al. 2010; Khalid et al. 2020; Teughels et al. 2006; Sima et al. 2016; Xu et al. 2017). The study of a number of these modus operandi was restricted because of the capable pronouncements from the accessible sequence tip en route for the opportunity of making use of these methodologies to contest BFs. Titanium is an embedded substance regularly employed to imitate embed exteriors. Authentication of the veneered type of class of substances capable of performing the chosen modus operandi with medium support pulsed laser type of evaporation/deposition, in turn, permits the authentication of polymer thin-film materials that were thermally and chemically sensitive (Moya et al. 2014; Becerro et al. 2014; Hou et al. 2017; Lin et al. 2019; Waghule 2000; Singh et al. 2010; Khalid et al. 2020; Teughels et al. 2006; Sima et al. 2016; Xu et al. 2017; Mair et al. 2017). Results demonstrate that covering titanium substances with antimicrobe composites for anti-BF activity is capable of managing embed-correlated contagions.

5.6.2.3 Microtexturing, Micropattern-Based Zones with Microrods, Microswimmers, and Microneedle Effectiveness

The microtexturing and micropatterning of the zones or surface-level impacts employ biological mimetic methodologies to construct anti-BF surfaces. Various relevances for these exteriors, the tubes and lobes and mechanisms were properly utilized to restrain bacteria connection, colonizing, and BF patterns without antimicrobes. Earlier discoveries illustrate competent outcomes of integrate microtexturing or micropatterning surface impacts for medicinal equipment-correlated contaminations. The micropatterning of surfaces exhibited a noteworthy decrease in bacteria colonizing and transmission through customary in vitro mechanisms. A more rapid way of in vivo examining confirmed an appreciably inferior bacteria burdening in models entrenched through micropatterned exteriors put side by side to the smooth level of surface control. Largely, the concluding section acquires an indicative track of the vicinity of micropatterning and microtextured exteriors and was continuous and capable of additional progress to advance the anti-BF action in surrounding areas. Magnetically rotating the microrods interrupted *A. fumigatus* BF and improved the antifungal action. Gold–iron–gold (Au–Fe–Au) microrods of about more than 1 µm long were used in iron-permissible magnetic rotations. The efficiency of the microrods was tested separately and in groups in opposition to *A. fumigatus* BF. No noteworthy decline was found in healing clusters in contrast to the managing except for the permutation exhibiting a 90%-plus eradicating rate. The microrods affected BF reliability in fungi hyphae at the same time as the eradication of the fungi cells throughout the magnetically rotated methodology. Appropriateness to the restricted characterization studies on microrods, and future studies to incorporate biocompatibility are needed (Mair et al. 2017; Johnson 2008; Petrova 2012).

5.6.3 BF Matrix Patterns and Organization of the BF

This phase shows that the planktonic cells turn out to be outstandingly further encrusted and methodical microcolonies with streaming watery controls build an irretrievable linkage. Colonizing, a characteristic of BFs, plays a crucial role in causing damage to the host. Once the cells were steadily remain to the pertinent face innumerable microbe's mound and attachment of microorganisms. After these coordinated levels, the microcolonies were produced. The extracellular polysaccharides created by the support forming a medium surrounded by the cells assemble their neighborhood and accomplish the utmost density of the cells. The extracellular polysaccharides summarizing the cells in a BF was an incorporation of components, together with extracellular DNA proteins, lipids, and polysaccharides. The polysaccharides in the medium make available vigor to the cells inside the BF, such as observance, protection, and structural stiffness (Sriramulu et al. 2005; Hooshdar et al. 2020; Flemming et al. 2010; Decho et al. 2017; Nishanth et al. 2021; Limoli et al. 2015; Karygianni et al. 2020; Asadi et al. 2019; Ghilini et al. 2019).

5.7 UTILITY OF PRESENT CASE

5.7.1 Anti-BF Representatives with Bacteria Exterior Connection Inhibition, Examination with Quorum Sensing

Quorum quenching is the process outlined with disruption caused by the bacterial commuting scheme. BF is an assembly of surface-associated microbial cells covered by a polymer matrix. Anti-BF is the process of obstructing and is on host surface impact. It was recognized that some of the *Pseudomonous* species and *Providencia* species are able to increase the pH of urinal constituents to the utmost assessment and are not capable of causing crystal authentication in BF. The main explicit mode is the dilution of urine and augmenting of citrates by way of pH >8. Catheter covering was inhibited and specified which bacteri is organizing the predicament. Bacterial attachment similar to flagella assists the attached ones to exteriors; consequently, reticence of the attachments can move to turn away linkage. Surface covering or amendment with mediators encompasses antibacterial studies and was an upcoming modus operandi to antagonize microbe linkage and propagation. Inhibition of bacterial linkage can be accomplished by surface veneer through biocide representatives or using explicit polymers including a capability toward inhibition of the cells. Microbial cell-level contact at the molecules facilitates the microorganisms to respond to neighboring transforms and was allowed by quorum sensing. QS was dependent on the obligatory of an autoinducer to an equivalent gene controlling, which triggers the consequent transcripts. The steps of formation are shown in Figures 5.1a and 5.1b and the elimination of BF in Figure 5.2 (Rodrigues et al. 2011; Pathak et al. 2018; Tuson et al. 2013; Fleitas Martínez et al. 2019; Reuter et al. 2016; Wu et al. 2021; Jiang et al. 2019; Fong et al. 2018; Khoshnood et al. 2020; Besharova et al. 2016).

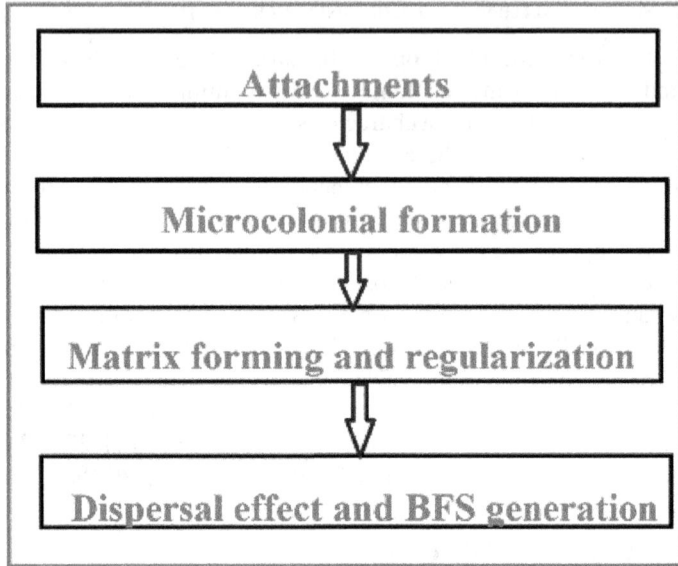

FIGURE 5.1 (a) Flowchart of BFS-forming mechanism.

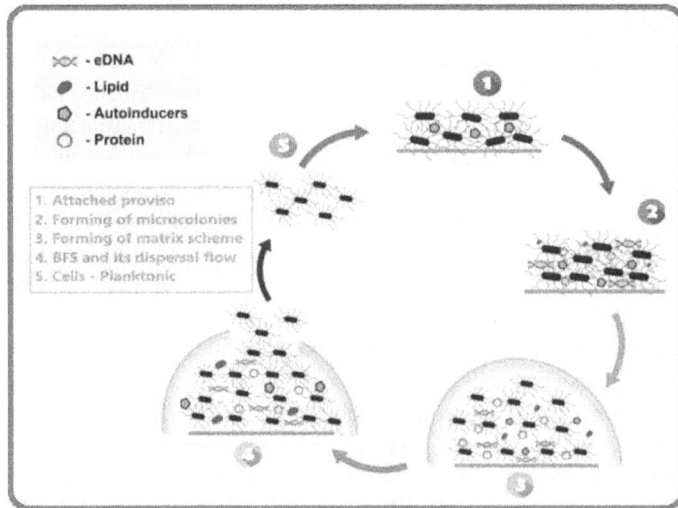

FIGURE 5.1 (b) Pictorial representation of BFS-forming mechanism.

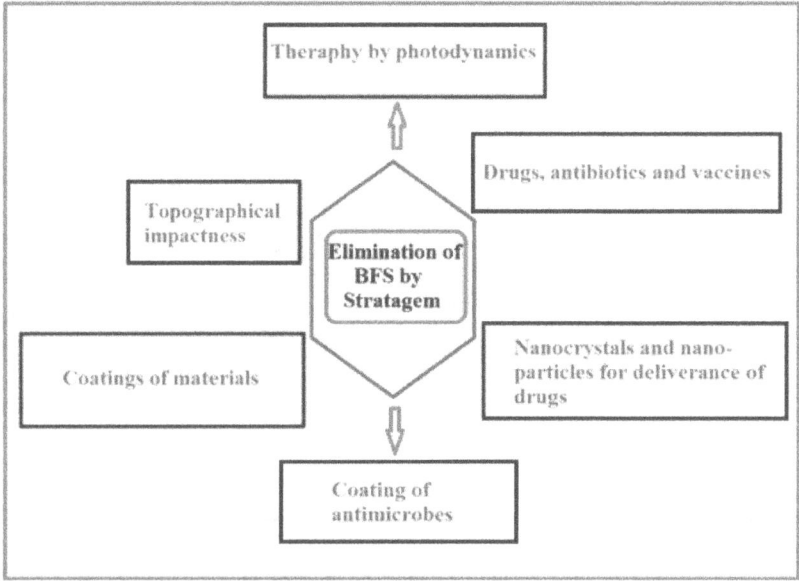

FIGURE 5.2   Elimination of BFS by stratagems.

5.7.2   INHIBITION BY BIODIVERSIFICATION AND BF DISTRIBUTION STIMULATORS

The genetics of biodiversification in bacteria show the way to materialization of a novelty level of subordinate populaces to attribute resistance to antibiotic treatment and ecological stressing sites. Horizontal gene transfer through pairing up takes part in a vital functionality in the expanded term of the resistance in a BF colony. The social evolution theory anticipates that inhibiting shared traits among the subpopulations could be a feasible way to exterminate BF. Organisms in subordinate populaces depend on a joint extracellular polysaccharide formulate and is a fascinating objective to contest genetically diversified proviso. BF distribution was commenced by the interruption of the extracellular polysaccharide medium to discharge the microcolonies. Anti-BF mediators that can encourage the progression of eliminating BF with stratagems for new-fangled BF dispersion stimulators are being investigated. The development of antibiotic resistance among species of bacteria is specified in Figure 5.3 (Blazanin and Turner 2021; Kaplan 2010; Guilhen et al. 2017; Wille and Coenye 2020; Boles and Horswill 2008; Stewart 2002; Mah et al. 2001; Fleitas Martínez et al. 2019; Cepas et al. 2019).

5.8   BACTERIAL RESISTANCE, UPCOMING ANTI-BF AGENTS, QUORUM-QUENCHING REPRESENTATIVES, AND ANTIMICROBIAL PEPTIDES

Antibiotics expected to withstand BF influxing must have the capability to target the cells entrenched inside. The majority of current antibiotics are unable to

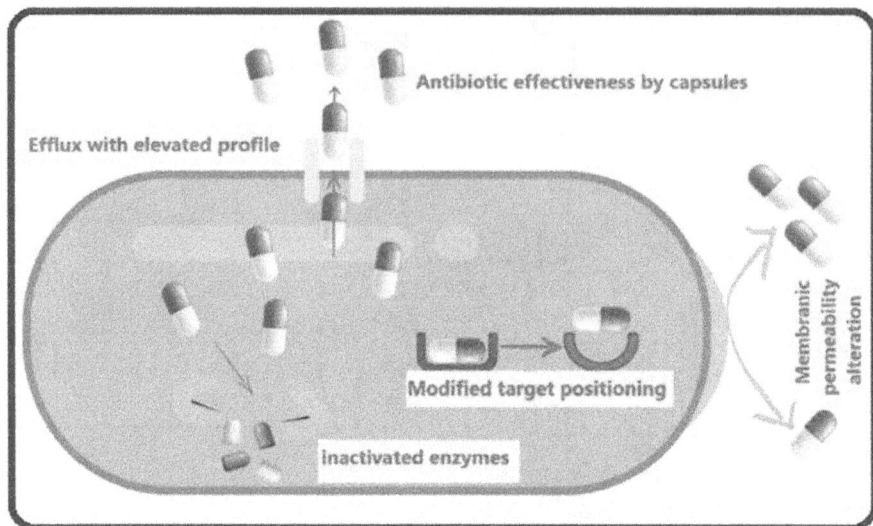

FIGURE 5.3 Development of antibiotic resistance among species of bacteria.

traverse the BF extracellular matrix appropriate to the peripheral amendment of the BF to decline influx. The methodology through which antibiotic resistance extends is a vital deterministic feature in the endurance of microbes of BFs. The microbes essentially experienced an elevated transformation to allow them to progress resistant methods to develop enzymes. The main functions were amending cell permeability to control the invasion of the antibiotics into the cells, changing the cellular intentions. Horizontal gene transfer, the movable nature of human being transporters resulted in the declaration of medicinal resistance over a large microbial subordinate allotment and microenvironment. BF can resist and endure inconsiderate ecological stipulations and overcome the host-resistant method, enabling the need for the investigation of innovative anti-BF mediators and confronters. Persister cells can converse surrounded by themselves to the severe effect and cause of the disease and the creation of resistance. Varied quorum quenching representatives were surveyed to assist in the healing. These studies denote the intention of the subsequent cohort of antimicrobes to restrain the BF-interrelated resistance exposed by contemporary antibiotics. This peptide demonstrates extraordinary abolition of preformed BF within 900 seconds (Ahmad et al. 2018; Tu et al. 2019; Shrout 2011; Abebe 2020; Davies 2023; Yan et al. 2020; Festa et al. 2021; SenthilKannan 2022).

5.9 SCOPE FOR FUTURE EFFECTIVENESS OF A CONTINUUM OF BFS AND ANTI-BF INTERIM RELATION

The nitrile groups ($-C{\equiv}N$) hydrolyze bacterial projection with proper growth as well as resisting the toxicity and bioimpacting. 2-Benzyl-amino-4-p-tolyl-6,7-di-hyd ro5H-cyclo-penta–[b]pyridine-3-carbonitrile (BAPTDHCPCN) of the micro- and nanoscale can be proceeded for BF entrusted proficient usage based on pyridine and nitriles in the specimen. As synthesized new molecular crystal of 2-amino-4-methylpyridinium fumarate (AMPF) (SenthilKannan 2022) of micro- and nanoscale can be of better use as the compound has pyridine clustering and the literature shows the scope for pyridine for anti-BF properties by using *Staphylococcus aureus* (gram-positive bacteria), *Escherichia coli* (gram-negative bacteria), *Candida albicans* (yeast), and *Aspergillus niger* (fungus).

5.10 CONCLUSIONS

A large amount of characterizations for microtechnology and nanotechnology in in vitro phases is prospective for the management as well as scheming and, perhaps, the abolition of bacterial and fungi-type BF. They demonstrate enhanced effectiveness and abridged contaminations using the slightest level of possibility to resistance in intensified microorganisms, principally when used in groups of antimicrobes. Additional results may necessitate ensuring the security of these deliverance arrangements so they be employed in healthcare. Nevertheless, the statistics from the results so designate that the operation of these microtechnology- and nanotechnology-based improvements will significantly progress the healing and supervision of BF-correlated diseases. The advancements in technology comprise alarming and potential anti-BF caches to contest AMR in future endeavors. The outcome acquired exposed two composites that could be engaged for future research of pharma modus operandi with BAPTDHCPCN and AMPF to prevail over evolved multidrug resistance performances by microscopic organisms.

REFERENCES

Abebe, G.M. The role of bacterial biofilm in antibiotic resistance and food contamination. *Int. J. Microbiol.* 2020, 2020, e1705814.

Acharya, G.; Mitra, A.K.; Cholkar, K. Nanosystems for diagnostic imaging, biodetectors, and biosensors. In *Emerging Nanotechnologies for Diagnostics, Drug Delivery and Medical Devices*, 1st ed.; Elsevier Inc.: Amsterdam, The Netherlands; Oxford; Cambridge, 2017; pp. 217.

Ahmad, I.; Nawaz, N.; Dermani, F.K.; Kohlan, A.K.; Saidijam, M.; Patching, S.G. Bacterial multidrug efflux proteins: A major mechanism of antimicrobial resistance. *Curr. Drug Targets* 2018, 19, 1.

Akins, R.A. An update on antifungal targets and mechanisms of resistance in Candida albicans. *Med. Mycol.* 2005, 43, 285.

Albuquerque, P.; Casadevall, A. Quorum sensing in fungi—A review. *Med. Mycol.* 2012, 50, 337.

Al-Dhaheri, R.S.; Douglas, L.J. Apoptosis in Candida biofilms exposed to Amphotericin B. *J. Med. Microbiol.* 2010, 59, 149.

Al-Fattani, M.A.; Douglas, L.J. Biofilm matrix of Candida albicans and Candida tropicalis: Chemical composition and role in drug resistance. *J. Med. Microbiol.* 2006, 55, 999.

Aparna, M.S.; Yadav, S. Biofilms: Microbes and disease. *Braz. J. Infect. Dis.* 2008, 12, 526.

Armstead, A.L.; Li, B. Nanomedicine as an emerging approach against intracellular pathogens. *Int. J. Nanomed.* 2011, 6, 3281.

Asadi, A.; Razavi, S.; Talebi, M.; Gholami, M. A review on anti-adhesion therapies of bacterial diseases. *Infection* 2019, 47, 13.

Bahar, O.; De La Fuente, L.; Burdman, S. Assessing adhesion, biofilm formation and motility of Acidovorax citrulli using microfluidic flow chambers. *FEMS Microbiol. Lett.* 2010, 312, 33.

Baillie, G.S.; Douglas, L.J. Iron-limited biofilms of Candida albicans and their susceptibility to Amphotericin B. *Antimicrob. Agents Chemother.* 1998, 42, 2146.

Beauvais, A.; Schmidt, C.; Guadagnini, S.; Roux, P.; Perret, E.; Henry, C.; Paris, S.; Mallet, A.; Prévost, M.-C.; Latgé, J.P. An extracellular matrix glues together the aerial-grown hyphae of Aspergillus fumigatus. *Cell. Microbiol.* 2007, 9, 1588.

Becerro, S.; Paredes, J.; Arana, S. Multiparametric biosensor for detection and monitoring of bacterial biofilm adhesion and growth. In Proceedings of the 6th European Conference of the International Federation for Medical and Biological Engineering, IFMBE Proceedings, Dubrovnik, Croatia, 7–11 September 2014; Springer: Cham, Switzerland; Volume 45, pp. 333.

Besharova, O.; Suchanek, V.M.; Hartmann, R.; Drescher, K.; Sourjik, V. Diversification of gene expression during formation of static submerged biofilms by Escherichia coli. *Front. Microbiol.* 2016, 7, 1568.

Bhattacharya, K.; Mukherjee, S.P.; Gallud, A.; Burkert, S.C.; Bistarelli, S.; Bellucci, S.; Bottini, M.; Star, A.; Fadeel, B. Biological interactions of carbon-based nanomaterials: From coronation to degradation. *Nanomed. Nanotechnol. Biol. Med.* 2016, 12, 333.

Bink, A.; VandenBosch, D.; Coenye, T.; Nelis, H.; Cammue, B.P.A.; Thevissen, K. Superoxide dismutases are involved in Candida albicans biofilm persistence against miconazole. *Antimicrob. Agents Chemother.* 2011, 55, 4033.

Blazanin, M.; Turner, P.E. Community context matters for bacteria-phage ecology and evolution. *ISME J.* 2021, 15, 3119.

Boda, S.K.; Bajpai, I.; Basu, B. Inhibitory effect of direct electric field and HA-ZnO composites on S. aureus biofilm formation. *J. Biomed. Mater. Res B Appl. Biomater.* 2016, 104, 1064.

Boles, B.R.; Horswill, A.R. agr-Mediated dispersal of Staphylococcus aureus biofilms. *PLoS Pathog.* 2008, 4, e1000052.

Brauner, A.; Fridman, O.; Gefen, O.; Balaban, N.Q. Distinguishing between resistance, tolerance and persistence to antibiotic treatment. *Nat. Rev. Genet* 2016, 14, 320.

Briones, E.; Colino, C.I.; Lanao, J.M. Delivery systems to increase the selectivity of antibiotics in phagocytic cells. *J. Control. Release* 2008, 125, 210.

Bryers, J.D. Medical biofilms. *Biotechnol. Bioeng.* 2008, 100, 1.

Cao, W.; Zhang, Y.; Wang, X.; Li, Q.; Xiao, Y.; Li, P.; Wang, L.; Ye, Z.; Xing, X. Novel resin-based dental material with anti-biofilm activity and improved mechanical property by incorporating hydrophilic cationic copolymer functionalized nanodiamond. *J. Mater. Sci. Mater. Med.* 2018, 29, 162.

Cao, Y.Y.; Cao, Y.-B.; Xu, Z.; Ying, K.; Li, Y.; Xie, Y.; Zhu, Z.-Y.; Chen, W.-S.; Jiang, Y.-Y. cDNA microarray analysis of differential gene expression in Candida albicans biofilm exposed to farnesol. *Antimicrob. Agents Chemother.* 2005, 49, 584.

Carlson, R.P.; Taffs, R.; Davison, W.M.; Stewart, P.S. Anti-biofilm properties of chitosan-coated surfaces. *J. Biomater. Sci. Polym. Ed.* 2008, 19, 1035.

Caza, M.; Kronstad, J.W. The cAMP/protein kinase A pathway regulates virulence and adaptation to host conditions in Cryptococcus neoformans. *Front. Cell. Infect. Microbiol.* 2019, 9, 212.

Centers for Disease Control (CDC). Healthcare-Associated Infections (HAI). 2020. Available online: https://www.cdc.gov/drugresistance/biggest-threats.html (accessed on 12 April 2020).

Centre for Disease Control and Prevention (CDC). Antibiotic/Antimicrobial resistance. 2020. Available online: https://www.cdc.gov/drugresistance/ biggest-threats.html (accessed on 13 February 2021).

Cepas, V.; López, Y.; Muñoz, E.; Rolo, D.; Ardanuy, C.; Martí, S.; Xercavins, M.; Horcajada, J.P.; Bosch, J.; Soto, S.M. Relationship between biofilm formation and antimicrobial resistance in Gram-negative bacteria. *Microb. Drug Resist.* 2019, 25, 72.

Chang, Y.-R.; Lee, H.-Y.; Chen, K.; Chang, C.-C.; Tsai, D.-S.; Fu, C.-C.; Lim, T.-S.; Tzeng, Y.-K.; Fang, C.-Y.; Han, C.-C.; et al. Mass production and dynamic imaging of fluorescent nanodiamonds. *Nat. Nanotechnol.* 2008, 3, 284.

Chen, M.; Pierstorff, E.D.; Lam, R.; Li, S.-Y.; Huang, H.; Osawa, E.; Ho, D. Nanodiamond-mediated delivery of water-insoluble therapeutics. *ACS Nano* 2009, 3, 2016.

Cohen, N.R.; Lobritz, M.A.; Collins, J.J. Microbial persistence and the road to drug resistance. *Cell Host Microbe.* 2013, 13, 632.

Costa-Orlandi, C.B.; Sardi, J.C.O.; Pitangui, N.S.; De Oliveira, H.C.; Scorzoni, L.; Galeane, M.C.; Medina-Alarcón, K.P.; Melo, W.C.M.A.; Marcelino, M.Y.; Braz, J.D.; et al. Fungal biofilms and polymicrobial diseases. *J. Fungi* 2017, 3, 22.

Cramton, S.E.; Gerke, C.; Schnell, N.F.; Nichols, W.W.; Götz, F. The intercellular adhesion (ica) locus is present in Staphylococcus aureus and is required for biofilm formation. *Infect. Immun.* 1999, 67, 5427.

Davey, M.E. Tracking dynamic interactions during plaque formation. *J. Bacteriol.* 2008, 190, 7869.

Davies, D. Understanding biofilm resistance to antibacterial agents. *Nat. Rev. Drug Discov.* 2003, 2, 114.

De La Fuente-Núñez, C.; Korolik, V.; Bains, M.; Nguyen, U.; Breidenstein, E.B.M.; Horsman, S.; Lewenza, S.; Burrows, L.; Hancock, R.E.W. Inhibition of bacterial biofilm formation and swarming motility by a small synthetic cationic peptide. *Antimicrob. Agents Chemother.* 2012, 56, 2696.

De Melo, W.C.M.A.; Avci, P.; de Oliveira, M.N.; Gupta, A.; Vecchio, D.; Sadasivam, M.; Chandran, R.; Huang, Y.-Y.; Yin, R.; Perussi, L.R.; et al. Photodynamic inactivation of biofilm: Taking a lightly colored approach to stubborn infection. *Expert. Rev. Anti Infect. Ther.* 2013, 11, 669.

De Prijck, K.; De Smet, N.; Rymarczyk-Machal, M.; Van Driessche, G.; Devreese, B.; Coenye, T.; Schacht, E.; Nelis, H.J. Candida albicans biofilm formation on peptide functionalized polydimethylsiloxane. *Biofouling* 2010, 26, 269.

Decho, A.W.; Gutierrez, T. Microbial extracellular polymeric substances (EPSs) in ocean systems. *Front. Microbiol.* 2017, 26, 922.

Deep, A.; Chaudhary, U.; Gupta, V. Quorum sensing and bacterial pathogenicity: From molecules to disease. *J. Lab. Physicians* 2011, 3, 4.

Delarze, E.; Sanglard, D. Defining the frontiers between antifungal resistance, tolerance and the concept of persistence. *Drug Resist. Updat.* 2015, 23, 12.

Delattin, N.; De Brucker, K.; De Cremer, K.; Cammue, B.P.; Thevissen, K. Antimicrobial peptides as a strategy to combat fungal biofilms. *Curr. Top. Med. Chem.* 2016, 17, 604.

Deorukhkar, S.C.; Saini, S.; Mathew, S. Non-albicans Candida infection: An emerging threat. *Interdiscip. Perspect. Infect. Dis.* 2014, 2014, 615958.

Dominguez, E.G.; Zarnowski, R.; Choy, H.L.; Zhao, M.; Sanchez, H.; Nett, J.E.; Andes, D.R. Conserved role for biofilm matrix polysaccharides in Candida auris drug resistance. *mSphere* 2019, 4, e00680–18.

Dong, Y.-H.; Wang, L.-H.; Xu, J.-L.; Zhang, H.-B.; Zhang, X.-F.; Zhang, L.-H. Quenching quorum-sensing-dependent bacterial infection by an N-acyl homoserine lactonase. *Nat. Cell Biol.* 2001, 411, 813.

Donnelly, R.F.; McCarron, P.A.; Tunney, M.M.; Woolfson, A.D. Potential of photodynamic therapy in treatment of fungal infections of the mouth. Design and characterisation of a mucoadhesive patch containing toluidine blue O. *J. Photochem. Photobiol. B Biol.* 2007, 86, 59.

Dos Santos Ramos, M.A.; Da Silva, P.B.; Spósito, L.; De Toledo, L.G.; Bonifácio, B.V.; Rodero, C.F.; Dos Santos, K.C.; Chorilli, M.; Bauab, T.M. Nanotechnology-based drug delivery systems for control of microbial biofilms: A review. *Int. J. Nanomed.* 2018, 13, 1179.

Dou, Y.; Song, F.; Guo, F.; Zhou, Z.; Zhu, C.; Xiang, J.; Huan, J. Acinetobacter baumanii quorum-sensing signalling molecule induces the expression of drug-resistance genes. *Mol. Med. Rep.* 2017, 15, 4061.

Dumitru, R.; Hornby, J.M.; Nickerson, K.W. Defined anaerobic growth medium for studying Candida albicans basic biology and resistance to eight antifungal drugs. *Antimicrob. Agents Chemother.* 2004, 48, 2350.

Eleraky, N.E.; Allam, A.; Hassan, S.B.; Omar, M.M. Nanomedicine fight against antibacterial resistance: An overview of the recent pharmaceutical innovations. *Pharmaceutics* 2020, 12, 142.

Festa, R.; Ambrosio, R.L.; Lamas, A.; Gratino, L.; Palmieri, G.; Franco, C.M.; Cepeda, A.; Anastasio, A. A study on the antimicrobial and antibiofilm peptide 1018-K6 as potential alternative to antibiotics against food-pathogen Salmonella enterica. *Foods* 2021, 10, 1372.

Fleitas Martínez, O.; Cardoso, M.H.; Ribeiro, S.M.; Franco, O.L. Recent advances in anti-virulence therapeutic strategies with a focus on dismantling bacterial membrane microdomains, toxin neutralization, quorum-sensing interference and biofilm inhibition. *Front. Cell. Infect. Microbiol.* 2019, 9, 74.

Fleitas Martínez, O.; Rigueiras, P.O.; Pires, Á.D.S.; Porto, W.F.; Silva, O.N.; de la Fuente-Nunez, C.; Franco, O.L. Interference with quorum-sensing signal biosynthesis as a promising therapeutic strategy against multidrug-resistant pathogens. *Front. Cell Infect. Microbiol.* 2019, 8, 444.

Flemming, H.C.; Wingender, J. The biofilm matrix. *Nat. Rev. Microbiol.* 2010, 8, 623.

Fong, J.; Zhang, C.; Yang, R.; Boo, Z.Z.; Tan, S.K.; Nielsen, T.E.; Givskov, M.; Liu, X.W.; Bin, W.; Su, H.; et al. Combination therapy strategy of quorum quenching enzyme and quorum sensing inhibitor in suppressing multiple quorum sensing pathways of P. aeruginosa. *Sci. Rep.* 2018, 8, 1155.

Francolini, I.; Donelli, G. Prevention and control of biofilm-based medical-device-related infections. *FEMS Immunol. Med. Microbiol.* 2010, 59, 227.

Galdiero, E.; Lombardi, L.; Falanga, A.; Libralato, G.; Guida, M.; Carotenuto, R. Biofilms: Novel strategies based on antimicrobial peptides. *Pharmaceutics* 2019, 11, 322.

Gao, Y.; Wang, J.; Chai, M.; Li, X.; Deng, Y.; Jin, Q.; Ji, J. Size and charge adaptive clustered nanoparticles targeting the biofilm microenvironment for chronic lung infection management. *ACS Nano* 2020, 14, 5686.

Garcia, I.M.; Leitune, V.C.B.; Visioli, F.; Samuel, S.M.W.; Collares, F.M. Influence of zinc oxide quantum dots in the antibacterial activity and cytotoxicity of an experimental adhesive resin. *J. Dent.* 2018, 73, 57.

Garcia, I.M.; Souza, V.S.; Scholten, J.D.; Collares, F.M. Quantum dots of tantalum oxide with an imidazolium ionic liquid as antibacterial agent for adhesive resin. *J. Adhes. Dent.* 2020, 22, 207.

Ge, Y.; Ren, B.; Zhou, X.; Xu, H.H.K.; Wang, S.; Li, M.; Weir, M.D.; Feng, M.; Cheng, L. Novel dental adhesive with biofilm-regulating and remineralization capabilities. *Materials* 2017, 10, 26.

Ghannoum, M.A.; Isham, N.; Jacobs, M.R. Antimicrobial activity of B-lock against bacterial and Candida spp. causing catheter-related bloodstream infections. *Antimicrob. Agents Chemother.* 2011, 55, 4430.

Ghilini, F.; Pissinis, D.E.; Miñán, A.; Schilardi, P.L.; Diaz, C. How functionalized surfaces can inhibit bacterial adhesion and viability. *ACS Biomater. Sci. Eng.* 2019, 5, 4920.

Guilhen, C.; Forestier, C.; Balestrino, D. Biofilm dispersal: Multiple elaborate strategies for dissemination of bacteria with unique properties. *Mol. Microbiol.* 2017, 105, 188.

Han, X.; Liu, Y.; Ma, Y.; Zhang, M.; He, Z.; Siriwardena, T.N.; Xu, H.; Bai, Y.; Zhang, X.; Reymond, J.-L.; et al. Peptide dendrimers G3KL and TNS18 inhibit Pseudomonas aeruginosa biofilms. *Appl. Microbiol. Biotechnol.* 2019, 103, 5821.

Held, K.; Gasper, J.; Morgan, S.; Siehnel, R.; Singh, P.; Manoil, C. Determinants of extreme β-lactam tolerance in the Burkholderia pseudomallei complex. *Antimicrob. Agents Chemother.* 2018, 62, e00068–18.

Hong, S.H.; Hegde, M.; Kim, J.; Wang, X.; Jayaraman, A.; Wood, T.K. Synthetic quorum-sensing circuit to control consortial biofilm formation and dispersal in a microfluidic device. *Nat. Commun.* 2012, 3, 613.

Hooshdar, P.; Kermanshahi, R.K.; Ghadam, P.; Darani, K.K. A review on production of exopolysaccharide and biofilm in probiotics like Lactobacilli and methods of analysis. *Biointerface Res. Appl. Chem.* 2020, 10, 6058.

Hou, J.; Liu, Z.; Zhou, Y.; Chen, W.; Li, Y.; Sang, L. An experimental study of pH distributions within an electricity-producing biofilm by using pH microelectrode. *Electrochim. Acta* 2017, 251, 187.

Jiang, Q.; Chen, J.; Yang, C.; Yin, Y.; Yao, K. Quorum sensing: A prospective therapeutic target for bacterial diseases. *BioMed Res. Int.* 2019, 2015978.

Johansson, E.M.V.; Crusz, S.A.; Kolomiets, E.; Buts, L.; Kadam, R.U.; Cacciarini, M.; Bartels, K.-M.; Diggle, S.P.; Camara, M.; Williams, P.; et al. Inhibition and dispersion of Pseudomonas aeruginosa biofilms by glycopeptide dendrimers targeting the fucose-specific lectin LecB. *Chem. Biol.* 2008, 15, 1249.

Johnson, L.R. Microcolony and biofilm formation as a survival strategy for bacteria. *J. Theor. Biol.* 2008, 251, 24.

Jones, K.E.; Patel, N.G.; Levy, M.A.; Storeygard, A.; Balk, D.; Gittleman, J.L.; Daszak, P. Global trends in emerging infectious diseases. *Nat. Cell Biol.* 2008, 451, 990.

Justo, J.A.; Bookstaver, P.B. Antibiotic lock therapy: Review of technique and logistical challenges. *Infect. Drug Resist.* 2014, 7, 343.

Kaplan, J.B. Biofilm dispersal. *J. Dent. Res.* 2010, 89, 205.

Karygianni, L.; Ren, Z.; Koo, H.; Thurnheer, T. Biofilm matrixome: Extracellular components in structured microbial communities. *Trends Microbiol.* 2020, 28, 668.

Keane, P.A.; Ruiz-Garcia, H.; Sadda, S.R. Advanced imaging technologies. *Retina* 2013, 133.

Keyt, H.; Faverio, P.; Restrepo, M.I. Prevention of ventilator-associated pneumonia in the intensive care unit: A review of the clinically relevant recent advancements. *Indian J. Med. Res.* 2014, 139, 814.

Khalid, K.; Tan, X.; Mohd Zaid, H.F.; Tao, Y.; Chew, C.L.; Chu, D.-T.; Lam, M.K.; Ho, Y.-C.; Lim, J.W.; Wei, L.C. Advanced in developmental organic and inorganic nanomaterial: A review. *Bioengineered* 2020, 11, 328.

Khan, H.A.; Baig, F.K.; Mehboob, R. Nosocomial infections: Epidemiology, prevention, control and surveillance. *Asian Pac. J. Trop. Biomed.* 2017, 7, 478.

Khanal, M.; Larsonneur, F.; Raks, V.; Barras, A.; Baumann, J.-S.; Martin, F.A.; Boukherroub, R.; Ghigo, J.-M.; Mellet, C.O.; Zaistev, V.; et al. Inhibition of Type 1 fimbriae-mediated Escherichia coli adhesion and biofilm formation by trimeric cluster thiomannosides conjugated to diamond nanoparticles. *Nanoscale* 2015, 7, 2325.

Khatoon, Z.; McTiernan, C.D.; Suuronen, E.J.; Mah, T.-F.; Alarcon, E.I. Bacterial biofilm formation on implantable devices and approaches to its treatment and prevention. *Heliyon* 2018, 4, e01067.

Khoshnood, S.; Savari, M.; Montazeri, E.A.; Sheikh, A.F. Survey on genetic diversity, biofilm formation, and detection of colistin resistance genes in clinical isolates of Acinetobacter baumannii. *Infect. Drug Resist.* 2020, 13, 1547.

Kim, K.P.; Kim, Y.-G.; Choi, C.-H.; Kim, H.-E.; Lee, S.-H.; Chang, W.-S.; Lee, C.-S. In situ monitoring of antibiotic susceptibility of bacterial biofilms in a microfluidic device. *Lab Chip* 2010, 10, 3296.

Kim, Y.W.; Mosteller, M.P.; Subramanian, S.; Meyer, M.T.; Bentley, W.E.; Ghodssi, R. An optical microfluidic platform for spatiotemporal biofilm treatment monitoring. *J. Micromechanics Microengineering* 2015, 26, 015013.

Kirby, A.E.; Garner, K.; Levin, B.R. The relative contributions of physical structure and cell density to the antibiotic susceptibility of bacteria in biofilms. *Antimicrob. Agents Chemother.* 2012, 56, 2967.

Kuan, C.-Y.; Wai, Y.-F.; Yuen, K.-H.; Liong, M.-T. Nanotech: Propensity in foods and bioactives. *Crit. Rev. Food Sci. Nutr.* 2012, 52, 55.

LaFleur, M.D.; Kumamoto, C.A.; Lewis, K. Candida albicans biofilms produce antifungal-tolerant persister cells. *Antimicrob. Agents Chemother.* 2006, 50, 3839.

Lazzell, A.L.; Chaturvedi, A.K.; Pierce, C.G.; Prasad, D.; Uppuluri, P.; Lopez-Ribot, J.L. Treatment and prevention of Candida albicans biofilms with caspofungin in a novel central venous catheter murine model of candidiasis. *J. Antimicrob. Chemother.* 2009, 64, 567.

Lederberg, J.; Zinder, N. Concentration of biochemical mutants of bacteria with penicillin. *J. Am. Chem. Soc.* 1948, 70, 4267.

Lee, J.-H.; Kaplan, J.B.; Lee, W.Y. Microfluidic devices for studying growth and detachment of Staphylococcus epidermidis biofilms. *Biomed. Microdevices* 2008, 10, 489.

Lee, S.H.; Sung, J.H. Microtechnology-based multi-organ models. *Bioengineering* 2017, 4, 46.

Li, X.; Yeh, Y.-C.; Giri, K.; Mout, R.; Landis, R.F.; Prakash, Y.S.; Rotello, V.M. Control of nanoparticle penetration into biofilms through surface design. *Chem. Commun.* 2015, 51, 282.

Li, Y.; Zhang, L.; Zhou, Y.; Zhang, Z.; Zhang, X. Survival of bactericidal antibiotic treatment by tolerant persister cells of Klebsiella pneumoniae. *J. Med. Microbiol.* 2018, 67, 273.

Li, Z.; Chen, Y.; Liu, D.; Zhao, N.; Cheng, H.; Ren, H.; Guo, T.; Niu, H.; Zhuang, W.; Wi, J.; et al. Involvement of glycolysis/gluconeogenesis and signaling regulatory pathways in Saccharomyces cerevisiae biofilms during fermentation. *Front. Microbiol.* 2015, 6, 139.

Limoli, D.H.; Jones, C.J.; Wozniak, D.J. Bacterial extracellular polysaccharides in biofilm formation and function. *Microbiol. Spectr.* 2015, 3.

Lin, C.-J.; Wu, C.-Y.; Yu, S.-J.; Chen, Y.-L. Protein kinase A governs growth and virulence in Candida tropicalis. *Virulence* 2018, 9, 331.

Lin, J.; Wang, Z.; Zang, Y.; Zhang, D.; Xin, Q. Detection of respiration changes inside biofilms with microelectrodes during exposure to antibiotics. *J. Environ. Sci. Health Part A* 2019, 54, 202.

Liu, L.; Yu, B.; Sun, W.; Liang, C.; Ying, H.; Zhou, S.; Niu, H.; Wang, Y.; Liu, D.; Chen, Y. Calcineurin signaling pathway influences Aspergillus niger biofilm formation by affecting hydrophobicity and cell wall integrity. *Biotechnol. Biofuels* 2020, 13, 54.

Mah, T.-F.C.; O'Toole, G.A. Mechanisms of biofilm resistance to antimicrobial agents. *Trends Microbiol.* 2001, 9, 34.

Mair, L.O.; Nacev, A.; Hilaman, R.; Stepanov, P.Y.; Chowdhury, S.; Jafari, S.; Hausfeld, J.; Karlsson, A.J.; Shirtliff, M.E.; Shapiro, B.; et al. Biofilm disruption with rotating microrods enhances antimicrobial efficacy. *J. Magn. Magn. Mater.* 2017, 427, 81.

Malik, A.A.; Martiny, J.B.H.; Brodie, E.L.; Martiny, A.C.; Treseder, K.K.; Allison, S.D. Defining trait-based microbial strategies with consequences for soil carbon cycling under climate change. *ISME J.* 2020, 14, 1.

Mangal, U.; Kim, J.-Y.; Seo, J.-Y.; Kwon, J.-S.; Choi, S.-H. Novel poly (methyl methacrylate) containing and fungal resistance. *Materials* 2019, 12, 3438.

Martinez, L.R.; Casadevall, A. Cryptococcus neoformans biofilm formation depends on surface support and carbon source and reduces fungal cell susceptibility to heat, cold, and UV light. *Appl. Environ. Microbiol.* 2007, 73, 4592.

Martinez, L.R.; Casadevall, A. Cryptococcus neoformans cells in biofilms are less susceptible than planktonic cells to antimicrobial molecules produced by the innate immune system. *Infect. Immun.* 2006, 74, 6118.

Martins, M.; Uppuluri, P.; Thomas, D.P.; Cleary, I.A.; Henriques, M.; Lopez-Ribot, J.L.; Oliveira, R. Presence of extracellular DNA in the Candida albicans biofilm matrix and its contribution to biofilms. *Mycopathologia* 2009, 169, 323.

Martin-Serrano, Á.; Gómez, R.; Ortega, P.; De La Mata, F.J. Nanosystems as vehicles for the delivery of antimicrobial peptides (AMPs). *Pharmaceutics* 2019, 11, 448.

Miyaue, S.; Suzuki, E.; Komiyama, Y.; Kondo, Y.; Morikawa, M.; Maeda, S. Bacterial memory of persisters: Bacterial persister cells can retain their phenotype for days or weeks after withdrawal from colony–biofilm culture. *Front. Microbiol.* 2018, 9, 1396.

Molina, A.; González, J.; Laborda, E.; Compton, R. Analytical solutions for fast and straight-forward study of the effect of the electrode geometry in transient and steady state voltammetries: Single- and multi-electron transfers, coupled chemical reactions and electrode kinetics. *J. Electroanal. Chem.* 2015, 756, 1.

Morrow, J.B.; Arango, C.P.; Holbrook, R.D. Association of quantum dot nanoparticles with Pseudomonas aeruginosa Biofilm. *J. Environ. Qual.* 2010, 39, 1934.

Moya, A.; Guimerà, X.; Del Campo, F.J.; Alfonso, E.P.; Dorado, A.D.; Baeza, M.; Villa, R.; Gabriel, D.; Gamisans, X.; Gabriel, G. Biofilm oxygen profiling using an array of microelectrodes on a microfabricated needle. *Procedia Eng.* 2014, 87, 256.

Moya, A.; Guimerà, X.; Del Campo, F.J.; Prats-Alfonso, E.; Dorado, A.D.; Baeza, M.; Villa, R.; Gabriel, D.; Gamisans, X.; Gabriel, G. Profiling of oxygen in biofilms using individually addressable disk microelectrodes on a microfabricated needle. *Microchim. Acta* 2014, 182, 985.

Nimesh, S. Dendrimers. In *Gene Therapy: Potential Applications of Nanotechnology*, 1st ed.; Woodhead Publishing Limited: Cambridge; Philadelphia, PA; New Delhi, 2013; pp. 259.

Nishanth, S.; Bharti, A.; Gupta, H.; Gupta, K.; Gulia, U.; Prasanna, R. Cyanobacterial extra-cellular polymeric substances (EPS): Biosynthesis and their potential applications. In *Microbial and Natural Macromolecules Synthesis and Applications*; Das, S., Dash, H.R., Eds.; Academic Press: London, 2021, pp. 349.

Nowakowska, J.; Landmann, R.; Khanna, N. Foreign body infection models to study host-pathogen response and antimicrobial tolerance of bacterial biofilm. *Antibiotics* 2014, 3, 378.

Papenfort, K.; Bassler, B.L. Quorum sensing signal–response systems in Gram-negative bacteria. *Nat. Rev. Genet.* 2016, 14, 576.

Pathak, R.; Bierman, S.F.; d'Arnaud, P. Inhibition of bacterial attachment and biofilm formation by a novel intravenous catheter material using an in vitro percutaneous catheter insertion model. *Med. Devices Evid. Res.* 2018, 11, 427.

Paul, W.; Sharma, C. Inorganic nanoparticles for targeted drug delivery. In *Biointegration of Medical Implant Materials: Science and Design*, 1st ed.; Woodhead Publishing Limited: Cambridge; New Delhi, India; Boca Raton, FL, 2010, pp. 204.

Percival, S.L. Importance of biofilm formation in surgical infection. *BJS* 2017, 104, e85–e94.

Percival, S.L.; Suleman, L.; Vuotto, C.; Donelli, G. Healthcare-associated infections, medical devices and biofilms: Risk, tolerance and control. *J. Med. Microbiol.* 2015, 64, 323.

Pereira, C.S.; Thompson, J.A.; Xavier, K.B. AI-2-mediated signalling in bacteria. *FEMS Microbiol. Rev.* 2013, 37, 156.

Perumal, P.; Mekala, S.; Chaffin, W.L. Role for cell density in antifungal drug resistance in Candida albicans biofilms. *Antimicrob. Agents Chemother.* 2007, 51, 2454.

Petrova, O.E.; Schurr, J.R.; Schurr, M.J.; Sauer, K. Microcolony formation by the opportunistic pathogen Pseudomonas aeruginosa requires pyruvate and pyruvate fermentation. *Mol. Microbiol.* 2012, 86, 819.

Pierce, C.G.; Srinivasan, A.; Ramasubramanian, A.K.; López-Ribot, J.L. From biology to drug development: New approaches to combat the threat of fungal biofilms. *Microbiol. Spectr.* 2015, 3.

Raghupathi, P.K.; Liu, W.; Sabbe, K.; Houf, K.; Burmølle, M.; Sørensen, S.J. Synergistic interactions within a multispecies biofilm enhance individual species protection against grazing by a pelagic protozoan. *Front. Microbiol.* 2018, 8, 2649.

Raheem, N.; Straus, S.K. Mechanisms of action for antimicrobial peptides with antibacterial and antibiofilm functions. *Front. Microbiol.* 2019, 10, 2866.

Rajendran, R.; Williams, C.; Lappin, D.F.; Millington, O.; Martins, M.; Ramage, G. Extracellular DNA release acts as an antifungal resistance mechanism in mature Aspergillus fumigatus biofilms. *Eukaryot. Cell* 2013, 12, 420.

Ramage, G.; Rajendran, R.; Gutierrez-Correa, M.; Jones, B.; Williams, C. Aspergillus biofilms: Clinical and industrial significance. *FEMS Microbiol. Lett.* 2011, 324, 89.

Ramage, G.; Rajendran, R.; Sherry, L.; Williams, C. Fungal biofilm resistance. *Int. J. Microbiol.* 2012, 2012, 1.

Reuter, K.; Steinbach, A.; Helms, V. Interfering with bacterial quorum sensing. *Perspect. Med. Chem.* 2016, 8, PMC-S13209.

Robbins, N.; Uppuluri, P.; Nett, J.; Rajendran, R.; Ramage, G.; Lopez-Ribot, J.L.; Andes, D.; Cowen, L.E. Hsp90 governs dispersion and drug resistance of fungal biofilms. *PLoS Pathog.* 2011, 7, e1002257.

Rodrigues, L.R. Inhibition of bacterial adhesion on medical devices. *Adv. Exp. Med. Biol.* 2011, 715, 351.

Römling, U.; Balsalobre, C. Biofilm infections, their resilience to therapy and innovative treatment strategies. *J. Intern. Med.* 2012, 272, 541.

Rosa, L.P.; de Silva, F.C. Antimicrobial photodynamic therapy: A new therapeutic option to combat infections. *J. Med. Microb. Diagn.* 2014, 3, 158.

Ross, P.; Mayer, R.; Benziman, M. Cellulose biosynthesis and function in bacteria. *Microbiol. Rev.* 1991, 55, 35.

Ruiz-Ruigomez, M.; Badiola, J.; Schmidt-Malan, S.M.; Greenwood-Quaintance, K.; Karau, M.J.; Brinkman, C.L.; Mandrekar, J.N.; Patel, R. Direct electrical current reduces bacterial and yeast biofilm formation. *Int. J. Bacteriol.* 2016, 2016, 9727810.

Sadekuzzaman, M.; Yang, S.; Mizan, M.; Ha, S. Current and recent advanced strategies for combating biofilms. *Compr. Rev. Food Sci. Food Saf.* 2015, 14, 491.

Sandvik, E.L.; McLeod, B.R.; Parker, A.E.; Stewart, P.S. Direct electric current treatment under physiologic saline conditions kills Staphylococcus epidermidis biofilms via electrolytic generation of hypochlorous acid. *PLoS ONE* 2013, 8, e55118.

Santajit, S.; Indrawattana, N. Mechanisms of antimicrobial resistance in ESKAPE pathogens. *BioMed Res. Int.* 2016, 2016, 1–8.

Schinabeck, M.K.; Long, L.A.; Hossain, M.A.; Chandra, J.; Mukherjee, P.K.; Mohamed, S.; Ghannoum, M.A. Rabbit model of Candida albicans biofilm infection: Liposomal Amphotericin B antifungal lock therapy. *Antimicrob. Agents Chemother.* 2004, 48, 1727.

Scorzoni, L.; De Paula e Silva, A.C.A.; Marcos, C.M.; Assato, P.A.; De Melo, W.C.M.A.; De Oliveira, H.C.; Costa-Orlandi, C.B.; Mendes-Giannini, M.J.S.; Fusco-Almeida, A.M. Antifungal therapy: New advances in the understanding and treatment of mycosis. *Front. Microbiol.* 2017, 8, 36.

SenthilKannan, K. Crystallographic, structural elucidation and electronic interactions of novel AMPF crystals for biomedicinal use by theory and practice as an anti-diabetic agent. *Results Chem.* 2022, 4, 100424. https://doi.org/10.1016/j.rechem.2022.100424.

Septimus, E.J.; Moody, J. Prevention of device-related healthcare-associated infections. *F1000Research* 2016, 5, 65.

Shaikh, A.F.; Tamboli, M.S.; Patil, R.H.; Bhan, A.; Ambekar, J.D.; Kale, B.B. Bioinspired carbon quantum dots: An antibiofilm agents. *J. Nanosci. Nanotechnol.* 2019, 19, 2339.

Shrout, J.D.; Tolker-Nielsen, T.; Givskov, M.; Parsek, M.R. The contribution of cell-cell signaling and motility to bacterial biofilm formation. *MRS Bull.* 2011, 36, 367–373.

Shumi, W.; Kim, S.H.; Lim, J.; Cho, K.-S.; Han, H.; Park, S. Shear stress tolerance of Streptococcus mutans aggregates determined by microfluidic funnel device (μFFD). *J. Microbiol. Methods* 2013, 93, 85.

Silva, S.; Henriques, M.; Martins, A.; Oliveira, R.; Williams, D.; Azeredo, J. Biofilms of non-Candida albicans Candida species: Quantification, structure and matrix composition. *Med. Mycol.* 2009, 47, 681.

Sima, F.; Ristoscu, C.; Duta, L.; Gallet, O.; Anselme, K.; Mihailescu, I. Laser thin films deposition and characterization for biomedical applications. In *Laser Surface Modification of Biomaterials*; Elsevier Inc.: Amsterdam, The Netherlands; Oxford; Cambridge, 2016; pp. 77.

Singh, M.N.; Hemant, K.S.Y.; Ram, M.; Shivakumar, H.G. Microencapsulation: A promising technique for controlled drug delivery. *Res. Pharm. Sci.* 2010, 5, 65.

Smith, K.F.; Goldberg, M.; Rosenthal, S.; Carlson, L.; Chen, J.; Chen, C.; Ramachandran, S. Global rise in human infectious disease outbreaks. *J. R. Soc. Interface* 2014, 11, 20140950.

Sriramulu, D.D.; Lünsdorf, H.; Lam, J.S.; Römling, U. Microcolony formation: A novel biofilm model of Pseudomonas aeruginosa for the cystic fibrosis lung. *J. Med. Microbiol.* 2005, 54, 667.

Steinberg, N.; Kolodkins-Gal, I. The matrix reloaded: How sensing the extracellular matrix synchronizes bacterial communities. *J. Bacteriol.* 2015, 197, 2092.

Stewart, P.S. Mechanisms of antibiotic resistance in bacterial biofilms. *Int. J. Med. Microbiol.* 2002, 292, 107.

Sturme, M.H.J.; Kleerebezem, M.; Nakayama, J.; Akkermas, A.D.L.; Vaugha, E.E.; de Vos, W.M. Cell to cell communication by autoinducing peptides in Gram-positive bacteria. *Antonie Leeuwenhoek* 2002, 81, 233.

Szunerits, S.; Barras, A.; Boukherroub, R. Antibacterial applications of nanodiamonds. *Int. J. Environ. Res. Public Health* 2016, 13, 413.

Taraszkiewicz, A.; Fila, G.; Grinholc, M.; Nakonieczna, J. Innovative strategies to overcome biofilm resistance. *BioMed Res. Int.* 2012, 2013, 1.

Teughels, W.; Van Assche, N.; Sliepen, I.; Quirynen, M. Effect of material characteristics and/or surface topography on biofilm development. *Clin. Oral Implants Res.* 2006, 17 (Suppl. 2), 68.

Tsai, H.-C.; Imae, T. Fabrication of dendrimers toward biological application. *Prog. Mol. Biol. Transl. Sci.* 2011, 104, 101.

Tu, C.; Wang, Y.; Yi, L.; Wang, Y.; Liu, B.; Gong, S. Roles of signaling molecules in biofilm formation. *Sheng Wu Gong Cheng Xue Bao Chin. J. Biotechnol.* 2019, 35, 558.

Turan, N.B.; Chormey, D.S.; Büyükpınar, Ç.; Engin, G.O.; Bakirdere, S. Quorum sensing: Little talks for an effective bacterial coordination. *TrAC Trends Anal. Chem.* 2017, 91, 1.

Tuson, H.H.; Weibel, D.B. Bacteria-surface interactions. *Soft Matter* 2013, 9, 4368.

Uppuluri, P.; Nett, J.; Heitman, J.; Andes, D. Synergistic effect of calcineurin inhibitors and fluconazole against Candida albicans biofilms. *Antimicrob. Agents Chemother.* 2008, 52, 1127.

Vergidis, P.; Patel, R. Novel approaches to the diagnosis, prevention, and treatment of medical device-associated infections. *Infect. Dis. Clin. N. Am.* 2012, 26, 173.

Vincent, B.M.; Lancaster, A.K.; Scherz-Shouval, R.; Whitesell, L.; Lindquist, S. Fitness trade-offs restrict the evolution of resistance to Amphotericin B. *PLoS Biol.* 2013, 11, e1001692.

Waghule, T.; Singhvi, G.; Dubey, S.K.; Pandey, M.M.; Gupta, G.; Singh, M.; Dua, K. Microneedles: A smart approach and increasing potential for transdermal drug delivery system. *Biomed. Pharmacother.* 2019, 109, 1249.

Walraven, C.J.; Lee, S.A. Antifungal lock therapy. *Antimicrob. Agents Chemother.* 2012, 57, 1.

Walters, M.C., III; Roe, F.; Bugnicourt, A.; Franklin, M.J.; Stewart, P.S. Contributions of antibiotic penetration, oxygen limitation, and low metabolic activity to tolerance of Pseudomonas aeruginosa biofilms to ciproflaxin and tobramycin. *Antimicrob. Agents Chemother.* 2003, 47, 317.

Wille, J.; Coenye, T. Biofilm dispersion: The key to biofilm eradication or opening Pandora's box? *Biofilm* 2020, 2, 100027.

Wu, S.; Liu, C.; Feng, J.; Yang, A.; Guo, F.; Qiao, J. QSIdb: Quorum sensing interference molecules. *Brief. Bioinform.* 2021, 22, bbaa218.

Wuyts, J.; Van Dijck, P.; Holtappels, M. Fungal persister cells: The basis for recalcitrant infections? *PLoS Pathog.* 2018, 14, e1007301.

Xu, B.; Wei, Q.; Mettetal, M.R.; Han, J.; Rau, L.; Tie, J.; May, R.M.; Pathe, E.T.; Reddy, S.T.; Sullivan, L.; et al. Surface micropattern reduces colonization and medical device-associated infections. *J. Med. Microbiol.* 2017, 66, 1692.

Yadav, H.K.S.; Raizaday, A. Inorganic nanobiomaterials for medical imaging. In *Nanobiomaterials in Medical Imaging*; Elsevier Inc.: Amsterdam, The Netherlands; Oxford; Cambridge, 2016; pp. 365.

Yan, Z.; Huang, M.; Melander, C.; Kjellerup, B.V. Dispersal and inhibition of biofilms associated with infections. *J. Appl. Microbiol.* 2020, 128, 1279.

Yin, W.; Wang, Y.; Liu, L.; He, J. Biofilms: The microbial "protective clothing" in extreme environments. *Int. J. Mol. Sci.* 2019, 20, 3423.

Zander, Z.K.; Becker, M.L. Antimicrobial and antifouling strategies for polymeric medical devices. *ACS Macro Lett.* 2018, 7, 16.

Zeng, Z.; Yu, D.; He, Z.; Liu, J.; Xiao, F.-X.; Zhang, Y.; Wang, R.; Bhattacharyya, D.; Tan, T.T.Y. Graphene oxide quantum dots covalently functionalized PVDF membrane with significantly enhanced bactericidal and antibiofouling performances. *Sci. Rep.* 2016, 6, 20142.

Zhang, J.; Chen, K.; Fan, Z. Circulating tumor cell isolation and analysis. In *Advances in Applied Microbiology*; Elsevier Inc.: Amsterdam, The Netherlands; Oxford; Cambridge, 2016; Volume 75, pp. 1.

Zhang, X.-Q.; Chen, M.; Lam, R.; Xu, X.; Osawa, E.; Ho, D. Polymer-functionalized nanodiamond platforms as vehicles for gene delivery. *ACS Nano* 2009, 3, 2609.

Zimmerli, W.; Trampuz, A.; Ochsner, P.E. Prosthetic-joint infections. *New. Engl. J. Med.* 2004, 351, 1645.

6 Ecological Relevance of Quorum Quenching

Carolina M. Viola[*], Mariela A. Torres[*],
Alejandra L. Valdez[*], Mariano J. Lacosegliaz,
Lucía I. Castellanos de Figueroa,
and Carlos G. Nieto-Peñalver

6.1 INTRODUCTION

Quorum sensing (QS) is a microbial communication mechanism first described in the 1970s during studies on bioluminescence in *Vibrio harveyi* MAV, a marine bacterium previously known as *Photobacterium fischeri* MAV, in which the LuxI/LuxR QS system mediates the cell density-dependent expression of the *lux* operon, which is involved in bioluminescence production (Nealson, 2020). Subsequently, homologous systems were revealed experimentally in other species regulating the most diverse processes and cellular functions, including bioluminescence, pathogenesis, virulence, biofilm formation, and antibiotic production and resistance (Papenfort & Bassler, 2016). For instance, in *Agrobacterium fabrum* (from. *tumefaciens*), the TraI/TraR QS system is involved in the conjugative transfer of pTi plasmid (L. Zhang, Murphy, Kerr, & Tate, 1993). In *Pseudomonas aeruginosa*, the expression of many virulence factors is controlled by three interconnected QS systems (Soukarieh, Williams, Stocks, & Cámara, 2018). QS systems allow microorganisms to communicate with members of their species, with other species, and with their eukaryotic hosts, that is, the intra- and interspecies interactions (Clinton & Rumbaugh, 2016).

In QS mechanisms, the accumulation of small diffusible signaling molecules called autoinducers (AIs) allows a cell to sense the population density. Synthesized in the intracellular space, these molecules are liberated and concentrated in the extracellular environment through passive diffusion across the membrane (Kaplan & Greenberg, 1985), efflux pumps, or specific transporters (Riedel et al., 2009). A sufficiently high concentration of autoinducers allows the activation of a cognate response regulator within the local cell population, resulting in synchronized gene expression (Fuqua & Greenberg, 2002).

In general, all QS systems show a common organization, comprising the following three steps: (1) intracellular production and extracellular secretion of AI; (2) reentry of extracellular AI into the cells either actively (via membrane-bound carrier proteins) or passively (via diffusion through the cell membrane) and binding to

---

[*] These authors contributed equally to this job

DOI: 10.1201/9781003297826-6

specific membrane or cytoplasmic receptors; and (3) signal transduction through IA receptors that activates downstream signaling pathways regulating the expression of target genes (Fuqua & Greenberg, 2002).

6.2   DIVERSITY OF AUTOINDUCER SIGNALS

Each AI signal molecule is detected and counteracted by specific detection machinery and regulatory networks. However, based on the structure of the AI signal, most QS systems in bacteria fall into three main categories: (1) present in several Alpha-, Beta-, and Gammaproteobacteria, LuxI/LuxR-type QS systems employ *N*-acyl-homoserine lactones (AHLs) as signal molecules; (2) most gram-positive bacteria where QS has been described, utilize small modified peptides called autoinducer peptides (AIPs), with the Actinobacteria phylum being the exception whose QS systems relies on gamma-butyrolactones (Polkade, Mantri, Patwekar, & Jangid, 2016; Takano et al., 2000); and (3) autoinducer-2 (AI-2), a furanosyl borate diester molecule synthesized and detected by both gram-positive (Yu, Zhao, Xue, & Sun, 2012) and gram-negative (Yu et al., 2012) bacteria.

6.2.1 *N*-ACYL-HOMOSERINE LACTONES (AHLs)

AHLs are small molecules featuring a homoserine lactone ring linked to a fatty acyl chain that varies in length (C4–C14), in the oxidation state at β-position, and in the saturation degree. For instance, C6-HSL refers to *N*-hexanoyl-L-homoserine lactone (Figure 6.1A); and 3OC12-HSL refers to *N*-3-oxododecanoyl-L-homoserine lactone (Figure 6.1B). With few exceptions, AHLs are typically

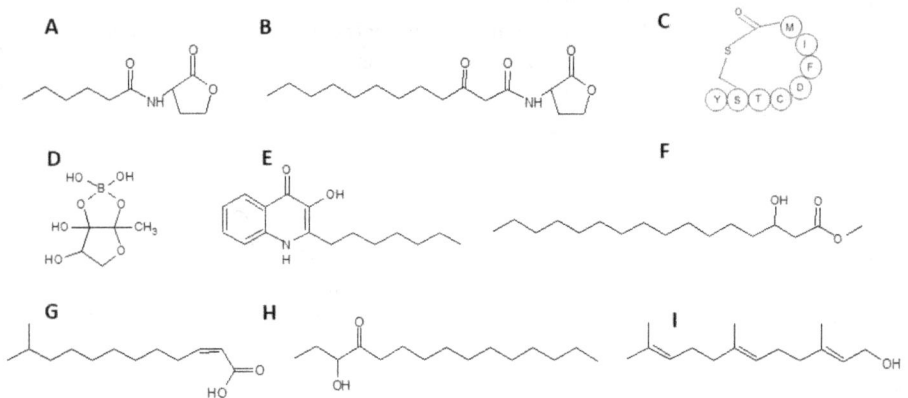

FIGURE 6.1   Structure of quorum sensing signals. (A) C6-HSL (*N*-hexanoyl-L-homoserine lactone). (B) 3OC12-HSL (*N*-3-oxododecanoyl-L-homoserine lactone). (C) AIP-I (autoinducer peptide I). (D) AI-2 (autoinducer-2). (E) PQS (2-heptyl-3-hydroxy-4(1*H*)-quinolone). (F) 3-OH PAME (3-hydroxy palmitic acid methyl ester). (G) DSF (diffusible signal factor). (H) LAI-1 (3-hydroxypentadecane-4-one). (I) Farnesol.

synthesized by LuxI-type AHL synthases that catalyze the condensation between *S*-adenosylmethionine (SAM) and an acylated acyl carrier protein (acyl-ACP) (Parsek, Val, Hanzelka, Cronan, & Greenberg, 1999). AHLs are detected by their cognate cytoplasmic LuxR receptor, where the specificity is determined by the characteristics (i.e., length and substitutions at the third position) of their acyl side chains (Vannini et al., 2002). Many pathogenic and nonpathogenic behaviors of gram-negative bacteria, including host adhesion, exoenzyme production, toxin secretion, biofilm formation, siderophores, and pigment production are regulated by AHL-mediated QS systems (Papenfort & Bassler, 2016). To note, putative *luxI* and *luxR* homologues have been predicted in the genomes of gram-positive bacteria and archaea (Rajput & Kumar, 2017a, 2017b).

6.2.2 AUTOINDUCER PEPTIDES (AIPS)

AIPs are modified oligopeptides that can range from 5 to 17 amino acids. AIPs are synthesized in the cytosol as pro-AIPs, and then processed to form mature AIPs either in the intracellular or the extracellular environment, depending on the species. Due to their inability to passively diffuse across the cell membrane, AIPs are chaperoned by specialized membrane transporters. AIPs are detected and bound by transmembrane histidine kinases when their extracellular concentration reaches the threshold concentration. This binding results in the phosphorylation of a downstream response regulator, which regulates the expression of target genes. In *Staphylococcus aureus*, one of the best characterized QS systems in gram-positive bacteria, AIP is produced after a precursor AgrD is processed and exported by the transpeptidase AgrB (Ji, Beavis, & Novick, 1995; Saenz et al., 2000). At a threshold concentration, AIP is sensed by the histidine kinase sensor AgrC (Lina et al., 1998), which then phosphorylates the response regulator AgrA. Once activated, AgrA induces modifications in the expressions of genes highly relevant for the virulence (Queck et al., 2008). Four AIPs (AIP-I, AIP-II, AIP-III, and AIP-IV) have been described in *S. aureus* (Figure 6.1C). Among other gram-positive bacteria, AIP-based QS systems have also been characterized in *Enterococcus faecalis*, (Ali et al., 2017) *Bacillus subtilis* (Kalamara, Spacapan, Mandic-Mulec, & Stanley-Wall, 2018), *Listeria monocytogenes* (Riedel et al., 2009), and *Clostridium perfringens* (Ma, Li, & McClane, 2015).

6.2.3 AUTOINDUCER-2 (AI-2)

Autoinducer-2 is the name of a family of QS signals represented by borated furanone derivatives (Miller et al., 2004), originated from DPD (4,5-dihydroxy-2,3-pentanedione) and synthesized by LuxS synthase in the *S*-adenosyl-methionine (SAM) recycling pathway (Surette, Miller, & Bassler, 1999). For instance, while the AI-2 in *V. harveyi* is a boron ester of (2R,4S)-2-methyl-2,3,3,4-tetrahydroxytetrahydro-furan (Figure 6.1D), in *Salmonella enterica* serovar Typhimurium, AI-2 lacks the borate (Miller et al., 2004). AI-2 is imported and bound by its cognate receptor leading to a cascade of phosphorylation signaling pathways that regulate phenotypes including virulence and bioluminescence (Neiditch & Hughson, 2007).

6.2.4 OTHER SIGNALING MOLECULES

Beyond those previously mentioned, other molecules have been also found to function as bacterial QS signals.

Alkylquinolones are synthesized by the PqsABCDH system and detected by PqsR. 4-Hydroxy-2-alkylquinolines (HAQs) are a class of QS signals that have been reported for several species of *Pseudomonas* (Diggle et al., 2007) and *Burkholderia* (Diggle et al., 2006). QS quinolones include derivatives of 4-hydroxy-2-heptyl-quinoline (HHQ) and the corresponding dihydroxylated derivatives, as 2-heptyl-3-hydroxy-4(1*H*)-quinolone (also known as PQS, *Pseudomonas* quinolone signal) (Figure 6.1E). PQS integrates physiological information, including low iron and oxidative stress, into the main LasI/LasR and RhlI/RhlR QS systems for fine-tuning virulence expression and biofilm formation (Diggle et al., 2006). In addition to altering the global transcriptional profile of genes via the PqsR-dependent pathway, PQS can also function independently by binding to hundreds of different cellular receptors, which modulates host immune responses, cytotoxicity, and key virulence pathways (Dandela, Mantin, Cravatt, Rayo, & Meijler, 2018; Rampioni et al., 2010).

Fatty acid derivatives as QS signals have been described in several proteobacteria. For instance, (*R*)-methyl 3-hydroxymyristate (3-OH MAME) (Kai et al., 2015) and (*R*)-methyl 3-hydroxypalmitate (3-OH PAME) (Figure 6.1F) (Flavier, Clough, Schell, & Denny, 1997) are employed as QS signals by the *Ralstonia solanacearum* species complex. 3-OH MAME and 3-OH PAME are synthesized by the methyltransferase PhcB and then sensed by the histidine kinase PhcS, which in turn phosphorylates the response regulators PhcR/PhcQ (Ujita, Sakata, Yoshihara, Hikichi, & Kai, 2019).

The diffusible signal factor (DSF) family of QS molecules is a group of *cis*-2-unsaturated fatty acids broadly present in *Xanthomonas* and *Burkholderia* spp. (Ryan, An, Allan, McCarthy, & Dow, 2015). One of the best described DSFs is *cis*-11-methyl-2-dodecenoic acid from *Xanthomonas campestris* pv. *campestris* (Figure 6.1G), which is synthesized by the enoyl CoA hydratase RpfF and the long-chain fatty acyl-CoA ligase RpfB (Dow, Feng, Barber, Tang, & Daniels, 2000). DSF in *X. campestris* pv. *campestris* is sensed by both the membrane-bound histidine kinase RpfC and the soluble histidine kinase RpfS. The response regulators RpfG and XC_2578 complete the QS system in this phytopathogen (Ryan et al., 2015).

α-Hydroxyketones have also been described as QS molecules. In *V. cholera* and *Legionella pneumophila*, the main QS signals are (S)-3-hydroxytridecan-4-one (CAI-1) and 3-hydroxypentadecane-4-one (LAI-1) (Figure 6.1H), respectively (Tiaden & Hilbi, 2012). In both microorganisms, the respective QS systems also differ from the well-known AHL-dependent QS mechanisms in that CAI-1 and LAI-1 are sensed by the sensor kinases CqsS and LqsS, respectively.

To date, fungal QS molecules are mainly represented by alcohol derivatives. The best characterized fungal QS system is that of the yeast *Candida albicans*, where the sesquiterpene farnesol (Figure 6.1I) farnesoic acid, and the aromatic alcohols tyrosol, 1-phenylethanol, and tryptophol are the QS signals. In addition, 2-phenylethanol, tyrosol, and tryptophol have been described in *Saccharomyces cerevisiae* (Jagtap, Bedekar, & Rao, 2020).

6.3   THE QUORUM-QUENCHING PHENOMENON

Small signaling molecules that are concentrated in the extracellular medium mediate QS in both fungi and bacteria. QS is involved in the regulation of not only virulence but also in beneficial traits in a broad spectrum of microorganisms. However, the necessity of finding novel manners for combating pathogens has boosted the research on the quorum quenching phenomenon as an alternative to antibiotics. The term "quorum quenching" (QQ) was coined to describe all processes that interfere with QS (Dong et al., 2001). QQ molecular actors are diverse in nature (enzymes or chemical compounds), mode of action (QS-signal cleavage or competitive inhibition), and targets, as all steps of the QS pathway (synthesis, diffusion, accumulation, and perception of the QS signals) may be affected. Chemical or enzymatic interference in QS inhibits microbial communication and subsequently reduces QS-regulated behaviors (Grandclément, Tannières, Moréra, Dessaux, & Faure, 2016). Of note, the enzymes that inactivate QS signals are named QQ enzymes, while the chemicals disrupting QS pathways are called QS inhibitors (QSIs) (Grandclément et al., 2016). Regulation and disruption of QS, therefore, presents an attractive opportunity to mitigate undesirable signaling-controlled microbial traits, including virulence and biofilm formation associated with infectious diseases. QQ strategies do not aim to kill the bacteria or limit their growth. Rather, they affect the expression of a specific function. This is an important feature because these strategies exert a more limited selective pressure for microbial survival than biocide treatments, which is a valuable trait for the development of sustainable biocontrol or therapeutic procedures in the present context of rising antibiotic resistance.

Beyond the diverse biotechnological applications of the interruption of QS signaling, the QQ phenomenon has ecological implications due to the modulations of microbial interactions in virtually any niche. One of the most illustrative examples is the production of halogenated furanones by *Delisea pulchra*. This red alga produces halogenated furanones with chemical structures resembling AHLs that induce the turnover of the LuxR receptors (Manefield et al., 2002). The capacity for quenching QS systems of these compounds has been explored against several pathogens, including *P. aeruginosa* (Wu et al., 2004), *Serratia liquefaciens* (Rasmussen et al., 2000), and *Pectobacterium carotovorum* (Manefield, Welch, Givskov, Salmond, & Kjelleberg, 2001). However, in nature, *D. pulchra* benefits from the QQ activities of its own furanones to avoid AHL-dependent biofilm formation on the algal surface (Givskov et al., 1996).

6.4   ENZYMATIC INACTIVATION OF AHLS

The first description of an enzymatic inactivation of QS signals showed that AiiA from *Bacillus* sp. 240B1 could effectively interfere with the AHL accumulation in the phytopathogen *P. carotovorum* (form. *E. carotovora*), preventing virulence in planta (Dong, Xu, Li, & Zhang, 2000). Since this first report, most of the scientific work has focused on the study of those activities that inactivate AHLs, even if the QS systems of several pathogens rely on signals other than AHLs. PQS in *P. aeruginosa*,

DSF in *Burkholderia* spp., and 3-OH PAME in *R. solanacearum* are just a few examples. This bias can be explained, at least partially, in the facility for screening QQ activities on AHLs by means of biosensor strains, including *Chromobacterium violaceum* CV026 (McClean et al., 1997), *Agrobacterium tumefaciens* NT1 (pZLR4) (Shaw et al., 1997), and *P. putida* F117 (pKR-C12) (McClean et al., 1997).

The production of enzymes with the capacity for inactivating AHLs is exemplified in different species of Bacteria, Archaea, and Eukaryotes. Though numerous enzymes involved in the degradation or modification of AHL have been reported, they can be grouped into three main catalytic classes: (1) lactonases, (2) amidases or acylases, and (3) oxidases and reductases.

6.4.1 LACTONASES

AHL-lactonases act on the AHL QS signal and hydrolyze the homoserine lactone ring rendering the corresponding *N*-acyl homoserine (Figure 6.2) (Kim et al., 2005). To date, four distinct families of QQ lactonases have been described: phosphotriesterase-like lactonases (PLLs), metallo-β-lactamase-like lactonases, α/β-hydrolase fold lactonases, and serum paraoxonases (PONs).

1. Phosphotriesterase-like lactonases (PLLs). PLLs exhibit a $(\alpha/\beta)_8$ fold (TIM barrel). PLLs are proficient lactonases that typically show a substrate preference for AHLs with long acyl chains. SsoPox, SacPox, and VmoLac (EC:3.1.8.1) from the archaea *Saccharolobus solfataricus*, *Sulfolobus acidocaldarius*, and *Vulcanisaeta moutnovskia,* respectively, are well-characterized PLL representatives (Bzdrenga et al., 2014; Ng, Wright, & Seah, 2011). However, PLLs have also been described in bacteria. For instance, QsdA from *Rhodococcus erythropolis* W2 (Uroz et al., 2008) is a PLL enzyme. Several of these metalloenzymes present desirable properties for biotechnological applications (e.g., thermostability, and resistance to pH and salinity), like moLRP lactonase, one of the last PLL described to date, which was obtained from a marine metagenome (Haramati et al., 2022).

2. Metallo-β-lactamase-like lactonases (MLLs). The main structural highlight of MLLs is a conserved metal binding motif [104]HXHXDH[109]~H[169] (positions according to AiiA from *Bacillus* sp. Strain 240B1). One of the first QQ enzymes to be characterized at the structural level was the MLL AiiA (EC:3.1.1.81) from *Bacillus thuringiensis*. The analysis of this enzyme showed a characteristic α β/β α fold bonded with two zinc cations (Kim

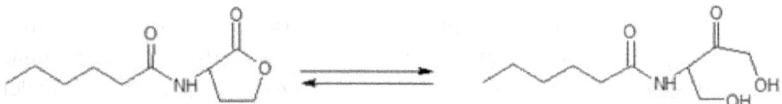

FIGURE 6.2 Enzymatic inactivation of AHLs by lactonases. In a reversible reaction, lactonases hydrolyze the lactone bond opening the ring, which rends the corresponding *N*-acyl homoserine. In the figure, C6-HSL is hydrolyzed to *N*-hexanoyl homoserine.

et al., 2005). Other representative MLLs that have been studied include AiiB from *Agrobacterium tumefaciens* (Liu et al., 2007) and GcL from *Geobacillus caldoxylosilyticus* (Bergonzi, Schwab, & Elias, 2016). To date, one of the last members reported in this group is Lrsl, a lactonase from *Labrenzia* sp. VG12 isolated from the Red Sea (Rehman et al., 2022).

3. α/β-Hydrolase fold lactonases. These enzymes (EC:3.1.1.81) also possess the characteristic α/β-hydrolase fold but, in contrast to MLLs, lack the conserved HXHXDH motif. AidH from *Ochrobactrum* sp. strain T63 was the first member of this group to be characterized (Mei, Yan, Turak, Luo, & Zhang, 2010). AiiM from *Microbacterium testaceum* is another member of this group (W.-Z. Wang, Morohoshi, Ikenoya, Someya, & Ikeda, 2010).

4. Paraoxonases (PONs). Largely studied in mammals, the activity on paraoxon gives the name to the group. The PON family is composed of three members—PON1, PON2, and PON3 (EC:3.1.1.2)—that show different prevalence in human tissues. These enzymes show a characteristic six-bladed β-propeller fold. Among the three members, PON2 degrades more efficiently AHLs (Draganov et al., 2005; Ozer et al., 2005). To note, PON enzymes hydrolyze not only AHLs, but also other substrates, including aryl esters, organophosphates, fatty acids, and diverse lactones (Draganov et al., 2005).

6.4.2 ACYLASES OR AMIDASES

Acylases or amidases interfere with bacterial QS cleaving the amide bond of AHLs (EC:3.5.1), which rend the homoserine lactone rings and the corresponding fatty acids (Figure 6.3). In contrast to lactonases, the inactivation of AHLs by amidases is irreversible. AiiD from *Ralstonia* sp. XJ12B, the first acylase to be described, belongs to the N-terminal nucleophile aminohydrolase (Ntn hydrolases) superfamily (Lin et al., 2003). This is a common aspect of several acylases, including PvdQ from *P. aeruginosa* (Bokhove, Nadal, Quax, & Dijkstra, 2009). Similar to other enzymes in this group, PvdQ shows a preference for AHLs with long acyl chains. In the structure of PvdQ, a large and hydrophobic binding pocket for the acyl part of the AHL explains this substrate specificity (Bokhove et al., 2009). However, AiiD degrades equally well short- and long-chain AHLs (Lin et al., 2003). An interesting feature is that most of them are dimmers, are cleaved to attain an active state, and are not secreted. The acylase group of enzymes is enlarged with the dienelactone hydrolase DlhR from *Sinorhizobium* sp. NGR234 (Krysciak et al., 2011) and

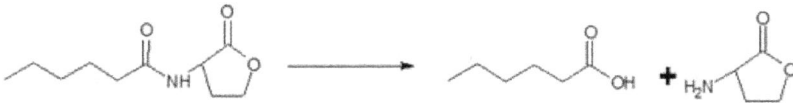

FIGURE 6.3 Enzymatic inactivation of AHLs by amidases or acylases. In a reversible reaction, amidases or acylases cleave the amide bond. As a result, the homoserine lactone ring and the corresponding fatty acid are produced. The reaction is irreversible, in contrast to those catalyzed by lactonases. In the figure, hexanoic acid and homoserine lactone are obtained from C6-HSL.

the α/β-hydrolase-like acylase AiiO from *Ochrobacterium* sp. A44 (Czajkowski et al., 2011). Recently, AHL acylase activity has been shown in GqqA, a bifunctional enzyme from *Komagataeibacter europaeus* CECT 8546, that also presents prephenate dehydratase activity (Werner et al., 2021).

6.4.3 OXIDASES AND REDUCTASES

Oxidases and reductase enzymes interfere with QS activity via the oxidation or reduction of the acyl side chain of AHLs, which reduces its capacity to be bound to its cognate receptor. Noteworthy, this group of enzymes has remained, to date, the least explored. Similar to other fatty acid–related compounds, cytochrome P450 CYP102A1 from *Bacillus megaterium* (EC:1.6.2.4) oxidizes the acyl side chain of AHLs at the ω -1, ω -2, and ω -3 position introducing a hydroxyl group (Figure 6.4A). The resulting products are not recognized by AHL receptors, which quenches the QS systems (Chowdhary et al., 2007). Due to the other substrates described for this enzyme, it is not expected that cytochrome P450 CYP102A1 oxidizes AHLs with short acyl side chains (Chowdhary et al., 2007). To date, this is the only example described in this group of QQ enzymes.

The carbonyl group of 3-oxo–substituted AHLs is also possible of being reduced. The NADP-dependent short-chain dehydrogenase/reductase BpiB09 obtained from a soil metagenome reduces 3OC12-HSL to 3OHC12-HSL (Figure 6.4B) (Bijtenhoorn et al., 2011). Similar activities have been identified in protein extracts from *R. erythropolis* W2 (Uroz et al., 2005) and *Burkholderia* sp. GG4 (Chan et al., 2011), though the corresponding enzymes were not identified.

6.4.4 ENZYMATIC INACTIVATION OF OTHER QS SIGNALS

Besides AHLs, other QS signals can be biologically degraded. The first report showing the inactivation of a QS signal other than AHLs presented evidence of

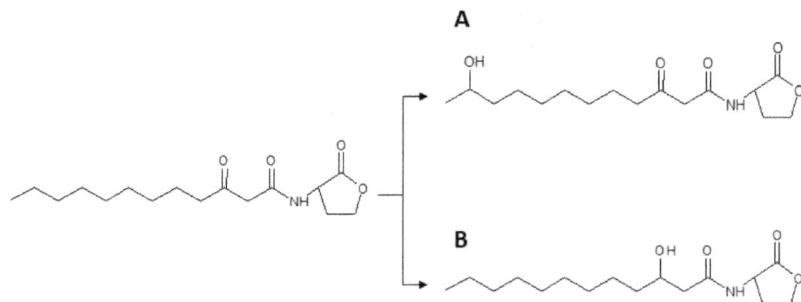

FIGURE 6.4 Oxidation and reduction of AHLs by oxidases and reductases. (A) Cytochrome P450 CYP102A1 from *B. megaterium* introduces a hydroxyl group at the ω -1, ω -2, and ω -3 positions of the acyl side chain of AHLs. In the figure, the position ω -1 of 3OC12-HSL is oxidized. (B) Reductases reduce the carbonyl group of 3-oxo-substituted AHLs. As a result, 3-hydroxy AHLs are formed. In the figure, 3OC12-HSL is reduced to 3OHC12-HSL.

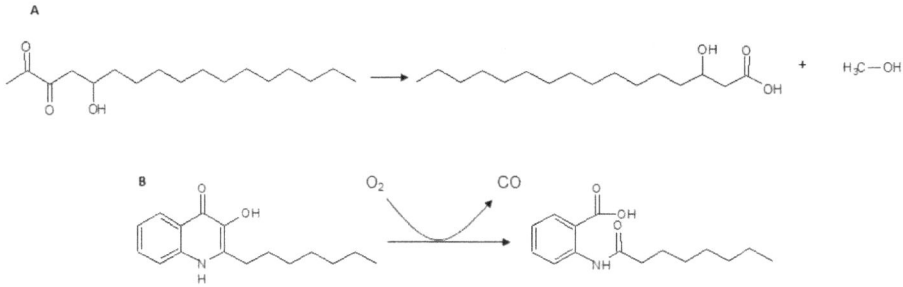

FIGURE 6.5 Inactivation of other QS molecules. (A) 3-OH PAME degradation by β-hydroxypalmitate methyl ester hydrolase from *Ideonella* sp. 0-0013. 3-OH palmitic acid and methanol are produced. (B) PQS degradation by 2,4-dioxygenases like HodC from *A. nitroguajacolicus* produces *N*-octanoylanthranilic acid.

an extracellular β-hydroxypalmitate methyl ester hydrolase with the capacity for degrading 3-OH PAME, the main QS signal in *R. solanacearum*. Employing a culture medium with 3-OH PAME as the main carbon source, *Ideonella* sp. 0-0013 was isolated from agricultural soils and served as the source for this esterase (Shinohara, Nakajima, & Uehara, 2007). As a result of the esterase activity on 3-OH PAME, 3-OH palmitic acid is produced, and methanol is liberated (Figure 6.5A). Similar activities were later found in clones from a soil metagenome (Lee et al., 2018).

The DSF produced by *Xanthomonas* spp. is also susceptible to being enzymatically inactivated by several bacterial species. However, the biochemical reactions involved in its degradation are not conserved. For instance, the corresponding QQ activity from *Pseudomonas* sp. strain G was attributed to the gene products of the *carAB* operon that are involved in the synthesis of carbamoyl phosphate (Newman, Chatterjee, Ho, & Lindow, 2008). In contrast, the inactivation of DSF by *X. campestris* pv. *campestris* is due to the fatty acyl-CoA ligase RpfB, which is a homologue to FadD in *E. coli* (Zhou et al., 2015). Similar to the reaction catalyzed by FadD, the degradation of DSF by RpfB produces fatty acyl-CoA, which is subsequently degraded through a β-oxidation process (H. Wang, Liao, Chen, & Zhang, 2020). The description of RpfB as a QQ enzyme with activity on DSF is relevant. Beyond being related to the inactivation of DSF, at the same time RpfB is involved in the production of DSF (Zhou et al., 2015). In this way, RpfB is part of the tuning of the QS system, similar to AttM and AiiB from *Agrobacterium fabrum* C58, as discussed later (Haudecoeur et al., 2009). The capacity to interfere with the virulence of *X. campestris* pv. *campestris* by means of the heterologous expression of RpfB homologues has been shown (H. Wang et al., 2020). Though to date it is not known whether this activity alters the pathogenesis in situ, this scenario is highly plausible, considering that the capacity to inactivate DSF is present in different species that inhabit the same plants infected by *X. campestris* pv. *campestris* (H. Wang et al., 2020).

As previously mentioned, *P. aeruginosa* also utilizes QS signals other than AHLs. 2-Heptyl-3-hydroxy-4(1*H*)-quinolone (PQS), the best characterized of these alternative signals, can also be inactivated. In a reaction catalyzed by

3-hydroxy-2-methyl-4(1H)-quinolone 2,4-dioxygenase HodC from *Arthrobacter nitroguajacolicus* Rü61a, one of the rings in PQS can be cleaved, which inactivates the QS signal. This 2,4-dioxygenolytic ring rupture produces *N*-octanoylanthranilic acid (Figure 6.5B), which cannot participate in the PQS QS system, and carbon monoxide. Nod is a member of the α/β-hydrolase fold superfamily that shows the particularity of not requiring metal ions or organic cofactors (Pustelny et al., 2009). In addition to PQS, dioxygenases AqdC1 and AqdC2 from *R. erythropolis* (Müller, Birmes, Rückert, Kalinowski, & Fetzner, 2015) are capable of inactivating 2-heptyl-4(1H)-quinolone (HHQ), which is a precursor of PQS synthesis that also has activity in this *P. aeruginosa* QS system. Recently, dioxygenases active on PQS have been characterized in *Nocardia farcinica* and *Streptomyces bingchenggensis* (Arranz San Martín, Vogel, Wullich, Quax, & Fetzner, 2022). It is interesting to note that other modifications of these molecules have also been reported. For instance, a vanadium-dependent haloperoxidase from *Microbulbifer* sp. HZ11 can brominate HHQ (Ritzmann et al., 2019). However, a loss of QS activity of this modified compound has not been reported.

Together with AHLs, AI-2 is one of the QS signals that has received much attention. First described in *V. harveyi* (Bassler, Wright, & Silverman, 1994), QS systems based on AI-2 have been described in several gram-positive and gram-negative bacteria (Pereira, Thompson, & Xavier, 2013). Surprisingly, the enzymatic inactivation of AI-2 has remained largely unexplored, though the capacity to inactivate this QS signal seems to be present in several microorganisms (Xu, Cho, Ng, Huang, & Ng, 2022). An interesting report showed that the LsrK kinase from *E. coli* can phosphorylate AI-2. The resulting phospho-AI-2 is spontaneously degraded to 2-phosphoglycolic acid, which cannot participate in the QS system (Roy, Fernandes, Tsao, & Bentley, 2010).

6.5   ECOLOGICAL RELEVANCE OF QUORUM QUENCHING

The examples of AHL degradation activities described earlier show that QQ enzymes are widespread in the natural environment. The necessity of new strategies for fighting infections has enormously driven the search for new QQ enzymes with particular properties. Unlike QS inhibitor compounds, QQ enzymes are significantly more potent than them and lack their cytotoxicity (Guendouze et al., 2017). Several industrial applications based on QQ enzymes have also been developed, in particular those related to antifouling strategies (Huang et al., 2016). In contrast, relatively little is known about the implications of QQ in nature. QS is more than a simple communication mechanism for the signaling cells. QS molecules are multifunctional, can exert detrimental effects on other organisms, and, in general, have broader ecological relevance. Relatively few reports have analyzed the "natural" relevance of the QQ phenomenon. However, as will be discussed in the following sections, the conclusions presented in those reports from specific cases can be extrapolated to broader scenarios.

6.5.1   QQ as a Strategy for Niche Colonization

Bacillus thuringiensis is an endospore-forming gram-positive bacterium largely utilized as a biocontrol agent due to its capacity to produce Cry and Cyt toxins that lyse midgut cells of Lepidoptera, Coleoptera, and Diptera (Bravo, Gill, & Soberón, 2007). Beyond this important biotechnological application, *B. thuringiensis* is prevalent in soils, where a high diversity of microorganisms, some of them also possessing AHL-based QS systems, are also present. AiiA lactonase from *B. thuringiensis*, one of the first QQ enzymes to be characterized at a structural level, has broad substrate specificity (Kim et al., 2005; Liu et al., 2005). Several reports have shown the potentiality of AiiA to interfere with QS systems of phytopathogens and, in consequence, the virulence (S.-J. Park, Park, Ryu, Park, & Lee, 2008). However, AiiA has a relevant role in the ecology of *B. thuringiensis*. The analysis of a Δ *aiiA* mutant of *B. thuringiensis* showed a lower capacity for colonizing the rhizosphere of pepper roots. Indeed, 30 days after the inoculation of the strains, the population of the mutant was more than 1100-fold lower than the wild type (S.-J. Park et al., 2008). To date, it is not clear how AiiA increases the colonization of *B. thuringiensis*. The relationship between the production of AHLs and the biofilm formation in the rhizosphere-associated bacteria could explain, at least partially, the lower competition capacities of *B. thuringiensis* Δ *aiiA*. Supporting this hypothesis, it was recently reported that the lactonase YtnP from *B. subtilis* strain UD1022 quenches the QS of *Sinorhizobium meliloti* strain Rm8530 (Rosier, Beauregard, & Bais, 2020). QS is involved in the regulation of several relevant traits in *S. meliloti* 8530, including the production of exopolysaccharide II required for symbiosis with the plant host (Rinaudi & González, 2009). The co-inoculation of *Medicago truncatula* with *B. subtilis* UD1022 and *S. meliloti* Rm8530 causes an altered nodulation of the plant, which can be correlated with the lower biofilm production by Rm8530 and the degradation of its QS molecules by YtnP from UD1022 (Rosier et al., 2020). However, it has to be remembered that in nature, microorganisms are not found as pure or dual cultures, but form complex multispecies communities. Considering this heterogeneity, it is interesting to note how the presence of a QQ activity may alter the microbiota. Utilizing a recirculating system, researchers managed to pump a diluted culture medium through silica beads containing SsoPox W263I to study the influence of the QQ activity on the profile of a soil microbial community and its biofilm formation (Schwab et al., 2019). SsoPox W263I is a derivative of the wild-type SsoPox lactonase from *S. acidocaldarius* (Bzdrenga et al., 2014). Results showed that the enzyme decreases the biofilm formation and alters the composition of the community. Changes were observed not only in genera reported as AHL producers (e.g., *Pseudomonas* and *Aeromonas*) but also in non-AHL producers, like *Clostridium* (Schwab et al., 2019).

Other factors related to microbial interactions can also be involved. It is plausible that the QQ activity of a particular microorganism modifies the QS regulatory mechanism of others, altering their physiology and the microbial interactions they are involved in. This could lead to a modulation of the colonization of the host and the associated microbiota. *Lysobacter daejeonensis* strain GH1-9 is a plant-beneficial rhizobacterium that colonizes the roots of tobacco plants. Its genome lacks a *luxI* homologue for the synthesis of AHLs but harbors a *luxR* gene, which suggests the capacity to bind and respond to AHLs produced by neighbor bacteria in the rhizosphere (Bejarano, Perazzolli, Pertot, & Puopolo, 2021). A mixture of AHLs (C6-HSL, 3OC8-HSL, and 3OC12-HSL) produces a modification in the antimicrobial activities of *L. daejeonensis* GH1-9. In addition, 20 and 4 genes are up- and downregulated, respectively, after exposure to AHLs (Bejarano et al., 2021). Similar behavior can be expected from other inhabitants of the root surfaces.

The QQ activity of *R. erythropolis* illustrates the relevance of AHL inactivation in the biocontrol potential of this bacterium, not only directly through the interference in the virulence of phytopathogens but also indirectly for the colonizer of a niche. *R. erythropolis* strain R138 is a versatile microorganism with several biotechnological applications. One is the inhibition of phytopathogens like *P. atrosepticum*, which utilizes QS to regulate the expression of several exoenzymes required for the colonization and maceration of plant tissues and for obtaining nutrients. The QQ activity of *R. erythropolis* R138 is partially due to the QsdA lactonase enzyme coded in the *qsd* operon together with *qsdC*, which codes for the fatty acyl-CoA ligase QsdC (Kwasiborski, Mondy, Beury-Cirou, & Faure, 2014). In addition, an amidase coded outside the *qsd* operon also provides QQ activity to *R. erythropolis* R138 (Latour, Barbey, Chane, Groboillot, & Burini, 2013). The amidase cleaves the AHLs produced by a phytopathogen with the concomitant production of the homoserine lactone ring. This gamma-lactone is bound by the TerR-family transcriptional repressor QsdR, which allows the expression of the *qsd* operon. In turn, the lactonase QsdA hydrolyzes the lactone ring of AHLs (Barbey et al., 2018). Co-inoculation experiments showed that *R. erythropolis* R138 quenches the QS activity of *P. atrosepticum*. In addition, the presence of the phytopathogen is also reduced, probably as a consequence of a reduced amount of nutrients due to the lack of enzyme production (Chane et al., 2019).

6.5.2 QQ as a Regulatory Mechanism of QS

As previously mentioned in this work, the paradigm QS system is that of *V. fischeri*. The colonization of the symbiosis organs in certain squid and fish allows the increase in the population density and, in consequence, the concentration of the QS signals. The attainment of the threshold concentration is the key event permitting the expression of the *lux* operon, the autoinduction loop, and the "switch-on" of the bioluminescence production. However, as any other regulatory mechanism, QS requires its "switching-off." In *V. fischeri*, this step is naturally produced when the bacterium is free in seawater and, high cell densities are usually not attained. Other microorganisms have developed QQ-based strategies for switching-off their QS systems. Probably, *A. fabrum* is one of the best described examples.

- *A. fabrum* is considered one of the most relevant phytopathogens (Mansfield et al., 2012). Most of the isolates are commensal; however, those harboring the oncogenic pTi plasmid cause the characteristic crown gall tumors in dicotyledonous plants. The *A. fabrum* QS system is not directly involved in the virulence but in the conjugation of pTi (Hwang, Cook, & Farrand, 1995).

The characterization of the different layers of regulation in the *A. fabrum* QS system revealed the presence of two enzymes with QQ activities. Coded in the pAt plasmid as part of the *attKLM* operon, AttM is a lactonase of the Zn-hydrolase family, which is active on 3OC8-HSL (Aurélien Carlier, Chevrot, Dessaux, & Faure, 2004). Compounds like gamma-aminobutyrate (GABA), gamma-butyrolactone (GBL), and salicylic acid are accumulated in the characteristic crown gall tumors. These compounds induce the expression of *attM*, whose product hydrolyzes not only 3OC8-HSL but also converts GBL to gamma-hydroxybutyrate (Haudecoeur et al., 2009). AiiB, coded in the pTi plasmid, is also a lactonase of the same Zn-hydrolase family (A Carlier et al., 2003). AiiB is also active on 3OC8-HSL but, in contrast to AttM, is not active on GBL (Haudecoeur et al., 2009). Another important difference is the plant compounds that induce the *aiiB* expression. In this case, conjugative opines agrocinopines A and B synthesized from the agrobacterial T-DNA inserted in the plant genome upregulate *aiiB* (Haudecoeur et al., 2009). Agrocinopines A and B are required to modify the activity of AccR (Beck von Bodman, Hayman, & Farrand, 1992), a repressor of the *traR* gene. TraR is the LuxR homologue in *A. fabrum* that, after binding 3OC8-HSL, overexpresses the *traI* synthase gene (L. H. Zhang & Kerr, 1991). TraR also directs the synthesis of the conjugative machinery that allows the transfer of pTi plasmids to neighbor agrobacteria that lack this oncogenic plasmid (L. H. Zhang & Kerr, 1991). In this way, plant compounds modify the conjugative transfer of pTi through the expression of the lactonase coding genes *attM* and *aiiB* and, in consequence, the levels 3OC8-HSL.

The QQ mechanisms of *P. aeruginosa* is another interesting example of the involvement of QQ in the regulation of the respective QS system. PvdQ, QuiP, and HacB acylases decrease the levels of 3OC12-HSL when *P. aeruginosa* is grown in rich media, the latter being the main QQ enzyme responsible for the attenuation of the AHL levels under that culture conditions (Utari, Vogel, & Quax, 2017). In contrast, PvdQ seems to be more relevant in the utilization of AHLs as a carbon source, as discussed later.

6.5.3 QQ AS A DETOXIFYING MECHANISM

QS signals evolved to provide bacteria with information. Though largely present in the scientific literature that the information is the cell density, this point is still a matter of debate. Several reports suggest that microorganisms could be utilizing this particular sensing to obtain other kinds of information from the environment, including diffusion rates (Redfield, 2002) and the spatial distribution of the cells (Alberghini et al., 2009). Beyond those scientific discussions, the biological activity of the signal molecules is not argued. Concerning this point, it is to highlight that AHLs possess other biological activities beyond microbial signaling. Two aspects of the toxicity of AHLs and their relationship with QQ will be discussed.

An early report showed that 3OHC14:1-HSL (an unsaturated derivative of 3OHC14-HSL) from *Rhizobium leguminosarum* bv. *viciae* strain RBL1390 could act as a bacteriocin inhibiting the growth of the closely related *R. leguminosarum* bv. *viciae* strain 248 (Jan Schripsema et al., 1996). The effect was indeed due to an induction to enter into the stationary phase. However, that was probably one of the first observations suggesting other particular physiological functions for AHLs. Later, a true antimicrobial activity was discovered for AHLs. Under certain conditions, in particular in aqueous environments, the lactone ring of 3-oxo substituted AHLs with long side chains, like 3OC12-HSL, spontaneously opens forming two compounds: 3OC12-homoserine and 3-(1-hydroxydecylidene)-5-(2-hydroxyethyl) pyrrolidine-2,4-dione, a tetramic-acid derivative (Kaufmann et al., 2005). The former is the same obtained under the action of lactonases (see earlier). The latter is a tetramic-acid derivative with antimicrobial activities against gram-positive bacteria but not gram-negative bacteria, similar to other related compounds. It also forms complexes with iron in a ratio of 3:1 (Kaufmann et al., 2005). It has been suggested that the QQ enzymes protect bacteria from this toxic compound. In agreement with this hypothesis, it has been reported that a Δ *aiiA* mutant of *B. thuringiensis*, which lacks QQ activity, has a lower survival rate than the wild-type strain when it co-cultures with *E. carotovora* that produces AHLs (S.-J. Park et al., 2008).

6.5.4   QQ AS ALTERNATIVE FOR OBTAINING NUTRIENTS

Several reports indicate that QS signals may serve as a source of nitrogen and/or carbon and an energy reservoir. QS signals are chemically composed of carbon and other elements, including oxygen and nitrogen, all of which can serve as a source of nutrients. From a "signaling" point of view, the metabolism of a QS signal undoubtedly results in the loss of the signal for the microorganism that perceives it and, in consequence, in the establishment of a QQ phenomenon. The first report showing a relationship of QQ as a means for obtaining nutrients was related to the growth of *Variovorax paradoxus* with AHLs as the sole source of nitrogen and energy (Leadbetter & Greenberg, 2000). *V. paradoxus* is a beta-proteobacterium commonly found in close associations with plants where it exerts a growth-promotion effect. Due to its versatile metabolic capabilities, the role of this bacterium in soils is relevant for the degradation of compounds produced by other microorganisms and the cycle of nutrients. For instance, *V. paradoxus* can metabolize sulfonates and is then part of the sulfur cycle in agricultural soils (Schmalenberger et al., 2008). Analyzing the susceptibility of AHLs to biotic inactivation, *V. paradoxus* strain VAI-C was isolated from a turf soil employing a mineral medium supplemented with 3OC6-HSL (500 µg mL^{-1}) as the sole nitrogen and energy source. *V. paradoxus* VAI-C could also utilize a broad spectrum of AHLs, those with longer acyl side chains being the ones allowing the higher molar growth yields. It was shown that the AHL is cleaved by acylase activity and the acyl chain is metabolized for energy generation (Leadbetter & Greenberg, 2000). An AhlD acylase was later identified in *Arthrobacter* sp. strain IBN110, and was shown to degrade several AHLs, including C6-HSL, 3OC6-HSL, C8-HSL, and C12-HSL (S. Y. Park et al., 2003). Interestingly, it was shown that *Arthrobacter* sp. VAI-A could utilize the homoserine lactone ring left behind by the metabolism of the AHL by *V. paradoxus* VAI-C (Flagan, Ching, & Leadbetter, 2003). Later, other species utilizing AHLs as the nutrient source were also reported. For instance, *Nocardioides kongjuensis* A2-4 and *Chryseobacterium* sp. EM10 can also grow in a minima media with AHLs as the sole carbon source (Mahmoudi et al., 2011; Yoon et al., 2006). To note, the biotic mineralization of AHLs seems to be highly prevalent at least in certain niches. The utilization of

AHLs as nutrient sources has been largely discussed in the scientific literature since the early observations of the QQ phenomenon. Probably the main point of "conflict" is the low concentrations at which these QS signals are normally present. The activation of the *lux* operon in *V. fischeri*, for instance, only requires nanomolar concentrations of 3OC6-HSL (Kaplan & Greenberg, 1985). However, concentrations of AHLs 1000-fold higher can also be attained in certain niches (Flagan et al., 2003). In consequence, the growth of AHLs as the source of nutrients with the consequent interference with the QS signaling is highly plausible in the environment. In soil, for instance, C6-HSL and 3OC6-HSL are rapidly degraded by the microbial metabolism (Y.-J. Wang & Leadbetter, 2005).

6.6 FINAL REMARKS

Since the first description of a QS system in *V. fischeri*, a long road has been traveled in the field of microbial interactions by means of chemical signaling. The potentiality of a microorganism to interfere with these mechanisms represented a relevant hallmark for both the ecological and biotechnological implications. The first description of a QQ activity in a microorganism was already accompanied by its application in the prevention of a disease by a phytopathogen (Dong et al., 2000). However, the complete ecological relevance of QQ has still to be unveiled. For instance, whether nonproducing AHL microorganisms have evolved their QQ activities specifically to interfere with AHL-signaling bacteria or whether it is just a fortuitous cross-reaction of a biochemical pathway, remains to be elucidated. The advent of new technologies will allow us to respond to the ecological questions about QQ in nature.

ACKNOWLEDGMENTS

This work was supported by the Consejo Nacional de Investigaciones Científicas y Técnicas (CONICET, PIP 2015-0946, PIP 2021-2436, PUE 22920160100012CO), Agencia Nacional de Promoción Científica y Tecnológica (PICT 2016 no. 0532; PICT 2019 no. 03336), and Secretaría de Ciencia, Arte e Innovación Tecnológica from the Universidad Nacional de Tucumán (PIUNT D742 and D764).

REFERENCES

Alberghini, S., Polone, E., Corich, V., Carlot, M., Seno, F., Trovato, A., & Squartini, A. (2009). Consequences of relative cellular positioning on quorum sensing and bacterial cell-to-cell communication. *FEMS Microbiology Letters*, *292*(2), 149–161. https://doi .org/10.1111/j.1574-6968.2008.01478.x

Ali, L., Goraya, M. U., Arafat, Y., Ajmal, M., Chen, J.-L., & Yu, D. (2017). Molecular mechanism of quorum-sensing in *Enterococcus faecalis*: Its role in virulence and therapeutic approaches. *International Journal of Molecular Sciences*, *18*(5), 960. https://doi.org /10.3390/ijms18050960

Arranz San Martín, A., Vogel, J., Wullich, S. C., Quax, W. J., & Fetzner, S. (2022). Enzyme-mediated quenching of the Pseudomonas Quinolone Signal (PQS): A comparison between naturally occurring and engineered PQS-cleaving dioxygenases. *Biomolecules*, *12*(2), 170. https://doi.org/10.3390/biom12020170

Barbey, C., Chane, A., Burini, J.-F., Maillot, O., Merieau, A., Gallique, M., … Latour, X. (2018). A rhodococcal transcriptional regulatory mechanism detects the common lactone ring of AHL quorum-sensing signals and triggers the quorum-quenching response. *Frontiers in Microbiology, 9*, 2800. https://doi.org/10.3389/fmicb.2018.02800

Bassler, B. L., Wright, M., & Silverman, M. R. (1994). Multiple signalling systems controlling expression of luminescence in *Vibrio harveyi*: Sequence and function of genes encoding a second sensory pathway. *Molecular Microbiology, 13*(2), 273–286. https://doi.org/10.1111/j.1365-2958.1994.tb00422.x

Beck von Bodman, S., Hayman, G. T., & Farrand, S. K. (1992). Opine catabolism and conjugal transfer of the nopaline Ti plasmid pTiC58 are coordinately regulated by a single repressor. *Proceedings of the National Academy of Sciences of the United States of America, 89*(2), 643–647. https://doi.org/10.1073/pnas.89.2.643

Bejarano, A., Perazzolli, M., Pertot, I., & Puopolo, G. (2021). The perception of rhizosphere bacterial communication signals leads to transcriptome reprogramming in *Lysobacter capsici* AZ78, a plant beneficial bacterium. *Frontiers in Microbiology, 12*, 725403. https://doi.org/10.3389/fmicb.2021.725403

Bergonzi, C., Schwab, M., & Elias, M. (2016). The quorum-quenching lactonase from *Geobacillus caldoxylosilyticus*: Purification, characterization, crystallization and crystallographic analysis. *Acta Crystallographica. Section F, Structural Biology Communications, 72*(Pt 9), 681–686. https://doi.org/10.1107/S2053230X16011821

Bijtenhoorn, P., Mayerhofer, H., Müller-Dieckmann, J., Utpatel, C., Schipper, C., Hornung, C., … Streit, W. R. (2011). A novel metagenomic short-chain dehydrogenase/reductase attenuates *Pseudomonas aeruginosa* biofilm formation and virulence on *Caenorhabditis elegans. PloS One, 6*(10), e26278. https://doi.org/10.1371/journal.pone.0026278

Bokhove, M., Nadal, P., Quax, W. J., & Dijkstra, B. W. (2009). The quorum-quenching *N*-acyl homoserine lactone acylase PvdQ is an Ntn-hydrolase with an unusual substrate-binding pocket. *Proceedings of the National Academy of Sciences of the United States of America, 107*, 689–691. https://doi.org/10.1073/pnas.0911839107

Bravo, A., Gill, S. S., & Soberón, M. (2007). Mode of action of *Bacillus thuringiensis* Cry and Cyt toxins and their potential for insect control. *Toxicon, 49*(4), 423–435. https://doi.org/10.1016/j.toxicon.2006.11.022

Bzdrenga, J., Hiblot, J., Gotthard, G., Champion, C., Elias, M., & Chabriere, E. (2014). SacPox from the thermoacidophilic crenarchaeon *Sulfolobus acidocaldarius* is a proficient lactonase. *BMC Research Notes, 7*, 333. https://doi.org/10.1186/1756-0500-7-333

Carlier, A., Uroz, S., Smadja, B., Fray, R., Latour, X., Dessaux, Y., & Faure, D. (2003). The Ti plasmid of *Agrobacterium tumefaciens* harbors an *attM*-paralogous gene, *aiiB*, also encoding *N*-acyl homoserine lactonase activity. *Applied and Environmental Microbiology, 69*(8), 4989–4993. Retrieved from http://www.ncbi.nlm.nih.gov/pubmed/12902298

Carlier, A., Chevrot, R., Dessaux, Y., & Faure, D. (2004). The assimilation of gamma-butyrolactone in *Agrobacterium tumefaciens* C58 interferes with the accumulation of the *N*-acyl-homoserine lactone signal. *Molecular Plant-Microbe Interactions, 17*(9), 951–957. https://doi.org/10.1094/MPMI.2004.17.9.951

Chan, K.-G., Atkinson, S., Mathee, K., Sam, C.-K., Chhabra, S. R., Cámara, M., … Williams, P. (2011). Characterization of *N*-acylhomoserine lactone-degrading bacteria associated with the *Zingiber officinale* (ginger) rhizosphere: Co-existence of quorum quenching and quorum sensing in *Acinetobacter* and *Burkholderia. BMC Microbiology, 11*, 51. https://doi.org/10.1186/1471-2180-11-51

Chane, A., Barbey, C., Robert, M., Merieau, A., Konto-Ghiorghi, Y., Beury-Cirou, A., … Latour, X. (2019). Biocontrol of soft rot: Confocal microscopy highlights virulent pectobacterial communication and its jamming by rhodococcal quorum-quenching. *Molecular Plant-Microbe Interactions*, *32*(7), 802–812. https://doi.org/10.1094/MPMI -11-18-0314-R

Chowdhary, P. K., Keshavan, N., Nguyen, H. Q., Peterson, J. A., González, J. E., & Haines, D. C. (2007). *Bacillus megaterium* CYP102A1 oxidation of acyl homoserine lactones and acyl homoserines. *Biochemistry*, *46*(50), 14429–14437. https://doi.org/10.1021/ bi701945j

Clinton, A., & Rumbaugh, K. P. (2016). Interspecies and interkingdom signaling via quorum signals. *Israel Journal of Chemistry*, *56*(5), 265–272. https://doi.org/10.1002/ijch .201400132

Czajkowski, R., Krzyzanowska, D., Karczewska, J., Atkinson, S., Przysowa, J., Lojkowska, E., … Jafra, S. (2011). Inactivation of AHLs by *Ochrobactrum* sp. A44 depends on the activity of a novel class of AHL acylase. *Environmental Microbiology Reports*, *3*(1), 59–68. https://doi.org/10.1111/j.1758-2229.2010.00188.x

Dandela, R., Mantin, D., Cravatt, B. F., Rayo, J., & Meijler, M. M. (2018). Proteome-wide mapping of PQS-interacting proteins in *Pseudomonas aeruginosa*. *Chemical Science*, *9*(8), 2290–2294. https://doi.org/10.1039/c7sc04287f

Diggle, S. P., Lumjiaktase, P., Dipilato, F., Winzer, K., Kunakorn, M., Barrett, D. A., … Williams, P. (2006). Functional genetic analysis reveals a 2-Alkyl-4-quinolone signaling system in the human pathogen *Burkholderia pseudomallei* and related bacteria. *Chemistry & Biology*, *13*(7), 701–710. https://doi.org/10.1016/j.chembiol.2006.05.006

Diggle, S. P., Matthijs, S., Wright, V. J., Fletcher, M. P., Chhabra, S. R., Lamont, I. L., … Williams, P. (2007). The *Pseudomonas aeruginosa* 4-quinolone signal molecules HHQ and PQS play multifunctional roles in quorum sensing and iron entrapment. *Chemistry & Biology*, *14*(1), 87–96. https://doi.org/10.1016/j.chembiol.2006.11.014

Dong, Y. H., Wang, L. H., Xu, J. L., Zhang, H. B., Zhang, X. F., & Zhang, L. H. (2001). Quenching quorum-sensing-dependent bacterial infection by an *N*-acyl homoserine lactonase. *Nature*, *411*(6839), 813–817. https://doi.org/10.1038/35081101

Dong, Y. H., Xu, J. L., Li, X. Z., & Zhang, L. H. (2000). AiiA, an enzyme that inactivates the acylhomoserine lactone quorum-sensing signal and attenuates the virulence of *Erwinia carotovora*. *Proceedings of the National Academy of Sciences of the United States of America*, *97*(7), 3526–3531. https://doi.org/10.1073/pnas.060023897

Dow, J. M., Feng, J.-X., Barber, C. E., Tang, J.-L., & Daniels, M. J. (2000). Novel genes involved in the regulation of pathogenicity factor production within the rpf gene cluster of *Xanthomonas campestris*. *Microbiology*, *146*, 885–891. https://doi.org/10.1099 /00221287-146-4-885

Draganov, D. I., Teiber, J. F., Speelman, A., Osawa, Y., Sunahara, R., & La Du, B. N. (2005). Human paraoxonases (PON1, PON2, and PON3) are lactonases with overlapping and distinct substrate specificities. *Journal of Lipid Research*, *46*(6), 1239–1247. https://doi .org/10.1194/jlr.M400511-JLR200

Flagan, S., Ching, W.-K., & Leadbetter, J. R. (2003). *Arthrobacter* strain VAI-A utilizes acyl-homoserine lactone inactivation products and stimulates quorum signal biodegradation by *Variovorax paradoxus*. *Applied and Environmental Microbiology*, *69*(2), 909–916. https://doi.org/10.1128/AEM.69.2.909-916.2003

Flavier, A. B., Clough, S. J., Schell, M. A., & Denny, T. P. (1997). Identification of 3-hydroxypalmitic acid methyl ester as a novel autoregulator controlling virulence in *Ralstonia solanacearum*. *Molecular Microbiology*, *26*(2), 251–259.

Fuqua, C., & Greenberg, E. P. (2002). Listening in on bacteria: Acyl-homoserine lactone signalling. *Nature Reviews. Molecular Cell Biology*, *3*(9), 685–695. https://doi.org/10.1038/nrm907

Givskov, M., de Nys, R., Manefield, M., Gram, L., Maximilien, R., Eberl, L., ... Kjelleberg, S. (1996). Eukaryotic interference with homoserine lactone-mediated prokaryotic signalling. *Journal of Bacteriology*, *178*(22), 6618–6622. https://doi.org/10.1128/jb.178.22.6618-6622.1996

Grandclément, C., Tannières, M., Moréra, S., Dessaux, Y., & Faure, D. (2016). Quorum quenching: Role in nature and applied developments. *FEMS Microbiology Reviews*, *40*(1), 86–116. https://doi.org/10.1093/femsre/fuv038

Guendouze, A., Plener, L., Bzdrenga, J., Jacquet, P., Rémy, B., Elias, M., ... Chabrière, E. (2017). Effect of quorum quenching lactonase in clinical isolates of *Pseudomonas aeruginosa* and comparison with quorum sensing inhibitors. *Frontiers in Microbiology*, *8*, 227. https://doi.org/10.3389/fmicb.2017.00227

Haramati, R., Dor, S., Gurevich, D., Levy, D., Freund, D., Rytwo, G., ... Afriat-Jurnou, L. (2022). Mining marine metagenomes revealed a quorum-quenching lactonase with improved biochemical properties that inhibits the food spoilage bacterium *Pseudomonas fluorescens*. *Applied and Environmental Microbiology*, *88*(4), e0168021. https://doi.org/10.1128/AEM.01680-21

Haudecoeur, E., Tannières, M., Cirou, A., Raffoux, A., Dessaux, Y., & Faure, D. (2009). Different regulation and roles of lactonases AiiB and AttM in *Agrobacterium tumefaciens* C58. *Molecular Plant-Microbe Interactions*, *22*(5), 529–537.

Huang, J., Shi, Y., Zeng, G., Gu, Y., Chen, G., Shi, L., ... Zhou, J. (2016). Acyl-homoserine lactone-based quorum sensing and quorum quenching hold promise to determine the performance of biological wastewater treatments: An overview. *Chemosphere*, *157*, 137–151. https://doi.org/10.1016/j.chemosphere.2016.05.032

Hwang, I., Cook, D. M., & Farrand, S. K. (1995). A new regulatory element modulates homoserine lactone-mediated autoinduction of Ti plasmid conjugal transfer. *Journal of Bacteriology*, *177*(2), 449–458.

Jagtap, S. S., Bedekar, A. A., & Rao, C. V. (2020). Quorum sensing in yeast. In *Quorum Sensing: Microbial Rules of Life* (pp. 235–250). https://doi.org/10.1021/bk-2020-1374.ch013

Ji, G., Beavis, R. C., & Novick, R. P. (1995). Cell density control of staphylococcal virulence mediated by an octapeptide pheromone. *Proceedings of the National Academy of Sciences of the United States of America*, *92*(26), 12055–12059. https://doi.org/10.1073/pnas.92.26.12055

Kai, K., Ohnishi, H., Shimatani, M., Ishikawa, S., Mori, Y., Kiba, A., ... Hikichi, Y. (2015). Methyl 3-hydroxymyristate, a diffusible signal mediating *phc* quorum sensing in *Ralstonia solanacearum*. *Chembiochem*, *16*(16), 2309–2318. https://doi.org/10.1002/cbic.201500456

Kalamara, M., Spacapan, M., Mandic-Mulec, I., & Stanley-Wall, N. R. (2018). Social behaviours by *Bacillus subtilis*: Quorum sensing, kin discrimination and beyond. *Molecular Microbiology*, *110*(6), 863–878. https://doi.org/10.1111/mmi.14127

Kaplan, H. B., & Greenberg, E. P. (1985). Diffusion of autoinducer is involved in regulation of the *Vibrio fischeri* luminescence system. *Journal of Bacteriology*, *163*(3), 1210–1214. https://doi.org/10.1128/jb.163.3.1210-1214.1985

Kaufmann, G. F., Sartorio, R., Lee, S.-H., Rogers, C. J., Meijler, M. M., Moss, J. A., ... Janda, K. D. (2005). Revisiting quorum sensing: Discovery of additional chemical and biological functions for 3-oxo-*N*-acylhomoserine lactones. *Proceedings of the National Academy of Sciences of the United States of America*, *102*(2), 309–314. https://doi.org/10.1073/pnas.0408639102

Kim, M. H., Choi, W.-C., Kang, H. O., Lee, J. S., Kang, B. S., Kim, K.-J., … Lee, J.-K. (2005). The molecular structure and catalytic mechanism of a quorum-quenching *N*-acyl-L-homoserine lactone hydrolase. *Proceedings of the National Academy of Sciences of the United States of America*, *102*(49), 17606–17611. https://doi.org/10.1073/pnas .0504996102

Krysciak, D., Schmeisser, C., Preuß, S., Riethausen, J., Quitschau, M., Grond, S., & Streit, W. R. (2011). Involvement of multiple loci in quorum quenching of autoinducer I molecules in the nitrogen-fixing symbiont *Rhizobium* (*Sinorhizobium*) sp. strain NGR234. *Applied and Environmental Microbiology*, *77*(15), 5089–5099. https://doi.org/10.1128 /AEM.00112-11

Kwasiborski, A., Mondy, S., Beury-Cirou, A., & Faure, D. (2014). Genome sequence of the quorum-quenching *Rhodococcus erythropolis* strain R138. *Genome Announcements*, *2*(2), e00224–14. https://doi.org/10.1128/genomeA.00224-14

Latour, X., Barbey, C., Chane, A., Groboillot, A., & Burini, J.-F. (2013). *Rhodococcus erythropolis* and its γ-lactone catabolic pathway: An unusual biocontrol system that disrupts pathogen quorum sensing communication. *Agronomy*, *3*(4), 816–838. https://doi.org/10 .3390/agronomy3040816

Leadbetter, J. R., & Greenberg, E. P. (2000). Metabolism of acyl-homoserine lactone quorum-sensing signals by *Variovorax paradoxus*. *Journal of Bacteriology*, *182*(24), 6921–6926.

Lee, M. H., Khan, R., Tao, W., Choi, K., Lee, S. Y., Lee, J. W., … Lee, S.-W. (2018). Soil metagenome-derived 3-hydroxypalmitic acid methyl ester hydrolases suppress extracellular polysaccharide production in *Ralstonia solanacearum*. *Journal of Biotechnology*, *270*, 30–38. https://doi.org/10.1016/j.jbiotec.2018.01.023

Lin, Y.-H., Xu, J.-L., Hu, J., Wang, L.-H., Ong, S. L., Leadbetter, J. R., & Zhang, L.-H. (2003). Acyl-homoserine lactone acylase from *Ralstonia* strain XJ12B represents a novel and potent class of quorum-quenching enzymes. *Molecular Microbiology*, *47*(3), 849–860.

Lina, G., Jarraud, S., Ji, G., Greenland, T., Pedraza, A., Etienne, J., … Vandenesch, F. (1998). Transmembrane topology and histidine protein kinase activity of AgrC, the agr signal receptor in *Staphylococcus aureus*. *Molecular Microbiology*, *28*(3), 655–662. https:// doi.org/10.1046/j.1365-2958.1998.00830.x

Liu, D., Lepore, B. W., Petsko, G. A., Thomas, P. W., Stone, E. M., Fast, W., & Ringe, D. (2005). Three-dimensional structure of the quorum-quenching *N*-acyl homoserine lactone hydrolase from *Bacillus thuringiensis*. *Proceedings of the National Academy of Sciences of the United States of America*, *102*(33), 11882–11887. https://doi.org/10.1073 /pnas.0505255102

Liu, D., Thomas, P. W., Momb, J., Hoang, Q. Q., Petsko, G. A., Ringe, D., & Fast, W. (2007). Structure and specificity of a quorum-quenching lactonase (AiiB) from *Agrobacterium tumefaciens*. *Biochemistry*, *46*(42), 11789–11799. https://doi.org/10.1021/bi7012849

Ma, M., Li, J., & McClane, B. A. (2015). Structure-function analysis of peptide signaling in the *Clostridium perfringens* Agr-like quorum sensing system. *Journal of Bacteriology*, *197*(10), 1807–1818. https://doi.org/10.1128/JB.02614-14

Mahmoudi, E., Ahmadi, A., Sayed-Tabatabaei, B. E., Ghobadi, C., Akhavan, A., Hasanzadeh, N., & Venturi, V. (2011). A novel ahl-degrading rhizobacterium quenches the virulence of pectobacterium atrosepticum on potato plant. *Journal of Plant Pathology*, *93*, 587–594. https://doi.org/10.4454/jpp.v93i3.3641

Manefield, M., Welch, M., Givskov, M., Salmond, G. P., & Kjelleberg, S. (2001). Halogenated furanones from the red alga, *Delisea pulchra*, inhibit carbapenem antibiotic synthesis and exoenzyme virulence factor production in the phytopathogen *Erwinia carotovora*. *FEMS Microbiology Letters*, *205*(1), 131–138. https://doi.org/10.1111/j.1574-6968.2001 .tb10936.x

Manefield, M., Rasmussen, T. B., Henzter, M., Andersen, J. B., Steinberg, P., Kjelleberg, S., & Givskov, M. (2002). Halogenated furanones inhibit quorum sensing through accelerated LuxR turnover. *Microbiology, 148*(Pt 4), 1119–1127. https://doi.org/10.1099/00221287-148-4-1119

Mansfield, J., Genin, S., Magori, S., Citovsky, V., Sriariyanum, M., Ronald, P., ... Foster, G. D. (2012). Top 10 plant pathogenic bacteria in molecular plant pathology. *Molecular Plant Pathology, 13*(6), 614–629. https://doi.org/10.1111/j.1364-3703.2012.00804.x

McClean, K., Winson, M., Fish, L., Taylor, A., Chhabra, S., Cámara, C., ... Williams, P. (1997). Quorum sensing and *Chromobacterium violaceum*: Exploitation of violacein production and inhibition for the detection of *N*-acylhomoserine lactones. *Microbiology, 143*, 3703–3711.

Mei, G.-Y., Yan, X.-X., Turak, A., Luo, Z.-Q., & Zhang, L.-Q. (2010). AidH, an alpha/beta-hydrolase fold family member from an *Ochrobactrum* sp. strain, is a novel *N*-acylhomoserine lactonase. *Applied and Environmental Microbiology, 76*(15), 4933–4942. https://doi.org/10.1128/AEM.00477-10

Miller, S. T., Xavier, K. B., Campagna, S. R., Taga, M. E., Semmelhack, M. F., Bassler, B. L., & Hughson, F. M. (2004). *Salmonella typhimurium* recognizes a chemically distinct form of the bacterial Quorum-sensing signal AI-2. *Molecular Cell, 15*(5), 677–687. https://doi.org/10.1016/j.molcel.2004.07.020

Müller, C., Birmes, F. S., Rückert, C., Kalinowski, J., & Fetzner, S. (2015). *Rhodococcus erythropolis* BG43 genes mediating *Pseudomonas aeruginosa* quinolone signal degradation and virulence factor attenuation. *Applied and Environmental Microbiology, 81*(22), 7720–7729. https://doi.org/10.1128/AEM.02145-15

Nealson, K. H. (2020). On the 50th anniversary of the discovery of autoinduction and the ensuing birth of quorum sensing. *Environmental Microbiology, 22*(3), 801–807. https://doi.org/10.1111/1462-2920.14928

Neiditch, M. B., & Hughson, F. M. (2007). The regulation of histidine sensor kinase complexes by quorum sensing signal molecules. *Methods in Enzymology, 423*, 250–263. https://doi.org/10.1016/S0076-6879(07)23011-3

Newman, K. L., Chatterjee, S., Ho, K. A., & Lindow, S. E. (2008). Virulence of plant pathogenic bacteria attenuated by degradation of fatty acid cell-to-cell signaling factors. *Molecular Plant-Microbe Interactions, 21*(3), 326–334. https://doi.org/10.1094/MPMI-21-3-0326

Ng, F. S. W., Wright, D. M., & Seah, S. Y. K. (2011). Characterization of a phosphotriesterase-like lactonase from *Sulfolobus solfataricus* and its immobilization for disruption of quorum sensing. *Applied and Environmental Microbiology, 77*(4), 1181–1186. https://doi.org/10.1128/AEM.01642-10

Ozer, E. A., Pezzulo, A., Shih, D. M., Chun, C., Furlong, C., Lusis, A. J., ... Zabner, J. (2005). Human and murine paraoxonase 1 are host modulators of *Pseudomonas aeruginosa* quorum-sensing. *FEMS Microbiology Letters, 253*(1), 29–37. https://doi.org/10.1016/j.femsle.2005.09.023

Papenfort, K., & Bassler, B. L. (2016). Quorum sensing signal-response systems in Gram-negative bacteria. *Nature Reviews Microbiology, 14*(9), 576–588. https://doi.org/10.1038/nrmicro.2016.89

Park, S. Y., Lee, S. J., Oh, T. K., Oh, J. W., Koo, B. T., Yum, D. Y., & Lee, J. K. (2003). AhlD, an *N*-acylhomoserine lactonase in *Arthrobacter* sp., and predicted homologues in other bacteria. *Microbiology, 149*(6), 1541–1550. https://doi.org/10.1099/mic.0.26269-0

Park, S.-J., Park, S.-Y., Ryu, C.-M., Park, S.-H., & Lee, J.-K. (2008). The role of AiiA, a quorum-quenching enzyme from *Bacillus thuringiensis*, on the rhizosphere competence. *Journal of Microbiology and Biotechnology, 18*(9), 1518–1521.

Parsek, M. R., Val, D. L., Hanzelka, B. L., Cronan, J. E., & Greenberg, E. P. (1999). Acyl homoserine-lactone quorum-sensing signal generation. *Proceedings of the National Academy of Sciences of the United States of America, 96*(8), 4360–4365. https://doi.org /10.1073/pnas.96.8.4360

Pereira, C. S., Thompson, J. A., & Xavier, K. B. (2013). AI-2-mediated signalling in bacteria. *FEMS Microbiology Reviews, 37*(2), 156–181. https://doi.org/10.1111/j.1574-6976.2012 .00345.x

Polkade, A. V., Mantri, S. S., Patwekar, U. J., & Jangid, K. (2016). Quorum sensing: An under-explored phenomenon in the Phylum Actinobacteria. *Frontiers in Microbiology, 7*, 131. https://doi.org/10.3389/fmicb.2016.00131

Pustelny, C., Albers, A., Büldt-Karentzopoulos, K., Parschat, K., Chhabra, S. R., Cámara, M., … Fetzner, S. (2009). Dioxygenase-mediated quenching of quinolone-dependent quorum sensing in *Pseudomonas aeruginosa*. *Chemistry & Biology, 16*(12), 1259–1267. https://doi.org/10.1016/j.chembiol.2009.11.013

Queck, S. Y., Jameson-Lee, M., Villaruz, A. E., Bach, T.-H. L., Khan, B. A., Sturdevant, D. E., … Otto, M. (2008). RNAIII-independent target gene control by the agr Quorum-sensing system: Insight into the evolution of virulence regulation in *Staphylococcus aureus*. *Molecular Cell, 32*(1), 150–158. https://doi.org/10.1016/j.molcel.2008.08.005

Rajput, A., & Kumar, M. (2017a). Computational exploration of putative LuxR Solos in archaea and their functional implications in quorum sensing. *Frontiers in Microbiology, 8*, 798. https://doi.org/10.3389/fmicb.2017.00798

Rajput, A., & Kumar, M. (2017b). In silico analyses of conservational, functional and phylogenetic distribution of the LuxI and LuxR homologs in Gram-positive bacteria. *Scientific Reports, 7*(1), 6969. https://doi.org/10.1038/s41598-017-07241-5

Rampioni, G., Pustelny, C., Fletcher, M. P., Wright, V. J., Bruce, M., Rumbaugh, K. P., … Williams, P. (2010). Transcriptomic analysis reveals a global alkyl-quinolone-independent regulatory role for PqsE in facilitating the environmental adaptation of *Pseudomonas aeruginosa* to plant and animal hosts. *Environmental Microbiology, 12*(6), 1659–1673. https://doi.org/10.1111/j.1462-2920.2010.02214.x

Rasmussen, T. B., Manefield, M., Andersen, J. B., Eberl, L., Anthoni, U., Christophersen, C., … Givskov, M. (2000). How *Delisea pulchra* furanones affect quorum sensing and swarming motility in *Serratia liquefaciens* MG1. *Microbiology, 146*, 3237–3244. https://doi.org/10.1099/00221287-146-12-3237

Redfield, R. J. (2002). Is quorum sensing a side effect of diffusion sensing? *Trends in Microbiology, 10*(8), 365–370. https://doi.org/10.1016/s0966-842x(02)02400-9

Rehman, Z. U., Momin, A. A., Aldehaiman, A., Irum, T., Grünberg, R., & Arold, S. T. (2022). The exceptionally efficient quorum quenching enzyme LrsL suppresses *Pseudomonas aeruginosa* biofilm production. *Frontiers in Microbiology, 13*, 977673. https://doi.org /10.3389/fmicb.2022.977673

Riedel, C. U., Monk, I. R., Casey, P. G., Waidmann, M. S., Gahan, C. G. M., & Hill, C. (2009). AgrD-dependent quorum sensing affects biofilm formation, invasion, virulence and global gene expression profiles in *Listeria monocytogenes*. *Molecular Microbiology, 71*(5), 1177–1189. https://doi.org/10.1111/j.1365-2958.2008.06589.x

Rinaudi, L. V., & González, J. E. (2009). The low-molecular-weight fraction of exopolysaccharide II from *Sinorhizobium meliloti* is a crucial determinant of biofilm formation. *Journal of Bacteriology, 191*(23), 7216–7224. https://doi.org/10.1128/JB.01063-09

Ritzmann, N. H., Mährlein, A., Ernst, S., Hennecke, U., Drees, S. L., & Fetzner, S. (2019). Bromination of alkyl quinolones by *Microbulbifer* sp. HZ11, a marine Gammaproteobacterium, modulates their antibacterial activity. *Environmental Microbiology, 21*(7), 2595–2609. https://doi.org/10.1111/1462-2920.14654

Rosier, A., Beauregard, P. B., & Bais, H. P. (2020). Quorum quenching activity of the PGPR *Bacillus subtilis* UD1022 alters nodulation efficiency of *Sinorhizobium meliloti* on *Medicago truncatula. Frontiers in Microbiology, 11*, 596299. https://doi.org/10.3389/fmicb.2020.596299

Roy, V., Fernandes, R., Tsao, C.-Y., & Bentley, W. E. (2010). Cross species quorum quenching using a native AI-2 processing enzyme. *ACS Chemical Biology, 5*(2), 223–232. https://doi.org/10.1021/cb9002738

Ryan, R. P., An, S., Allan, J. H., McCarthy, Y., & Dow, J. M. (2015). The DSF family of cell–cell signals: An expanding class of bacterial virulence regulators. *PLOS Pathogens, 11*(7), e1004986. https://doi.org/10.1371/journal.ppat.1004986

Saenz, H. L., Augsburger, V., Vuong, C., Jack, R. W., Götz, F., & Otto, M. (2000). Inducible expression and cellular location of AgrB, a protein involved in the maturation of the staphylococcal quorum-sensing pheromone. *Archives of Microbiology, 174*(6), 452–455. https://doi.org/10.1007/s002030000223

Schmalenberger, A., Hodge, S., Bryant, A., Hawkesford, M. J., Singh, B. K., & Kertesz, M. A. (2008). The role of *Variovorax* and other *Comamonadaceae* in sulfur transformations by microbial wheat rhizosphere communities exposed to different sulfur fertilization regimes. *Environmental Microbiology, 10*(6), 1486–1500. https://doi.org/10.1111/j.1462-2920.2007.01564.x

Schripsema, J., De Rudder, K. E. E., Vanvliet, T. B., Lankhorst, P. P., De Vroom, E., Kijne, J. W., & Van Brussel, A. A. N. (1996). Bacteriocin *small* of *Rhizobium leguminosarum* belongs to the class of *N*-acyl-L -homoserine lactone molecules, known as autoinducers and as quorum sensing co-transcription factors. *Journal of Bacteriology, 178*(2), 366–371.

Schwab, M., Bergonzi, C., Sakkos, J., Staley, C., Zhang, Q., Sadowsky, M. J., … Elias, M. (2019). Signal disruption leads to changes in bacterial community population. *Frontiers in Microbiology, 10*, 611. https://doi.org/10.3389/fmicb.2019.00611

Shaw, P. D., Ping, G., Daly, S. L., Cha, C., Cronan, J. E., Rinehart, K. L., & Farrand, S. K. (1997). Detecting and characterizing *N*-acyl-homoserine lactone signal molecules by thin-layer chromatography. *Proceedings of the National Academy of Sciences of the United States of America, 94*(12), 6036–6041. https://doi.org/10.1073/pnas.94.12.6036

Shinohara, M., Nakajima, N., & Uehara, Y. (2007). Purification and characterization of a novel esterase (beta-hydroxypalmitate methyl ester hydrolase) and prevention of the expression of virulence by *Ralstonia solanacearum. Journal of Applied Microbiology, 103*(1), 152–162. https://doi.org/10.1111/j.1365-2672.2006.03222.x

Soukarieh, F., Williams, P., Stocks, M. J., & Cámara, M. (2018). *Pseudomonas aeruginosa* quorum sensing systems as drug discovery targets: Current position and future perspectives. *Journal of Medicinal Chemistry, 61*(23), 10385–10402. https://doi.org/10.1021/acs.jmedchem.8b00540

Surette, M. G., Miller, M. B., & Bassler, B. L. (1999). Quorum sensing in *Escherichia coli, Salmonella typhimurium*, and *Vibrio harveyi*: A new family of genes responsible for autoinducer production. *Proceedings of the National Academy of Sciences of the United States of America, 96*(4), 1639–1644. https://doi.org/10.1073/pnas.96.4.1639

Takano, E., Nihira, T., Hara, Y., Jones, J. J., Gershater, C. J., Yamada, Y., & Bibb, M. (2000). Purification and structural determination of SCB1, a gamma-butyrolactone that elicits antibiotic production in *Streptomyces coelicolor* A3(2). *The Journal of Biological Chemistry, 275*(15), 11010–11016. https://doi.org/10.1074/jbc.275.15.11010

Tiaden, A., & Hilbi, H. (2012). α-Hydroxyketone synthesis and sensing by *Legionella* and *Vibrio. Sensors (Basel), 12*(3), 2899–2919. https://doi.org/10.3390/s120302899

Ujita, Y., Sakata, M., Yoshihara, A., Hikichi, Y., & Kai, K. (2019). Signal production and response specificity in the *phc* quorum sensing systems of *Ralstonia solanacearum* species complex. *ACS Chemical Biology*, 2243–2251. https://doi.org/10.1021/acschembio.9b00553

Uroz, S., Chhabra, S. R., Cámara, M., Williams, P., Oger, P., & Dessaux, Y. (2005). *N*-acylhomoserine lactone quorum-sensing molecules are modified and degraded by *Rhodococcus erythropolis* W2 by both amidolytic and novel oxidoreductase activities. *Microbiology*, *151*(10), 3313–3322. https://doi.org/10.1099/mic.0.27961-0

Uroz, S., Oger, P. M., Chapelle, E., Adeline, M.-T., Faure, D., & Dessaux, Y. (2008). A *Rhodococcus qsdA*-encoded enzyme defines a novel class of large-spectrum quorum-quenching lactonases. *Applied and Environmental Microbiology*, *74*(5), 1357–1366. https://doi.org/10.1128/AEM.02014-07

Utari, P. D., Vogel, J., & Quax, W. J. (2017). Deciphering physiological functions of AHL quorum quenching acylases. *Frontiers in Microbiology*, *8*, 1123. https://doi.org/10.3389/fmicb.2017.01123

Vannini, A., Volpari, C., Gargioli, C., Muraglia, E., Cortese, R., De Francesco, R., … Di Marco, S. (2002). The crystal structure of the quorum sensing protein TraR bound to its autoinducer and target DNA. *EMBO Journal*, *21*(17), 4393–4401. https://doi.org/10.1093/emboj/cdf459

Wang, H., Liao, L., Chen, S., & Zhang, L.-H. (2020). A quorum quenching bacterial isolate contains multiple substrate-inducible genes conferring degradation of Diffusible Signal Factor. *Applied and Environmental Microbiology*, *86*(7), e02930–19. https://doi.org/10.1128/AEM.02930-19

Wang, W.-Z., Morohoshi, T., Ikenoya, M., Someya, N., & Ikeda, T. (2010). AiiM, a novel class of *N*-acylhomoserine lactonase from the leaf-associated bacterium *Microbacterium testaceum*. *Applied and Environmental Microbiology*, *76*(8), 2524–2530. https://doi.org/10.1128/AEM.02738-09

Wang, Y.-J., & Leadbetter, J. R. (2005). Rapid acyl-homoserine lactone quorum signal biodegradation in diverse soils. *Applied and Environmental Microbiology*, *71*(3), 1291–1299. https://doi.org/10.1128/AEM.71.3.1291-1299.2005

Werner, N., Petersen, K., Vollstedt, C., Garcia, P. P., Chow, J., Ferrer, M., … Streit, W. R. (2021). The *Komagataeibacter europaeus* GqqA is the prototype of a novel bifunctional *N*-acyl-homoserine lactone acylase with prephenate dehydratase activity. *Scientific Reports*, *11*(1), 12255. https://doi.org/10.1038/s41598-021-91536-1

Wu, H., Song, Z., Hentzer, M., Andersen, J. B., Molin, S., Givskov, M., & Høiby, N. (2004). Synthetic furanones inhibit quorum-sensing and enhance bacterial clearance in *Pseudomonas aeruginosa* lung infection in mice. *The Journal of Antimicrobial Chemotherapy*, *53*(6), 1054–1061. https://doi.org/10.1093/jac/dkh223

Xu, B., Cho, Q. A. C., Ng, T. C. A., Huang, S., & Ng, H. Y. (2022). Enriched autoinducer-2 (AI-2)-based quorum quenching consortium in a ceramic anaerobic membrane bioreactor (AnMBR) for biofouling retardation. *Water Research*, *214*, 118203. https://doi.org/10.1016/j.watres.2022.118203

Yoon, J.-H., Lee, J.-K., Jung, S.-Y., Kim, J.-A., Kim, H.-K., & Oh, T.-K. (2006). *Nocardioides kongjuensis* sp. nov., an *N*-acylhomoserine lactone-degrading bacterium. *International Journal of Systematic and Evolutionary Microbiology*, *56*(Pt 8), 1783–1787. https://doi.org/10.1099/ijs.0.64120-0

Yu, D., Zhao, L., Xue, T., & Sun, B. (2012). *Staphylococcus aureus* autoinducer-2 quorum sensing decreases biofilm formation in an *icaR*-dependent manner. *BMC Microbiology*, *12*, 288. https://doi.org/10.1186/1471-2180-12-288

Zhang, L. H., & Kerr, A. (1991). A diffusible compound can enhance conjugal transfer of the Ti plasmid in *Agrobacterium tumefaciens*. *Journal of Bacteriology, 173*(6), 1867–1872.

Zhang, L., Murphy, P. J., Kerr, A., & Tate, M. E. (1993). *Agrobacterium* conjugation and gene regulation by *N*-acyl-L-homoserine lactones. *Nature, 362*(6419), 446–448. https://doi.org/10.1038/362446a0

Zhou, L., Wang, X.-Y., Sun, S., Yang, L.-C., Jiang, B.-L., & He, Y.-W. (2015). Identification and characterization of naturally occurring DSF-family quorum sensing signal turnover system in the phytopathogen *Xanthomonas*. *Environmental Microbiology, 17*(11), 4646–4658. https://doi.org/10.1111/1462-2920.12999

7 Quorum Quenching in Biofilm Mitigation

Şuheda Reisoglu and Sevcan Aydin

7.1 INTRODUCTION

Bacteria emerge as a planktonic form, rarely exposed to damaging environmental factors, as they are protected against the external environment by a structure called biofilm, the extracellular matrix (EPS). Biofilm structure creates a serious problem caused by microorganisms in various environments, including wastewater treatment, food, aquaculture, corrosion, and the health/biomedical sectors. Controlling bacterial biofilms is challenging, and most species within the biofilm show high antibiotic resistance. To eradicate the matured biofilms, it is crucial to exploit compounds penetrating the biofilm layer or deteriorating it mechanically (Rewak-Soroczyńska et al., 2019).

Various methods, including antibiofilm agents, antibiotics, and biocides, clean and solve biofilm-related problems. Still, alternative approaches are required due to the rise of antibiotic-resistant microorganisms and traditional chemicals significantly impacting the environment. Biofilm formation by opportunistic pathogens is constructed by a quorum sensing (QS) communication system between microbial consortium members. Since QS is essential in biofilm production (Christiaen et al., 2013), the quorum quenching (QQ) mechanism that targets and inhibits QS provides a promising alternative to tackle biofilm structure and related issues. This chapter will briefly highlight the potential of QQ in biofilm mitigation and its applications in various fields in addition to reflecting QS mechanisms and inhibition strategies.

7.1.1 QS MECHANISMS

Bacteria were considered to have solely basic processes and were self-sufficient individual cells for decades. However, thorough studies have indicated that bacteria can construct large communities, cooperate in a multicellular manner, and exhibit coordinated behaviors including bioluminescence, DNA uptake, virulence factors, and biofilm production (Reuter et al., 2016). These are a few examples of bacterial coordinated behavior used as a survival strategy; however, achieving these tasks requires the coordination of individual bacterial cells. Bacteria have a special communication mechanism named "quorum sensing" to assess collective behavior, arrangement of population density, and gene expression through signal molecules. QS comprises the stages of the production, secretion, and sensing of extracellular chemical signal molecules termed autoinducers (AIs). Bacteria regulate group behavior, gene expression,

DOI: 10.1201/9781003297826-7

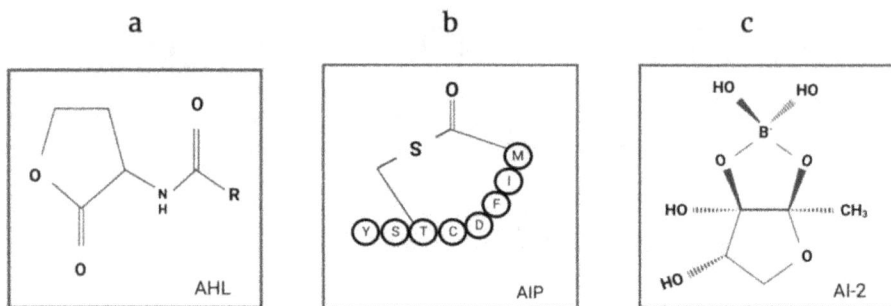

FIGURE 7.1 Representative chemical structures of autoinducers: (a) *N*-acyl-homoserine lactone (AHL), (b) autoinducing peptide (AIP), (c) autoinducer-2 (AI-2).

and information exchange with other bacterial cells through QS. At a lower cellular population density, bacteria generate and release autoinducers (AIs) into their adjacent environments. Diffusion diminishes the proximal concentration of AIs, rendering them undetectable to sustain individual bacterial activity. As bacteria proliferate, the localized concentration of AIs escalates commensurate with the population density. Upon reaching a critical concentration threshold, bacteria perceive the presence of AIs, prompting alterations in gene expression profiles to enact group behavior (Abisado et al., 2018).

Although QS controls the behavior of most bacterial classes, signaling molecules and transmission systems in gram-negative and gram-positive bacteria differ. Essential differences between these two systems are the signal peptide synthesis mechanism and the transduction pathway from sensing proteins to effectors. In this context, there are three central signaling systems and molecules (Figure 7.1). QS in gram-negative bacteria includes LuxI and LuxR as regulatory proteins. The best-known type of AIs in gram-negative bacterial QS systems is acyl-homoserine lactones (AHLs), and LuxI protein synthesizes AHL molecules. LuxR protein, on the other hand, is an AHL detector that arranges gene expression and alterations. In gram-positive bacteria, oligopeptides or briefly AIP molecules and bicomponent systems consisting of membrane-bound sensor kinase receptors and cytoplasmic transcription factors are involved in the gene expression by QS (Papenfort & Bassler, 2016). In addition, it has been demonstrated that QS signals are not only intraspecies channel specific; QS signals in interspecies have also been defined in bacteria. The third signaling molecule autoinducer-2 (AI-2) is observed in all bacteria, regardless of gram-negative and gram-positive distinction. This signal molecule, a universal channel for interspecies communication, is widely seen in bacterial species and ensures bacteria discern different culture conditions. The AI-2 in QS regulates biofilm formation and increases virulence factor expression (Plančak et al., 2015).

7.1.2 ROLE OF QS IN BIOFILM FORMATION

Regarding the coordinated behavior of bacteria, bacterial biofilms are the perfect model for a leading alteration in phenotype. This change is in charge of the rising

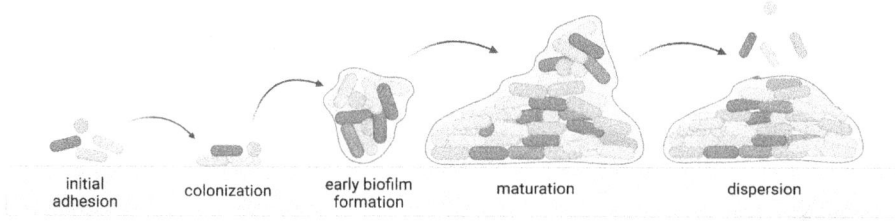

| initial adhesion | colonization | early biofilm formation | maturation | dispersion |

FIGURE 7.2 Five steps of the biofilm formation process. The first is the bacterial attachment onto the surface. Then, the cells start colonization, biofilm formation, and production of eDNA and EPS. The colonies construct a mature biofilm that has three-dimensional structures. The last step is biofilm dispersion, where each cell detaches from the biofilm.

adhesion onto the surfaces and ensures the bacteria's persistence. Biofilm structure is a multispecies bacterial community offering various advances in particular environments. A frequent bacterial characteristic of biofilm formation is the capacity to form an extracellular matrix that provides structural aid and is critical to tolerating antimicrobials. This matrix comprises polysaccharides, proteins, lipids, and extracellular DNA (Billings et al., 2013). The biofilm formation process has five foundational steps (Figure 7.2): initial adhesion, colonization, early biofilm formation, maturation, and dispersion.

The adhesion onto the surfaces and cohesion can be formed through bacterial appendages such as flagella and pili, van der Waal's forces, or electrostatic interactions. While biofilm can be constructed on abiotic and biotic surfaces, some surface features may provide better attachment (Jamal et al., 2018). After stable attachment, reproduction and cell division start through chemical signals within the EPS. The phase is followed by the forming of microbial colonies. At the production of the biofilm phase, cells associate with each other via AIs. This cell-to-cell interaction is a crucial activity in achieving the requisite cell density. It results in the secretion of AIs, and AIs ease quorum sensing. Specific gene products considered essential for forming EPS are expressed at maturation. At this stage, quick multiplication and dispersion of the microbial cells within the biofilm turn from sessile into motile condition. While the detachment process emerges in a natural pathway, various bacteria do not form extracellular polysaccharides, and these cells spread directly into the external environment. Then, microbial cells upregulate the protein expression required for flagella production to provide the bacteria movement to a different site. Thus, microbial detachment and transposition to a novel environment spread infections (Otto, 2013).

Bacterial biofilms account for more than 99% of microbial life, can occur on many surfaces, and strengthen cells against antimicrobials and the host's immune system. With the help of this resistance, various factors, including impotent diffusion of antimicrobials into biofilm structure and transmission of resistance genes, are provided for microbial life within the biofilm formation (Preda & Săndulescu, 2019). Most bacteria balance the production of biofilms via QS-based strategies. Davies et al. (1998) first reported the roles of QS in biofilm production. The complicated relation of QS and biofilm was first detected in a biofilm by a specific mutant of *P. aeruginosa*. This biofilm was thinner and more susceptible to antimicrobials than the biofilm formed by wild *P. aeruginosa* strains.

QS signals have been distinguished in biofilm structures both in situ and in vitro. A novel approach has been created in biofilm mitigation by understanding the crucial role of QS in biofilm formation. When comparing the QS-deficient *P. aeruginosa* strain obtained from implants to its wild counterpart, it was found that the QS-deficient one was more readily and rapidly eradicated. Results of previous studies have shown that QS has a substantial part in biofilm formation. Therefore, interfering with QS signaling is an efficacious method for hindering the biofilms formed by opportunistic pathogens, making pathogens susceptible to antibacterials, and creating a synergy with antibiotics (Ponnusamy et al., 2009).

7.2 QQ IN BIOFILM MITIGATION

In recent years, there has been an increase in deaths caused by antibiotic-resistant pathogenic bacterial infections. Antibiotics in treating pathogenic bacteria may pave the way for the evolution of drug-resistant strains while eliminating antibiotic-susceptible ones. Antimicrobials have a minimum bactericidal concentration required to kill bacteria. Some species may survive and form a biofilm below the minimum bactericidal concentration. Therefore, antibiofilm agents that hinder the production of biofilm layers by adhering to the surfaces of bacteria have gained great importance. In the fight against biofilm, which is formed by pathogenic bacteria and has undesirable results in various areas, preventing communication channels by targeting the QS components and the communication system between bacteria have gained significant interest. Also, studies have demonstrated that the QS could be associated with resistance mechanisms. Thus, preventing QS has been a favorable antibacterial approach, which not only hinders the progression of the resistance but also suppresses virulence factor gene expression (Haque et al., 2018).

Quorum quenching, disrupting the microbial QS system, can eliminate biofilm formation and covers all processes included in the disruption of QS. In QQ systems, enzymes inactivating QS signal molecules are named QQ enzymes, while the chemicals interfering with QS paths are termed QS inhibitors (QSIs) (Delalande et al., 2005). Figure 7.3 shows the main QQ strategies to disrupt microbial interactions: (1) blockage of the signal molecule synthesis, (2) signaling enzyme degradation, and (3) disruption of signaling receptors. Also, inducing the efficiency and development of QQ bacteria can impede the QS systems. The details of these strategies are mentioned in the following sections.

7.2.1 ENZYMATIC QQ

The World Health Organization (WHO) has highlighted antibiotic-resistant strains of various gram-negative bacteria, including those highly opportunistic, as an urgent problem that needs to be addressed (Tacconelli et al., 2018). Since AHL molecules regulate various bacterial behaviors, comprising the virulence factor production,

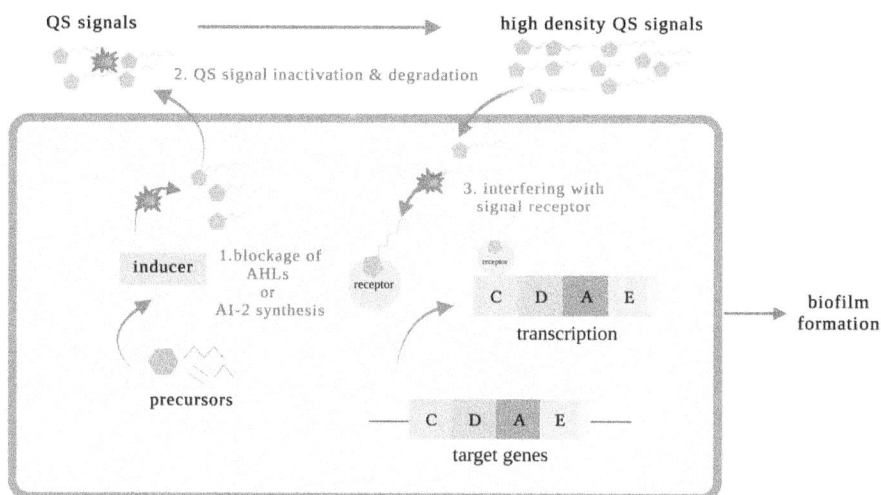

FIGURE 7.3 QS signal paths and QQ strategies for biofilm control.

biofilm, and antimicrobial resistance of most pathogens that harm human health, they form the basis of different enzymatic QQ research. QQ includes degrading signal chemicals by specific enzymes to prevent signal molecule accumulation and hinder gene expression alterations. In QQ, AHL degradation is an essential strategy, and the three main enzyme groups targeting AHL signals are lactonases, acylases, and oxidoreductases. Lactonases are proteins that cleave the ester bond in the homoserine lactone ring to expose the target acyl-homoserine molecule. Lactonases have broad AHL substrate specificity, as the homoserine lactone ring is conserved in AHLs and only makes nonspecific interactions.

QQ enzymes are able to disrupt AHL molecules with no penetration into the cells, making them more attractive QS inhibition strategies compared to others; thus, AHL-inhibiting enzymes have been thoroughly studied. QQ strategy contains four enzyme groups: lactonases, acylases, reductases, and oxidases. Lactonases and acylases hydrolyze AHL's homoserine lactone ring and amide bond; the lactonase enzyme can unlock the lactone ring, while acylase enzymes can cut the acyl side. Meanwhile, this lactone ring may recover the ring when acidic levels are maintained (<2). Reductases and oxidases modify the AHL molecule activity but are not responsible for degrading them; however, their activity, selectivity, and stability were rarely studied (Fetzner, 2015).

The secretion of QS signal molecules is related to multidrug efflux pumps. So, the prevention of QS by QQ enzymes is a logical approach to tackling the rising antimicrobial resistance crisis in various environments. Also, QQ enzymes were suggested as an efficacious approach for wastewater treatment. Opportunistic pathogen *P. aeruginosa* can produce biofilm in drinking water, imposing a threat to public health. Liu et al. (2020) exploited lactonase analogue AiiADH82 isolated from the marine bacterium *Bacillus velezensis* to examine its QQ activity for *P. aeruginosa* from pipelines. Their study showed that AiiADH82 displayed a substantial

TABLE 7.1

Studies using QQ enzymes in mitigating QS in biofilm formation

QQ enzyme	Bacteria	Effect	Reference
Acylase	Bacterial sludge	Mitigation of biofilm formation capability	Jiang et al. (2013)
Recombinant lactonase	Multidrug-resistant *A. baumannii*	Mitigation of biofilm	Chow et al. (2014)
Coatings acylase and α-amylase enzymes	*P. aeruginosa*	Biofilm inhibition	Ivanova et al. (2015)
Lactonases and acylases	*P. aeruginosa*	Reducing biofilm	Li et al. (2016)
SsoPox-W2631 lactonase	*P. aeruginosa* PA14	Reducing biofilm	Mion et al. (2019)

reduction in the early step of proliferation, biofilm production, and virulent factors of *P. aeruginosa*.

Additionally, when considering the health concerns and environmental issues related to the extreme usage of toxic chemicals, QQ is an environment-friendly approach to inhibiting microbial virulence and biofouling, especially in membrane filtration of wastewater treatment plants (WWTPs) (Syafiuddin et al., 2021). Nevertheless, studies of QSIs for eradicating bacterial colonization from solid material surfaces are still secondary to the ones in biomedical applications, therefore, studies need to use QSIs to handle biofilm-related issues in engineering materials. QQ enzymes are hopeful due to their possible usage in catalytic quantities and extracellularly degradation of QS signals. Table 7.1 briefly shows studies using QQ enzymes in mitigating QS in biofilm formation.

7.2.2 Bacterial QQ

Enzymatic QQ is an efficacious method for interfering with bacterial QS and biofilm mitigation However, relatively expensive costs and low stability restrict enzyme usage in enzymatic pathways. For adequate QQ in WWTPs, QQ bacteria-producing AHL-degrading QQ enzymes have been well isolated from activated sludge and performed successfully in membrane bioreactor (MBR) processes. *Rhodococcus spp.* BH4 and *Bacillus methylotrophicus* spp. WY isolates are QQ bacteria that produce lactonase enzymes to degrade various AHLs (Oh et al., 2012). In addition, *Pseudomonas spp.* 1A1-producing acylase enzymes were isolated from the activated sludge of a WWTP. Even though QQ bacterium is not as effective as directly joined QQ enzymes, the exploitation of QQ bacteria has a couple of benefits, including more robust stability and affordable cost (Lee et al., 2013).

As AI-2 works as a QS signal secreted by gram-negative and gram-positive bacteria, a novel strategy to disrupt the AI-2 QS approach was followed as an antibiofilm approach in an MBR for wastewater treatment. An indigenous bacterial isolate (*Acinetobacter spp.* DKY-1) was observed to inactivate DPD (4,5-dihydroxy-2,3-pentane dione: DPD,

AI-2) in the activated sludge of MBRs. Adding DKY-1-entrapping media (e.g., beads) in an MBR notably reduced the DPD concentration in the liquor, resulting in a noticeable decrement in biofouling (Lee et al., 2018).

7.2.3 FUNGAL QQ AGAINST AI-2 QS

The activated sludge of MBRs includes various microscale entities, such as algae, protozoa, and fungi, as well as bacteria. Therefore, other microorganisms besides bacteria are able to influence bacterial QS strategy. Apart from bacteria, fungi communicate with intraspecific and interspecific microorganisms via signaling molecules to regulate various changes, and their enzymes are reportedly capable of disrupting bacterial biofilms. The potential of fungal enzymes to mitigate the biofilm structure formed by bacteria has been reported. Enzymes obtained from three different fungal species (*A. niger*, *T. viride*, and *Penicillium*) effectively removed the biofilm formed by *P. fluorescens* (Gautam et al., 2013). A study indicated that the farnesol molecule obtained from *C. albicans* considerably mitigated biofouling due to QQ activity against bacterial QS. In another study, (RT-qPCR) analysis showed that farnesol removed biofilm structure by hampering luxS expression, which takes part in bacterial AI-2 molecule synthesis (Lee et al., 2016). Also, Fakhri et al. (2021) revealed that *P. restrictum* (a fungus) was efficacious in improving QQ activity to control biofouling in addition to adequate antibiotic removal in an aerobic membrane bioreactor that treats antibiotic-contaminated wastewater.

7.2.4 BACTERIOPHAGE QQ ENZYME

The coaction between bacteriophages and bacteria in biofilm formation has recently gained interest as an essential part of phage therapy in the West. Phages are natural entities that can kill host cells in mono- and mixed-species bacterial biofilm structures (Ji et al., 2021). Phages have been investigated as antimicrobial agents in various fields, such as phage therapy, biofilm-coated medical devices, and membrane filtration. Nevertheless, EPS limits the antibacterial activity of phages. A strategy developed through phages in the phage-bacteria race is the utilization of polysaccharide depolymerize enzymes to disrupt EPS, allowing phages to penetrate encapsulated host cells. Bhattacharjee et al. (2015) demonstrated that biofouling caused by an antibiotic-resistant bacterial strain was cleared in a membrane bioreactor using a lytic phage. Despite the limitation, both natural and engineered phage-producing polysaccharide depolymerizes ensured a model for biofilm mitigation that inspired Pei and Lamas-Samanamud (2014). They engineered T7 phage for encoding a lactonase enzyme that degrades AHLs, and the biofilm structure formed by different bacterial species was effectively mitigated with this engineered phage. Aydin et al. (2022) also reported that pyophage added to an MBR system exhibited improved performance in treating antibiotic-containing wastewater. Compared to the control, membrane biofouling decreased by 25% with pyophage augmentation. Their results show a strong synergy between phage-host bacterial communities regarding the QQ–QS strategies and highlight the phage potential as antibiofouling.

7.3   APPLICATIONS OF QQ

Recent publications have frequently reported the practical biotechnological applications of QS inhibitors (quorum quenchers). The usage of different QQ approaches has been reported so far. These approaches may be composed of bacterial products such as norspermidine, plants (secondary metabolites), and animals (acylases, lactonases, and oxidoreductase enzymes isolated from *Mus musculus* or *Danio rerio* (Kalia, 2013). QQ enzymes can be utilized in various fields, particularly medicine and wastewater treatment.

7.3.1   QQ APPLICATION IN MEDICINE

The dissemination of multidrug-resistant pathogens in healthcare environments is a vital issue that has to be tackled urgently. Opportunistic bacterial pathogens are serious etiological factors and tough-to-combat diseases. Such pathogens are known to secrete numerous resistance factors and produce difficult-to-eradicate biofilms. Searching for chemicals that can mitigate biofilm and prevent biofilm formation in advance is pivotal in various fields. One is health care, where diseases resulting from biofilms, such as oral cavities and cystic fibrosis, are a crucial problem. Stoodley et al. (2002) indicated that more than 80% of the bacteria could form a biofilm, contributing to various infectious diseases. Unlike free cells, cells capsulated with biofilm have higher antibiotic-resistant characteristics, increasing 100–1000 times in minimum inhibitory concentration. They also found that the antibiotic resistance in novel biofilms was not as strong as that of mature biofilms.

Successful inhibition of QS can benefit patients suffering from infectious conditions. QQ-based therapeutic approaches from antibacterial treatments aim to mitigate virulence factors and bacterial behaviors, including biofilm formation, instead of killing pathogens. Therefore, this ensures less selective pressure for the evolution of novel resistance mechanisms toward antibiotic treatment. As interest and studies on QQ mechanisms have increased, several innovative and environmentally friendly attempts have emerged from QQ strategies. Enzymatic QQ has shown efficacious results in controlling various bacterial infections. Promising results were also indicated by Castillo Juárez et al. (2018), who studied PvdQ acylase activity on AHL of *Pseudomonas aeruginosa* in a mouse model, resulting in a reduction in infection. The virulence of pathogen *P. aeruginosa* PAO1 was investigated by Vandeputte et al. (2011), and they showed that specific flavonoids could decrease signal perception, leading to lower virulence and biofilm mitigation. *Staphylococcus aureus* is a widespread pathogenic bacterium that is able to produce biofilm structure; thus, QQ molecule activation can be beneficial in mitigating its virulence (Ziemichód & Skotarczak, 2017). Lactonase enzyme from *Geobacillus kaustophilus* HTA426 is shown to have the potential to degrade lactone ring in the structure of AHL, affecting *Acinetobacter baumannii* through penetrating the biofilm structure (Chow et al., 2014).

In addition, several assessments of QQ strategies at the topical level have been made. The dissemination of *P. aeruginosa* in animals with burned skin was prevented via the topical application of lactonase from *Bacillus* spp. ZA12 and decreased skin burn mortality. The results were more efficacious in combining the lactonase enzyme with the antibiotic, demonstrating strong fitness and synergy between QQ molecules and antibiotics. The QQ strategy has also been applied to dental care. Various dental plaque biofilm-forming pathogens, such as *Aggregatibacter actinomycetemcomitans* and *Streptococcus* spp., have been successfully prevented via QQ strategies that provide favorable oral hygiene (Basavaraju et al., 2016). However, considering the lack of sufficient information about QSIs, QQ applications in dental health should be carried forward.

7.3.2   QQ Application in Agriculture

Due to the increasing world population, meeting the need for food and agricultural products has become a serious problem on a global scale. In addition, plant pathogens that result in serious economic losses in agriculture have recently made the process even more difficult. Although antibiotics traditionally used in the fight against plant pathogens are considered effective in controlling opportunistic pathogens, increasing drug resistance, environmental pollution caused by the release of antibiotics without being completely degraded, and the deterioration of the ecological balance with the inappropriate usage of antibiotics pose a vital problem. Thus, there is increasing interest in biological control in preventing and treating pathogenic plant diseases. In this context, studies with the QQ strategy have shown promising control in treating plant diseases through regulating gene expression related to plant pathogens, thereby increasing agricultural production efficiency. In line with these promising studies, QQ is considered a potential alternative to traditional approaches or a complementary strategy to antibiotics (Zhang et al., 2019).

Dong et al. (2000) transplanted a plasmid carrying the aiiA gene into strain *Erwinia carotovora* SCG1 and showed that aiiA gene expression could inhibit virulence factors by disrupting the QS system. A study using various plants, such as bok choy and potatoes, that were infected with recombinant pathogens showing no signs of soft rot was the first QQ application in biological disease control. *P. aureofaciens* 30–84 is a symbiotic bacterial species that arranges phenazine antibiotic production via AHL-mediated QS. In addition, it can protect the wheat plant against the pathogen *Gaeumannomyces graminis* var. *tritici*, while reducing the vulnerability of wheat to fungal infections.

The signal trade-off among bacteria mediates the coordination of diverse physiological activities. In leguminous rhizobia, the QS system actively provides and regulates symbiotic interactions between bacteria involved in nitrogen fixation and plant hosts. The potential of interspecies symbiotic interaction to increase nitrogen fixation through triggering the QS system of bacteria can reduce fertilizer needs and financial investment for crop hosts, thus protecting the environment and ecological equilibrium (Cao et al., 2009).

7.3.3   QQ Application in Wastewater Treatment

Biological treatment stands out as an environmentally friendly and economical strategy for removing pathogens and pollutants in wastewater. In biological wastewater treatment, bacteria control population density through QS, while many bacterial species cause membrane biofouling in the wastewater treatment process. The biofilm layers formed by these bacteria can be beneficial as biocatalysis in WWTPs or harmful to the system as a source of biological pollution. Thus, the main concern in this system is how to manage biofilm formation without harming the bacterial community survival rate and the growth kinetics of the microbial community (Huang et al., 2016). Sustaining a stable biofilm thickness in the wastewater treatment process is tough because limitations in mass transfer, fouling issues, and high fluid head loss are among the major biofilm-induced problems in membrane biofilm reactors, which collectively degrade the performance of the reactor at the end (Hwang et al., 2010).

In this context, various studies conducted that aim at taking advantage of the QQ mechanism reported QQ enzymes and QQ bacteria/fungi are efficient in disrupting the QS system in various WWTPs. Paul et al. (2009) revealed that the QQ enzyme (5 µg/mL acylase I) reduced the biofilm structure formed *by A. hydrophila* and *Pseudomonas putida* species by 60%–73%. However, they stated that QQ microorganisms are more efficacious than QQ enzymes due to the high enzyme production cost and short QQ enzyme half-life. Studies have been carried out to isolate indigenous QQ bacterium from WWTPs and to clear biofilm structures produced by bacteria sharing the same environment with these QQ bacteria. In the light of research, various QQ bacteria, including *Acinetobacter* spp., *Afipia* spp., *Microbacterium* spp., *Micrococcus* spp., *Pseudomonas* spp., and *Rhodococcus* spp., were isolated and found to be effective in mitigating biofilm formation at both the initial and maturation phases. QQ-based approaches have been thoroughly investigated and applied in membrane bioreactors, following successful results with QQ strategies leading to wider acceptance of QQ-based methods in WWTPs (Maddela et al., 2019).

In addition, AHLs are suitable environments for the coexistence of microorganisms that both produce and degrade AHL. One of the pieces of evidence for QS- and QQ-bacteria association is that induction of β-galactosidase was not observed in the *A. tumefaciens* KYC55 reporter strain incubated with AHL (3-oxo-C8-HSL), which indicates the presence of indigenous QQ activity (Song et al., 2014). Lastly, the higher population of signal-quenchers than signal generators in certain environments suggests the existence of excellent interaction between QQ and QS microorganisms (Hao Tan et al., 2015). Nevertheless, the detailed role of indigenous QQ in WWTPs must be clarified. In addition, the impact of numerous environmental factors in QQ communities should be visible. For these reasons, there is a need for extensive further studies of environmental factors and QQ communities to learn more about their distribution and coexistence, which could improve cooperation between the laboratory and commercial stages of QQ MBRs.

7.3.4   QQ Application in Food Safety

Foodborne microorganisms, which can cause decay and digestive disorders as a result of consumption, are of vital importance in terms of food safety. Various foodborne pathogens can produce biofilm structures, significantly impacting food processing and safety processes. In biofilm mitigation, QS is the pivotal element in biofilm formation, while biofilm formation creates synergistic effects by affecting QS regulation. In particular, *Salmonella*, one of the leading pathogens of foodborne diseases and among the most important public health issues worldwide, severely threatens human health and life. In addition, *Listeria monocytogenes* can rapidly produce biofilm structures in food production facilities and packaging containers. This protection method developed by opportunistic pathogens can form a more robust biofilm layer of mixed species with other pathogens that are hard to destroy and frequently lead to foodborne gastrointestinal diseases (Daneshvar Alavi & Truelstrup Hansen, 2013). Another serious foodborne pathogen, *Vibrio parahaemolyticus*, is a cause of gastroenteritis or poisoning when taken in through uncooked or inappropriately cooked products. Related studies have indicated that brominated furanone could hinder the AI-2 activity and luxS gene expression in *V. parahaemolyticus*. Studies have revealed that brominated furanone can inhibit the activity of AI-2 signaling molecules and luxS gene expression in *V. parahaemolyticus*. Also, the extracellular enzymatic activity of this pathogen and the biofilm structures it formed were influenced likewise (Phuvasate et al., 2012). QQ is a promising approach to prevent bacterial pathogenicity by acting on biofilm formation. Moreover, biofilm-forming microorganisms can decompose wastes in the food industry, help the remediation of environmental pollution, and increase the adaptation of beneficial microorganisms to stabilization (Singh et al., 2006). Thus, it is estimated that the practical problems in the food sector will be solved.

It has been stated that it would be possible to trigger the formation of certain probiotic biofilms and to control biofilm formation by decreasing microbial resistance through the QS system regulation to increase the synthesis of specific human metabolites. It has been reported that biofilms help increase environmental adaptation and steadiness of probiotics. The probiotic *Lactobacillus* can successfully break down lactic acid and various antibacterial substances, and its use is common in fermentative products such as yogurt, kefir, kimchi, and other products. Researchers reported that the production of bacteriostatic substances by *Lactobacillus plantarum* HE-1, AI-2 synthesis, and biofilm production nearly achieved the peak level in the metabolic process, stating that converting bacterial lactic acid metabolism to bacteriostatic substances may depend on the QS mechanism and biofilm production. Nevertheless, the details of the regulatory mechanisms have not yet been elucidated exactly (Risoen et al., 2000).

7.4   CONCLUDING REMARKS

With the rapid spread of multidrug-resistant opportunistic pathogens that complicate the activity in various areas by forming a biofilm layer and the ineffectiveness of new antibiotic development to eliminate these pathogens, studies have evolved toward developing new approaches to reduce the pathogenicity of pathogens. The expression of certain genes, including lethal ones, that cause bacterial pathogenicity depends on a well-ordered intercellular signaling system (QS) modulated by small molecules and can be attenuated without impairing cell viability. QQ, inhibition of QS, represents a promising strategy for clearing the biofilm structure developed by pathogens while offering a potent antimicrobial effect. The QQ approach reduces biofilm-forming bacterial pathogenicity and increases the biofilm's susceptibility to antibiotics while increasing antibiotic-mediated biofilm degradation. The discovery of QSIs can be a powerful weapon in target identification, pathogen specificity, drug delivery, and cellular toxicity against pathogenic microorganisms that threaten human health by forming biofilms in various fields, including medicine, agriculture, food safety, and wastewater treatment. Current knowledge about QQ enzymes and bacteria (and how best to use these enzymes and bacteria) still needs to be improved. This is important for an augmented comprehension of the risk and potential resistance mechanisms. Also, QQ enzymes can be more beneficial in prevention than treatment, as biofilm structures are more challenging to eliminate once fully formed. QQ bacteria and enzymes should be studied beforehand in media that are as closely compatible as possible with the environment in which they will be used. While QQ enzymes are promising antimicrobials in various applications, the potential issue in this approach is the development of resistance (Rasko & Sperandio, 2010). It has been hypothesized that QQ strategies do not kill pathogenic cells and display less selective pressures. Hence, resistance is less likely to develop. Further research is necessary before using these approaches in the clinic and various industrial fields.

REFERENCES

Abisado, R. G., Benomar, S., Klaus, J. R., Dandekar, A. A., & Chandler, J. R. (2018). Bacterial quorum sensing and microbial community interactions. In *mBio* (Vol. 9, Issue 3). American Society for Microbiology. https://doi.org/10.1128/mBio.02331-17

Aydin, S., Can, K., Çalışkan, M., & Balcazar, J. L. (2022). Bacteriophage cocktail as a promising bio-enhancer for methanogenic activities in anaerobic membrane bioreactors. *Science of the Total Environment, 832.* https://doi.org/10.1016/j.scitotenv.2022.154716

Basavaraju, M., Sisnity, V. S., Palaparthy, R., & Addanki, P. K. (2016). Quorum quenching: Signal jamming in dental plaque biofilms. In *Journal of Dental Sciences* (Vol. 11, Issue 4, pp. 349–352). Association for Dental Sciences of the Republic of China. https://doi .org/10.1016/j.jds.2016.02.002

Bhattacharjee, A. S., Choi, J., Motlagh, A. M., Mukherji, S. T., & Goel, R. (2015). Bacteriophage therapy for membrane biofouling in membrane bioreactors and antibiotic-resistant bacterial biofilms. *Biotechnology & Bioengineering, 112,* 1644–1654. https://doi.org/10.1002/bit.25574/abstract

Billings, N., Millan, M. R., Caldara, M., Rusconi, R., & Tarasova, Y. (2013). The extracellular matrix component Psl provides fast-acting antibiotic defense in pseudomonas aeruginosa biofilms. *PLoS Pathogens, 9*(8), 1003526. https://doi.org/10.1371/journal.ppat .1003526

Cao, H., Menghua, A. E., Ae, Y., Zheng, H., Jiang, A. E., Ae, Z., Zhong, Z., & Zhu, A. J. (2009). Complex quorum-sensing regulatory systems regulate bacterial growth and symbiotic nodulation in *Mesorhizobium tianshanense. Archives of Microbiology, 191,* 283–289. https://doi.org/10.1007/s00203-008-0454-7

Castillo Juárez, I., De Postgraduados, C., Quax, W. J., Utari, P. D., Setroikromo, R., & Melgert, B. N. (2018). PvdQ quorum quenching Acylase attenuates pseudomonas Aeruginosa virulence in a mouse model of pulmonary infection. *Frontiers in Cellular and Infection Microbiology | www.frontiersin.org, 1,* 119. https://doi.org/10.3389/fcimb.2018.00119

Chow, J. Y., Yang, Y., Tay, S. B., Chua, K. L., & Yew, W. S. (2014). Disruption of biofilm formation by the human pathogen Acinetobacter baumannii using engineered quorum-quenching lactonases. *Antimicrobial Agents and Chemotherapy*, *58*(3), 1802–1805. https://doi.org/10.1128/AAC.02410-13

Christiaen, S. E. A., Matthijs, N., Zhang, X.-H., Nelis, H. J., Bossier, P., & Coenye, T. (2013). Bacteria that inhibit quorum sensing decrease biofilm formation and virulence in Pseudomonas aeruginosa PAO1. *Pathogens and Diseases*, *70*(3), 271–279. https://doi.org/10.1111/2049-632X.12124

Daneshvar Alavi, H. E., & Truelstrup Hansen, L. (2013). Kinetics of biofilm formation and desiccation survival of Listeria monocytogenes in single and dual species biofilms with Pseudomonas fluorescens, Serratia proteamaculans or Shewanella baltica on food-grade stainless steel surfaces. *Biofouling*, *29*(10), 1253–1268. https://doi.org/10.1080/08927014.2013.835805

Davies, D. G., Parsek, M. R., Pearson, J. P., Iglewski, B. H., Costerton, J. W., & Greenberg, E. P. (1998). The involvement of cell-to-cell signals in the development of a bacterial biofilm. *Science*, *280*(5361), 295–298. https://doi.org/10.1126/science.280.5361.295

Delalande, L., Faure, D., Raffoux, A., Uroz, S., Dõangelo-Picard, C., Elasri, M., Carlier, A., Berruyer, R., Petit, A., Williams, P., & Dessaux, Y. (2005). N-hexanoyl-L L-homoserine lactone, a mediator of bacterial quorum-sensing regulation, exhibits plant-dependent stability and may be inactivated by germinating Lotus corniculatus seedlings. *FEMS Microbiology Ecology*, *52*, 13–20. https://doi.org/10.1016/j.femsec.2004.10.005

Dong, Y.-H., Xu, J.-L., Li, X.-Z., & Zhang, L.-H. (2000). AiiA, an enzyme that inactivates the acylhomoserine lactone quorum-sensing signal and attenuates the virulence of *Erwinia carotovora*. *PNAS*, *97*(7), 3526–3531. www.pnas.orgcgidoi10.1073pnas.060023897

Fakhri, H., Shahi, A., Ovez, S., & Aydin, S. (2021). Bioaugmentation with immobilized endophytic Penicillium restrictum to improve quorum quenching activity for biofouling control in an aerobic hollow-fiber membrane bioreactor treating antibiotic-containing wastewater. *Ecotoxicology and Environmental Safety*, *210*. https://doi.org/10.1016/j.ecoenv.2020.111831

Fetzner, S. (2015). Quorum quenching enzymes. *Journal of Biotechnology*, *201*, 2–14. https://doi.org/10.1016/j.jbiotec.2014.09.001

Hao Tan, C., Koh, K. S., Xie, C., Zhang, J., Tan, X. H., Lee, G. P., Zhou, Y., Ng, W. J., Rice, S. A., & Kjelleberg, S. (2015). ARTICLE community quorum sensing signalling and quenching: Microbial granular biofilm assembly. *NPJ Biofilms and Microbiomes*, *1*. https://doi.org/10.1038/npjbiofilms.2015.6

Haque, S., Ahmad, F., Dar, S. A., Jawed, A., Mandal, R. K., Wahid, M., Lohani, M., Khan, S., Singh, V., & Akhter, N. (2018). Developments in strategies for Quorum Sensing virulence factor inhibition to combat bacterial drug resistance. In *Microbial pathogenesis* (Vol. 121, pp. 293–302). Academic Press. https://doi.org/10.1016/j.micpath.2018.05.046

Huang, J., Shi, Y., Zeng, G., Gu, Y., Chen, G., Shi, L., Hu, Y., Tang, B., & Zhou, J. (2016). Acyl-homoserine lactone-based quorum sensing and quorum quenching hold promise to determine the performance of biological wastewater treatments: An overview. In *Chemosphere* (Vol. 157, pp. 137–151). Elsevier Ltd. https://doi.org/10.1016/j.chemosphere.2016.05.032

Hwang, J. H., Cicek, N., & Oleszkiewicz, J. A. (2010). Achieving biofilm control in a membrane biofilm reactor removing total nitrogen. *Water Research*, *44*(7), 2283–2291. https://doi.org/10.1016/j.watres.2009.12.022

Ivanova, K., Fernandes, M. M., Francesko, A., Mendoza, E., Guezguez, J., Burnet, M., & Tzanov, T. (2015). Quorum-quenching and matrix-degrading enzymes in multilayer coatings synergistically prevent bacterial biofilm formation on urinary catheters. *ACS Applied Materials and Interfaces*, *7*(49), 27066–27077. https://doi.org/10.1021/acsami.5b09489

Jamal, M., Ahmad, W., Andleeb, S., Jalil, F., Imran, M., Nawaz, M. A., Hussain, T., Ali, M., Rafiq, M., & Kamil, M. A. (2018). Bacterial biofilm and associated infections. In *Journal of the Chinese Medical Association* (Vol. 81, Issue 1, pp. 7–11). Elsevier Ltd. https://doi.org/10.1016/j.jcma.2017.07.012

Ji, M., Liu, Z., Sun, K., Li, Z., Fan, X., & Li, Q. (2021). Bacteriophages in water pollution control: Advantages and limitations. *Front Environ Sci Eng*, 15:84. https://doi.org/10.1007/s11783-020-1378-y

Jiang, W., Xia, S., Liang, J., Zhang, Z., & Hermanowicz, S. W. (2013). Effect of quorum quenching on the reactor performance, biofouling and biomass characteristics in membrane bioreactors. *Water Research*, *47*(1), 187–196. https://doi.org/10.1016/j.watres.2012.09.050

Kalia, V. C. (2013). Quorum sensing inhibitors: An overview. *Biotechnology advances*, *31*(2), 224–245. https://doi.org/10.1016/j.biotechadv.2012.10.004

Kumar Gautam, C., Kumar Srivastav, A., Bind, S., Madhav, M., & Shanthi, V. (2013). An insight into biofilm ecology and its applied aspects. *International Journal of Pharmacy and Pharmaceutical Sciences*, *5*(4), 69–73.

Lee, C. H., Cheong, W. S., Lee, C. H., Moon, Y. H., Oh, H. S., Kim, S. R., Lee, S. H., & Lee, J. K. (2013). Isolation and identification of indigenous quorum quenching bacteria, Pseudomonas sp. 1A1, for biofouling control in MBR. *Industrial and Engineering Chemistry Research*, *52*(31), 10554–10560. https://doi.org/10.1021/ie303146f

Lee, K., Kim, Y. W., Lee, S., Lee, S. H., Nahm, C. H., Kwon, H., Park, P. K., Choo, K. H., Koyuncu, I., Drews, A., Lee, C. H., & Lee, J. K. (2018). Stopping autoinducer-2 chatter by means of an indigenous bacterium (Acinetobacter sp. DKY-1): A new antibiofouling strategy in a membrane bioreactor for wastewater treatment. *Environmental Science and Technology*, *52*(11), 6237–6245. https://doi.org/10.1021/acs.est.7b05824

Lee, K., Lee, S., Lee, S. H., Kim, S. R., Oh, H. S., Park, P. K., Choo, K. H., Kim, Y. W., Lee, J. K., & Lee, C. H. (2016). Fungal quorum quenching: A paradigm shift for energy savings in Membrane Bioreactor (MBR) for wastewater treatment. *Environmental Science and Technology*, *50*(20), 10914–10922. https://doi.org/10.1021/acs.est.6b00313

Li, X. C., Wang, C., Mulchandani, A., & Ge, X. (2016). Engineering soluble human paraoxonase 2 for quorum quenching. *ACS Chemical Biology*, *11*(11), 3122–3131. https://doi.org/10.1021/acschembio.6b00527

Liu, J., Sun, X., Ma, Y., Zhang, J., Xu, C., & Zhou, S. (2020). Quorum quenching mediated bacteria interruption as a probable strategy for drinking water treatment against bacterial pollution. *ACS International Journal of Environmental Research and Public Health*, *17*(24), 9539. https://doi.org/10.3390/ijerph17249539

Maddela, N. R., Sheng, B., Yuan, S., Zhou, Z., Villamar-Torres, R., & Meng, F. (2019). Roles of quorum sensing in biological wastewater treatment: A critical review. In *Chemosphere* (Vol. 221, pp. 616–629). Elsevier Ltd. https://doi.org/10.1016/j.chemosphere.2019.01.064

Mion, Sonia, Remy, Benjamin, Plener, Laure, Bregeon, Fabienne, Chabriere, Eric, Daude, David. (2019). Quorum quenching lactonase strengthens bacteriophage and antibiotic arsenal against pseudomonas aeruginosa clinical isolates. *Front Microbiol*, 10:2049. https://doi.org/10.3389/fmicb.2019.02049

Oh, H. S., Yeon, K. M., Yang, C. S., Kim, S. R., Lee, C. H., Park, S. Y., Han, J. Y., & Lee, J. K. (2012). Control of membrane biofouling in MBR for wastewater treatment by quorum quenching bacteria encapsulated in microporous membrane. *Environmental Science and Technology*, *46*(9), 4877–4884. https://doi.org/10.1021/es204312u

Otto, M. (2013). Staphylococcal infections: Mechanisms of biofilm maturation and detachment as critical determinants of pathogenicity. *Annual Review of Medicine*, 64, 175–188. https://doi.org/10.1146/annurev-med-042711-140023

Papenfort, K., & Bassler, B. L. (2016). Quorum sensing signal-response systems in gram-negative bacteria. In *Nature Reviews Microbiology* (Vol. 14, Issue 9, pp. 576–588). Nature Publishing Group. https://doi.org/10.1038/nrmicro.2016.89

Paul, D., Kim, Y. S., Ponnusamy, K., & Kweon, J. H. (2009). *Application of quorum quenching to inhibit biofilm formation.*

Pei, R., & Lamas-Samanamud, G. R. (2014). Inhibition of biofilm formation by T7 bacteriophages producing quorum-quenching enzymes. *Applied and Environmental Microbiology*, *80*(17), 5340–5348. https://doi.org/10.1128/AEM.01434-14

Phuvasate, S., Chen, M. H., & Su, Y. C. (2012). Reductions of Vibrio parahaemolyticus in Pacific oysters (Crassostrea gigas) by depuration at various temperatures. *Food Microbiology*, *31*(1), 51–56. https://doi.org/10.1016/j.fm.2012.02.004

Plančak, D., Musić, L., & Puhar, I. (2015). Quorum sensing of periodontal pathogens. *Acta Stomatologica Croatica*, *49*(3), 234–241. https://doi.org/10.15644/asc49/3/6

Ponnusamy, K., Paul, D., & Kweon, J. H. (2009). *Inhibition of quorum sensing mechanism and aeromonas hydrophila biofilm formation by vanillin*, Environmental Engineering Science, 26(8),1359–1363.

Preda, V. G., & Săndulescu, O. (2019). Communication is the key: Biofilms, quorum sensing, formation and prevention. *Discoveries*, *7*(3), e10. https://doi.org/10.15190/d.2019.13

Rasko, D. A., & Sperandio, V. (2010). Anti-virulence strategies to combat bacteria-mediated disease. *Nature Reviews Drug Discovery*, *9*, 117–128. https://doi.org/10.1038/nrd3013

Reuter, K., Steinbach, A., & Helms, V. (2016). Interfering with bacterial quorum sensing. *Perspectives in Medicinal Chemistry*, *8*, 1–15. https://doi.org/10.4137/PMc.s13209

Rewak-Soroczyńska, J., Paluch, E., Siebert, A., Szałkiewicz, K., & Obłąk, E. (2019). Biological activity of glycine and alanine derivatives of quaternary ammonium salts (QASs) against micro-organisms. *Letters in Applied Microbiology*, *69*(3), 212–220. https://doi.org/10.1111/lam.13195

Singh, R., Paul, D., & Jain, R. K. (2006). Biofilms: Implications in bioremediation. In *Trends in microbiology* (Vol. 14, Issue 9, pp. 389–397). https://doi.org/10.1016/j.tim.2006.07.001

Stoodley, P., Sauer, K., Davies, D. G., & Costerton, J. W. (2002). Biofilms as complex differentiated communities. In *Annual review of Microbiology* (Vol. 56, pp. 187–209). https://doi.org/10.1146/annurev.micro.56.012302.160705

Tacconelli, E., Carrara, E., Savoldi, A., Harbarth, S., Mendelson, M., Monnet, D. L., Pulcini, C., Kahlmeter, G., Kluytmans, J., Carmeli, Y., Ouellette, M., Outterson, K., Patel, J., Cavaleri, M., Cox, E. M., Houchens, C. R., Grayson, M. L., Hansen, P., Singh, N., … Zorzet, A. (2018). Discovery, research, and development of new antibiotics: The WHO priority list of antibiotic-resistant bacteria and tuberculosis. *The Lancet Infectious Diseases*, *18*(3), 318–327. https://doi.org/10.1016/S1473-3099(17)30753-3

Vandeputte, O. M., Kiendrebeogo, M., Rasamiravaka, T., Stévigny, C., Duez, P., Rajaonson, S., Diallo, B., Mol, A., Baucher, M., & el Jaziri, M. (2011). The flavanone naringenin reduces the production of quorum sensing-controlled virulence factors in pseudomonas aeruginosa PAO1. *Microbiology*, *157*(7), 2120–2132. https://doi.org/10.1099/mic.0.049338-0

Zhang, J., Feng, T., Wang, J., Wang, Y., & Zhang, X. H. (2019). The mechanisms and applications of Quorum Sensing (QS) and Quorum Quenching (QQ). *Journal of Ocean University of China*, *18*(6), 1427–1442. https://doi.org/10.1007/s11802-019-4073-5

Ziemichód, A., & Skotarczak, B. (2017). QS – Systems communication of Gram-positive bacterial cells. *Acta Biologica*, *24*, 51–56. https://doi.org/10.18276/ab.2017.24-06

8 The Hypothalamic–Pituitary–Gonadal Axis in Drug Development for Androgens across Sex and Life Span

Gabriel Gbenga Babaniyi, Ulelu Jessica Akor, and Ebunoluwa Elizabeth Babaniyi

8.1 INTRODUCTION

The hypothalamus, pituitary gland, and gonadal glands are referred to as the hypothalamic–pituitary–gonadal axis (HPG axis) as if they were all one endocrine gland. There is a negative feedback loop that regulates the HPG axis. Gonadotropin-releasing hormone (GnRH) is released by the hypothalamus into the median eminence of the healthy brain, where it travels via the hypophyseal portal system to the anterior pituitary, where it acts on its receptor.[2] The HPG axis is essential for the growth and control of several bodily systems, including the immunological and reproductive systems. Changes in this axis alter the hormones each gland produces, which has a variety of local and systemic impacts on the body. Animal development, reproduction, and aging are all controlled by this axis. GnRH-expressing neurons in the brain secrete GnRH. Luteinizing hormone (LH) and follicle-stimulating hormone (FSH) are produced by the anterior pituitary gland, whereas estrogen and testosterone are produced by the gonads.[25] In oviparous creatures (such as fish, reptiles, amphibians, and birds), the hypothalamus–pituitary–gonadal–liver axis (HPGL axis) is the name given to this system in females. The liver produces a large number of chorionic and egg-yolk proteins that are essential for the growth and development of oocytes. These essential liver proteins include choriogenin and vitellogenin, for instance. The hypothalamus and pituitary control neuroendocrine activity through the hypothalamic–pituitary–adrenal (HPA), hypothalamic–pituitary–testicular (HPT), and HPG axes, three different pathways.[25,2]

However, with serum gonadotropin recovery, endocrine function finally becomes fully functional although slowly. Instead of indicating androgen shortage, a persistent mild, proportional drop in serum SHBG and T suggests long-lasting exogenous T effects

DOI: 10.1201/9781003297826-8

on hepatic SHBG secretion. This shows that rather than dose or length of androgen exposure, recovery from androgen-induced HPT axis suppression depends mostly on time following discontinuation.[55] However, early menopausal women have a distinct and distinctive pattern of "surges" of LH followed by pituitary "weariness," and was described as "oscillations" of LH excretion. The fact that this pattern has not been seen in nonvasomotor symptom (VMS) intermenstrual intervals supports the idea that a breakdown in the hypothalamic–pituitary–ovarian axis feedback loop results in extreme and cyclic variations in GnRH secretion, which in turn stimulates collateral nerves to change core body temperature. Regardless of the precise mechanism, Kuiri-Hänninen et al.[36] and Horstman et al.[32] found that a VMS algorithm may be developed and validated using the pattern of LH secretion as represented by oscillations in daily urine.

Furthermore, the activation of a neuroendocrine signaling cascade, known as the HPA axis, is necessary for all mammals to be able to respond to any environmental or homeostatic challenge (also known as a stressor) or to perceive threats to homeostasis. The adrenal glands produce and secrete glucocorticoids as a result of the HPA axis being activated in response to actual or perceived stimuli. To enable a body wide stress response, they affect almost all tissues. Glucocorticoids cause beneficial and necessary physiological and behavioral changes when acutely raised by stressors.[42,11,15] However, chronic stress or illness conditions that cause persistent glucocorticoid increases are harmful and raise the likelihood of stress-related pathology. Surprisingly, women have twice as high a chance of acquiring several of these disorders as men do, most likely because the HPA axis regulates and operates differently in each gender.[6] Understanding the nature and underlying factors causing these sex-specific variations in the HPA axis in response to stress has significant ramifications for comprehending sex-specific illness risk. Studies on rats have revealed a lot about the differences between sexes in the stress-induced activation of the HPA axis and their underlying processes. Such investigations have shown that sex variations in the HPA axis can be caused by the action of gonadal hormones in adulthood or during significant developmental times.[57,24] They also suggest that sex prejudices may be caused by sex chromosomal effects, albeit there is currently little data to support this.[5]

On the other hand, a paradox of aging is shown when older men and women are compared in terms of muscle loss. Hormones that men and women experience before, during, and after menopause and andropause may help to partially explain this paradox. Men and women experience muscle increase and loss at different rates and levels throughout their lives, for instance. Despite having a shorter life span than men, women have a faster rate of loss of muscular mass and strength as they get older.[58,11,57] In light of this, women are more vulnerable than men to age-related health issues, particularly reductions in muscle mass.[20] However, it has not been investigated if age-related reductions in sex hormones, muscle mass, and physical function are associated with increased longevity.

8.1.1 ACTIVATION OF THE HYPOTHALAMIC–PITUITARY–GONADAL (HPG) AXIS

The negative feedback effects mediated by the placental hormones force the HPG axis, which is active in the midgestational fetus but quiet toward term, to shut down.

At birth, this constraint is released, reactivating the axis and raising gonadotrophin levels. Except for FSH levels in girls, which stay elevated until three to four years of age, gonadotrophin levels are high during the first three months of life and start to decline around the age of six. Following this, the HPG axis is dormant until puberty.[7] The gonadal activation of both sexes is caused by the postnatal gonadotropin surge. At one to three months of age, testosterone levels in boys reach their peak and then fall in tandem with LH levels. Because postnatal HPG axis activation is linked to penile and testicular growth, it is thought to be crucial for the growth of male genitalia. Boys with congenital hypogonadotropic hypogonadism have underdeveloped penises and maldeveloped testicles at birth, which serve as proof of this. The development of ovarian follicles and an increase in estradiol levels occur in girls when gonadotropin levels are high.[36,66] The biological relevance of this minipuberty and its potential long-term effects, as well as the processes that keep the HPG axis dormant until puberty, are yet unknown. However, before pubertal development, the first few months of life offer a window of opportunity for functional research of the HPG axis.

8.1.1.1   Fetal HPG Axis Activity

Early in development, GnRH neurons move from the nasal placode to the hypothalamus, and at around 15 weeks of gestation, GnRH is found in the fetus's hypothalamus. Kisspeptin and KISS1R are components that regulate the activity of fetal GnRH neurons.[21] By 12–14 weeks of pregnancy, LH and FSH can be found in the anterior pituitary and blood circulation.[10,34] It is not entirely clear at what stage the pituitary gonadotrophin secretion starts to be controlled by the hypothalamus

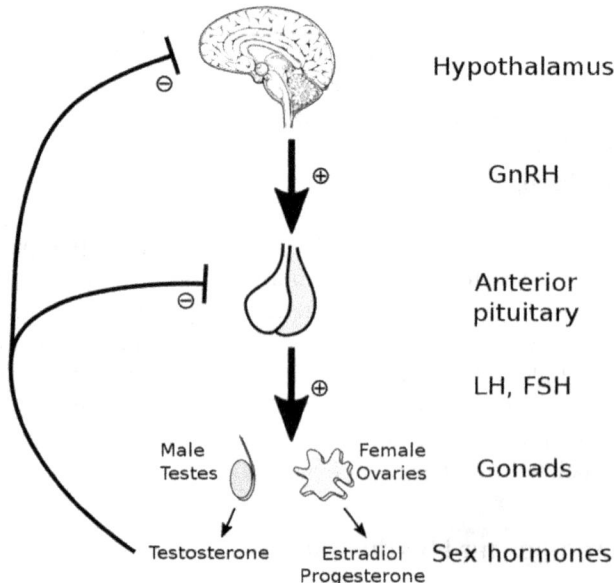

FIGURE 8.1   Hypogonadal axis.

GnRH. At the conclusion of the first trimester of pregnancy, vascular connections are already evident; nevertheless, the portal vascular system continues to develop after this point. Gonadotrope development is normal in anencephalic fetuses without the hypothalamus but with an intact pituitary until around 17 to 18 weeks of pregnancy, after which the cells become involuted.[53] They almost completely disappear after 32 weeks of gestation, indicating that hypothalamic input is necessary for the gonadotropes to be active after midgestation. Compared to male fetuses, female fetuses have greater pituitary gonadotrophin concentrations and serum LH and FSH levels throughout the first half of pregnancy.[36] The negative feedback effects of fetal testicular hormones have been hypothesized to be the cause of this sex difference.

LH and FSH levels in female fetuses are quite high at midgestation, comparable to those of agonadal adults or postmenopausal women.[21] LH levels are higher than FSH levels in male fetuses. The third gonadotrophin, hCG, has physiologic effects comparable to those of LH and is secreted by the placenta. According to Kuiri-Hänninen et al.,[36] the hCG levels in the fetus rise early in gestation, reach a peak at 8 to 12 weeks, and then start to decline as the baby approaches term but continue to be high into late gestation. Both sexes' LH and FSH levels are low at term and decline as the pregnancy progresses.[14] On the other hand, as gestation progresses, placental estrogen synthesis rises, and estrogen levels are high in both maternal and fetal circulation.[61] By the conclusion of gestation, there will likely be low levels of fetal gonadotrophin as a result of these high levels likely suppressing the activity of the fetal HPG axis. At the eighth week of gestation, the fetal testis begins to release testosterone and anti-Müllerian hormone (AMH). At this point, testosterone synthesis is crucial for the masculinization of the fetus, and testosterone also stimulates the growth of the male internal genitalia. The 5-reductase 2 (SRD5A2) enzyme produces the active testosterone metabolite dihydrotestosterone, which is necessary for the growth of the prostate, penis, and scrotum. The development of a uterus and fallopian tubes is inhibited by AMH because it causes the Müllerian ducts to retreat. The testosterone levels of male fetuses peak between 10 and 20 weeks of gestation, reaching adult levels, and then fall as they approach term.[21]

8.1.2   INHIBITION OF THE HYPOTHALAMIC–PITUITARY–GONADAL (HPG) AXIS

The HPG axis controls reproduction. Gonadotropin-releasing hormone is released to coordinate the hypothalamic control of reproduction (GnRH). A network of linked neurons in the brain controls the pulsatile release of GnRH. However, a large number of the crucial mechanisms and elements, such as modulation of GnRH pulsatile and surge modes of secretion, remain poorly understood. In the last ten years, it has been demonstrated that the neuropeptides kisspeptin and RFRP-3 have strong stimulatory or inhibitory effects on GnRH secretion in mammals, which modulate reproductive status.[1] There are numerous endocrine inputs that affect the gonadotrope, but none of them are more important than GnRH. The expression of the GnRH receptor (GnRHR) on the plasma membrane, as well as the production and secretion of LH and FSH, characterize the distinct phenotype of gonadotropes. It is widely known that GnRH causes the release of granules of LH secretory tissue into the bloodstream.[25] LH secretion is favored by an increase in GnRH pulse frequency and amplitude, whereas FSH secretion is favored by a decrease in frequency. The number of GnRHRs on the plasma membrane rises as a result of GnRH binding to its associated membrane receptor, and the expression of the various gonadotropin subunits also increases. The GnRHR is one of seven transmembrane domain G protein–coupled receptors that resemble rhodopsin (GPCR). Increases in GnRH pulsatility are necessary for the LH surge and ovulation, which makes this exquisite process especially crucial for female reproduction.[28] In response to hormone binding to the GnRHR, Gαq/11 is activated, and this sets off a series of phospholipase activities that result in the production of inositol 1,4,5- trisphosphate (IP3) and diacylglycerol.[25,1] In addition to increasing intracellular calcium concentrations, receptor activation activates protein kinase C (PKC) isoforms by releasing intracellular calcium stores and opening voltage-gated L-type calcium channels. The appropriate control of the HPG axis is regulated by a variety of factors, including neurological and hormonal ones. These aspects also present numerous intriguing study issues. Since reproduction and survival are essential for life, it makes sense that the two systems that support them, the HPG and HPA axes, would be connected. by conducting additional research on the HPG axis and the factors that control it. As a result, factors causing health problems and reproductive problems can be better understood.

8.2   SEX DIFFERENCES IN HYPOTHALAMIC–PITUITARY–GONADAL (HPG) AXIS ACTIVITY

Alzheimer's disease (AD) has been linked to gender as an independent risk factor. Age-adjusted odds ratios demonstrate that females have a higher risk of developing AD, whether familial or sporadic AD was acquired.[7] The changes in reproductive hormones that take place following menopause have been related to the higher prevalence and incidence of AD in women. As a result, women have increasingly been the subject of several studies on aging, such as the Women's Health Initiative Memory Study.[67,54] Hormone replacement therapy (HRT) is recommended to enhance cognition and lessen the risk of AD in postmenopausal women, since endocrinological assessments reveal decreased levels of estrogens in women with AD.[7] This theory is supported by a wealth of data showing the neuroprotective properties of estrogens in healthy cells. Axonal sprouting, regeneration, synaptic transmission, and the inhibition of cell death are all induced by estrogen signaling through a variety of mechanisms. Estrogen receptors can activate the production of brain-derived neurotrophic factor (BDNF), which has been shown to protect against ischemic injury in vitro and retain cognitive function as measured with passive avoidance in mice in vivo. Additionally, other in vitro studies have shown protective effects of estrogens from excitotoxicity by increasing the apoptosis regulator Bcl-2.[7] Moreover, estrogens have been shown to protect against oxidative stress induced by amyloid-β fibrils alone or in a complex with acetylcholinesterase, making estrogens a target for AD therapeutics. This study is relevant because the only available treatment for AD is cholinesterase inhibitors, which have only a modestly beneficial effect according to meta-analyses.[60] The absence of sex steroids causes significant increases in peripheral levels of LH, which works in concert with estrogens' role in cognition. LH and FSH levels rise by three- and fourfold, respectively, in aging women, while they rise by two- to threefold in aging men.[7] Given that gonadotropins only play a minor role in reproduction, the impact of altering gonadotropin levels during reproductive aging was largely overlooked until recently. A growing body of research, however, suggests that LH and activation of its receptor may play a significant role in cognitive function and neural plasticity in humans and rats, and in vitro.

Nevertheless, it has been demonstrated in some but not all studies that levels of LH and FSH are considerably elevated in AD patients compared to controls, and that increases in peripheral LH levels are associated with impaired cognition in both healthy men and women. For instance, it has been demonstrated that blood LH and FSH levels in both male and female patients are unaffected by the presence or absence of dementia.[12,53] Male AD status was found to be correlated with a tendency toward high serum LH levels, according to Hogervorst et al.[31] A study found a correlation between LH levels and amyloid levels, supporting the role of LH in the onset and progression of AD.[65] However, a receptor (LHCGR) shared by human chorionic gonadotropin (hCG) and LH is essential for reproductive processes like Leydig cell testosterone production and follicular maturation. The physiological and molecular function of LHCGR in reproduction is described in a substantial body of literature.[41] Following its identification and purification, it was discovered that LHCGR belongs to the rhodopsin-like class A GPCRs, which are expressed as a number of splice variants, all of which feature leucine-rich repeats in the extracellular domain.[41] G protein phosphorylates LHCGR, activating adenylyl cyclase, which then activates the cAMP/PKA and ERK pathways. Although LHCGR typically signals via the Gs/cAMP/PKA route, it can independently mediate phospholipase C (PLC) activation.[7]

Intriguingly, LH positivity has been shown in the hypothalamus, amygdala, septal area, preoptic area, thalamus caudate nucleus, and hippocampus by radioimmunoassay as well as immunocytochemistry.[30] Brain-derived LH has been demonstrated by rat brain extracts to have a similar chromatographic profile to pituitary LH and to be active in both the interstitial cell testosterone secretion bioassay and the testis LH radioligand receptor assay. Additionally, an adsorption dramatically decreased the immunoreactivity of LH in the rat brain. So, the central nervous system (CNS) contains LH and it is biologically active there. Studies involving the 3xTg AD mouse model have revealed LH immunoreactivity in areas of the brain associated with cognition. Importantly, ovariectomy lowers brain-derived LH levels, which are elevated in peripheral LH and positively correlated with enhanced performance in the Morris water maze.[49] This demonstrates an inverse relationship between serum (peripheral) LH levels and CNS LH levels. Importantly, this inverse relationship between peripheral and brain-derived LH may help explain the beneficial effects of hCG reported by Al-Hader et al.[3] in vitro and even the functional advantages of activation of LHCGR-dependent cascades by leuprolide acetate.[7]

As a result, the potential of sex hormone–binding globulin (SHBG) to diminish the bioactivity of sex steroids through binding and blocking action on their individual receptors confuses the age-dependent attenuation of sex steroid signaling in the HPG axis. Patients with AD have higher levels of SHBG and thus have decreased serum levels of bioactive sex steroids. Both male and female AD patients exhibit the resulting inverse association between cognition and SHBG.[7] It's crucial to take into account SHBG levels and how they relate to cognitive deterioration while evaluating the effectiveness of E2 and testosterone therapy. Importantly, SHBG levels might invalidate earlier research by turning off the sex steroid therapies. Although more research is required, pharmacological management of SHBG would maintain the bioactivity of endogenous estrogens and androgens and may lower the risk of cognitive decline.

8.2.1 ACTIVATIONAL EFFECTS OF GONADAL HORMONES

The interactions between the HPA axis and HPG axis, a parallel neuroendocrine network that regulates reproduction, are partly responsible for adult sex variations in the neuroendocrine response to acute stress.[64] In the testis and ovary, respectively, the HPG axis results in the generation of testosterone and the synthesis of estrogens from aromatizable androgens. In maturity, the HPA axis can be modulated by both testosterone and estrogen (i.e., they both have activational effects) and help to support its sex-dependent function. It's noteworthy that gonadal steroids also influence how the HPA axis functions in aging rodents. Receptors for gonadal hormones and where they are located by acting on estrogen receptors (ERs) and androgen receptors (ARs), respectively, estrogens and androgens affect HPA axis activity in adults.[24] While the powerful endogenous estrogen estradiol can activate any of the two primary ER subtypes, estrogen receptor alpha (ERα) or beta (ERβ), androgen testosterone and its metabolite, dihydrotestosterone (DHT), both bind the androgen receptor. The nuclear receptor subfamily 3, which also contains GR, MR, and the progesterone receptor (PR), includes the receptors AR, ERα, and ERβ. The traditional function of every receptor in this subfamily is as a ligand-activated transcription factor. They dwell in the nucleus or cytoplasm as multiprotein complexes until ligand interaction causes them to shuttle to chromatin DNA, where they can affect transcription.[50] These receptors interact with other transcriptional regulators or bind directly to DNA regions that contain hormone response elements to change transcription. ERs and ARs are membrane receptors that, like other nuclear receptor subfamily 3 members, have quicker (nonclassical) effects on neuronal function and/or transcriptional activity through modifying second messenger pathways and ion channels.[63,18] In addition, the membrane estrogen receptor G protein–coupled estrogen receptor (GPER), which has a high affinity for estradiol and can also mediate its immediate effects, has been discovered.[9] Therefore, gonadal hormone receptors allow gonadal hormones to alter HPA axis activity quickly and gradually through both classical and nonclassical activities. Gonadal steroids can alter the neuroendocrine response to stress in conjunction with changes in reproductive function because gonadal steroid hormone receptors are widely expressed in important regions of the brain circuitry governing the HPA axis. The cortex, hippocampus, MeA, bed nucleus of the stria terminalis (BNST), and various hypothalamic regions, including the medial preoptic area (MPOA), have been identified to express AR, ERα, and ERβ in the appropriate ways. The hippocampus and the hypothalamus both express GPER. However,

ERs and GPERs are strongly expressed in neuroendocrine paraventricular nucleus (PVN) neurons that control the activity of the HPA axis, whereas ARs are only weakly expressed. This suggests that gonadal steroids affect HPA activity in several ways.[25] Estradiol can affect HPA function directly by acting on neuroendocrine PVN neurons or indirectly by doing so through brain regions upstream of the PVN that project there; androgens, on the other hand, have been demonstrated to mostly have indirect effects. Because they have high levels of AR expression and project to the PVN and peri-PVN, the MPOA and BNST, for instance, are crucial mediators of the effects of androgens.[25]

The HPG-mediated fluctuations in estradiol levels that take place during a four-day estrus cycle in female rodents may have a significant impact on sex differences in the HPA axis activity. Early studies showed that basal and stress-induced activity of the HPA axis increases as estradiol concentrations do throughout the estrus cycle in female rats. Because of this, male and female rodents in diestrus (low estradiol) are similar in that they both have low resting glucocorticoid secretion and respond to stressors in a relatively quick on–off manner. Contrarily, females who have recently been exposed to peak estradiol are in estrus, which is characterized by elevated basal and stress-induced ACTH and CORT levels. Notably, increases in HPA production are greatest early in the proestrus cycle when estradiol levels are peaking but progesterone levels have not yet increased. Estradiol's effects on HPA production seem to be lessened by progesterone. Accordingly, estradiol treatment stimulates HPA activity more than estradiol and progesterone treatment combined in ovariectomized female rats replenished with physiological doses of estradiol with or without progesterone to imitate the estrus cycle.[25] Therefore, whether there is a high or low background amount of progesterone determines how much estradiol can raise HPA production during proestrus. This is consistent with animal research showing that progesterone therapy alone reduces HPA axis stress reactivity.[25] Additionally, after stress, glucocorticoid release in female rats in proestrus and estrus takes longer to return to baseline levels.[26] This might be because the glucocorticoid negative feedback on the HPA axis is less robust or because limbic areas that are known to suppress the HPA axis are not as active.[19,26] In fact, compared to diestrus females, proestrus and estrus females exhibit decreased levels of neural activation in the cortical and hippocampus areas.[19] Overall, research on how the HPA axis functions throughout the reproductive cycle has shown how crucial estradiol is to regulating the neuroendocrine reaction to stress.

8.2.2 Hormone Deficiencies, Therapies, and Longevity

All types of hormonal shortages can have a negative impact on health and longevity, which makes this debate more difficult. In order to promote function in older men and women, the use of testosterone treatments, and to a lesser extent estradiol and growth hormone replacement, has expanded significantly over the past few years. These therapies work by enhancing protein anabolism and reducing protein catabolism in skeletal muscle.[25] It is unclear if this strategy will result in longer life spans, but accumulating data points to the possibility that it could produce major health benefits through improved functional performance. In order to determine the efficacy and safety of hormone replacement with age and to clarify how it affects functional performance, health span, and life span, a more extensive large-scale study is required.

8.2.2.1 Androgens

A significant independent predictor of death in older men is the fall in anabolic hormone levels that comes with age. Beyond its impact on skeletal muscle and frailty, testosterone insufficiency has been associated with increased early mortality risk[2] and a range of comorbidities, including sexual problems, diabetes, and metabolic syndrome (including dyslipidemia, visceral obesity, hyperglycemia, hypertension, and thrombus formation process). Furthermore, low testosterone is linked to insulin resistance, which puts older men at risk for developing metabolic syndrome or type 2 diabetes. Additionally, given that these metabolic processes are probably connected, difficulties with cardiovascular disease in aging males are further complicated.[32] Nieschlag et al.[47] discovered no indication of a difference in life expectancy between intact and castrated singers. This could mean that orchiectomy did not affect men's longevity when they were prepubertal. But as the population ages, androgens may become more crucial to fend off weakness in the eighth, ninth, and tenth decades of life.

Irrespective of gender, testosterone replacement therapy may be successful in correcting age-related morbidity and body composition changes. Lean body mass and muscle strength increase as a result of testosterone administration, which also reduces body fat. However, not all research supports these (direct) changes in physical function or muscle strength.[32] To determine if androgens can have a positive or neutral influence on the morbidity and mortality associated with male cardiovascular disease, randomized controlled clinical trials evaluating testosterone therapy would be necessary. To ascertain the long-term dangers and advantages of testosterone administration in older adults, large-scale, long-term research on testosterone replacement in older men and women is required.[13,33] It would be extremely beneficial if it were possible to boost muscle strength through androgen injection, especially in people with limited or compromised functional ability. In order to gain fresh insights into the mechanisms behind the tissue-specific regulatory action of these protein complexes linked to sex hormones and steroid receptors, greater investigation into the bone-specific components of these complexes is required. These investigations may help identify new therapeutic targets and build more effective treatment plans for osteoporosis that develops as people age.

8.2.2.2 Estrogens

In postmenopausal women, estrogens improved muscle strength, as demonstrated by Lowe et al.,[40] whereas estrogen decreases have been linked to age-related declines in muscle strength. Two well-controlled studies demonstrate positive effects of hormone replacement therapy on skeletal muscle composition and function in postmenopausal women. However, the results on the effects of estradiol on muscle structure and contractile function in humans are conflicting and depend on the species examined, study type, age, muscle size, and fiber type, among other factors.[16,56] In older women, estrogens are also crucial for maintaining bone health. Older men who are estrogen deficient develop hypergonadotropism, osteoporosis, and elevated testosterone levels. The metabolism of carbohydrates and lipids is significantly impacted by estrogen deprivation, and estrogen resistance is linked to early coronary atherosclerosis in men. Cardiovascular events are linked to an elevated risk in both men and women with low estrogen levels. Hormone therapy based on estrogen helps maintain muscle strength.[22] Hormone replacement therapy is the first-line and most effective treatment for menopausal symptoms in older women, as well as for improving their low quality of life as a result of low estrogen.[2] However, Michael et al.[43] demonstrated that hormone therapy offered non-disabled postmenopausal women (aged 65–79) little overall protection against functional deterioration. Long-term postmenopausal estrogen replacement has the unfavorable effects of increasing cancer risk, venous thromboembolism rates, and the need for biliary tract surgery in older women with cardiovascular disease.[2] More research needs to be done in this area.

8.3 DRUG DEVELOPMENT FOR ANDROGENS ACROSS SEX

The gonads (the Leydig cells in the testes in men and the ovaries in women) are the primary organs responsible for producing testosterone. However, both sexes' adrenal glands also produce a trace amount of the hormone in both sexes. It increases the growth of male features because it is an androgen.[28,8] The genital tract, secondary sexual traits, and fertility are examples of reproductive tissues that can develop and maintain masculine qualities, and androgen is therefore characterized as a chemical that can do both while also promoting the anabolic status of somatic tissues. However, the main androgens found in mature male mammals' bloodstreams are testosterone and its powerful metabolite, dihydrotestosterone (DHT). As a result, Leydig cells, which are found in the interstitium of the testis between the seminiferous tubules, manufacture the majority of testosterone, which has a distinctive four-ring C18 steroid structure. In addition to maintaining blood levels of testosterone, Leydig cell secretion raises the local concentration of testosterone in the testis to extremely high levels, which has distinctive androgenic effects on distant androgen-sensitive target tissues.[2] The primary mechanism by which androgens exert their traditional biological effects is through binding to the androgen receptor, a member of the steroid nuclear receptor superfamily that is expressed by a single gene on the X chromosome. The androgen receptor then controls the transcription of a variety of androgen-responsive target genes, resulting in the expression of specific patterns of genes. A biochemical and pharmacological definition of an androgen as a substance that successfully competes with testosterone binding to the androgen receptor to stimulate post-receptor functions in isolated cells or cell-free systems has been added to this physiological definition of an androgen in the whole animal. Additionally, non-genomic methods of androgen action involving quick, membrane-mediated nontranscriptional processes in the cytoplasm have been described, but these have not yet been fully defined.[28,8]

Similar to how testosterone is used in androgen replacement therapy, testosterone or synthetic androgens based on their structural makeup are also utilized in pharmacologic androgen therapy at typically larger doses. Restoring a physiological pattern of androgen exposure to all tissues is the main objective of androgen replacement therapy. Such treatment is typically limited to the main androgen in nature, testosterone, and aims to mimic physiological levels of circulating testosterone, the full range of endogenous androgen effects on tissues (including activation of pre-receptor androgens), and the natural history of efficacy and safety. Pharmacologic androgen therapy takes advantage of the anabolic or other actions of androgens on bone, muscle, and other tissues as hormonal medications try to change the course of the underlying condition. Its effectiveness, safety, and relative cost efficiency are assessed like other therapeutic agents. For understanding and best utilization of androgen pharmacology, knowledge of the physiology of testosterone is a prerequisite.[48]

8.3.1 Testosterone Physiology

Within the 500 million Leydig cells, which make up about 5% of the mature testis and are found in the interstitial compartment of the testis between the seminiferous tubules, testosterone is produced through an enzymatic process from cholesterol. Although preformed cholesterol from intracellular cholesterol ester reserves or external supply from circulating low-density lipoproteins also contributes, de novo synthesis from acetate produces the majority of the cholesterol.[44]

8.3.1.1 Biosynthesis

Two multifunctional cytochrome P-450 complexes that involve hydroxylations and side-chain scissions are required for the production of testosterone. These include the 17-hydroxylase/17,20-lyase (CYP17A1 or P450c17), which hydroxylates the C17 and then excises two carbons (20 and 21), converting a 21- to a 19-carbon structure, and the 3- and 17-hydroxysteroid dehydrogenases.[44] A crucial branch point in the steroidogenic pathways is the extreme tissue-specific control of the 17,20-lyase activity, which is active in the gonads but dormant in the adrenals, independent of the 17-hydroxylase activity. The P450 oxidoreductase (POR), a membrane-bound flavoprotein with several functions as a reductase, and cytochrome b5 are two enzyme cofactors that affect the directionality of the route flux. Both activities are present in a single, multifunctional protein.[45,51] Additionally, it has been reported that the weak adrenal androgen precursor DHEA circulates in various tissues and is used in the extragonadal production of testosterone and dihydrotestosterone. Adrenal androgens do, however, provide a far bigger proportionate contribution to the amount of testosterone that is circulated in women than it does in men.[46] Although the exact physical state in which such high concentrations of intratesticular testosterone and related steroids exist in the testis is still unknown, the high testicular production rate of testosterone results in both high local concentrations of testosterone (up to 1 µg/g tissue, which is approximately 100 times higher than blood concentrations) and rapid turnover (200 times per day).

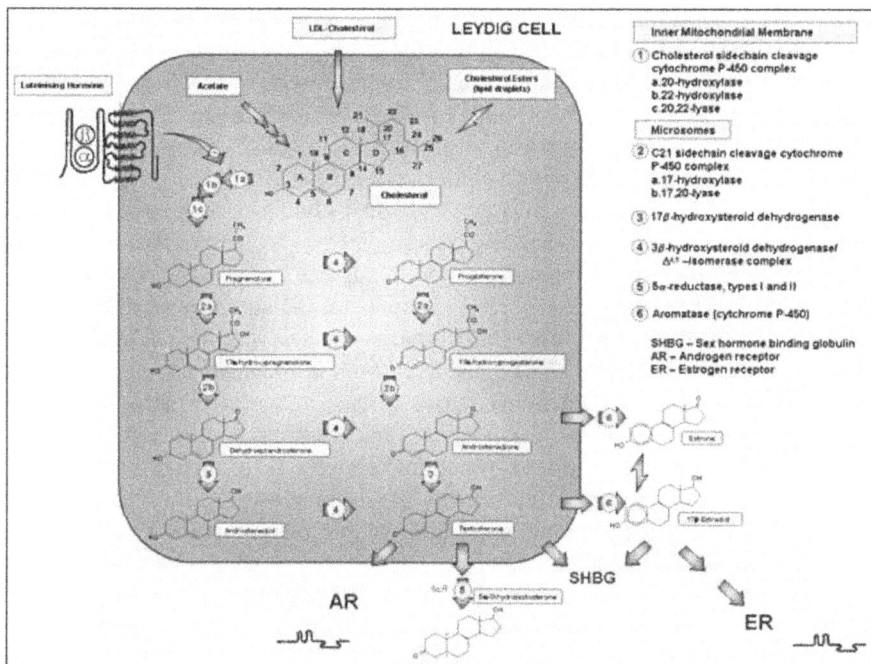

FIGURE 8.2 Pathways of testosterone biosynthesis and action.

By the enzyme sequences shown in Figure 8.2, testosterone production in men nearly entirely takes place in mature Leydig cells. Luteinizing hormone controls the rate-limiting step in the conversion of cholesterol to pregnenolone inside mitochondria. The remaining enzymatic steps take place in the smooth endoplasmic reticulum. Cholesterol is mostly produced by the de novo synthesis pathway from acetyl CoA. The left and right sides, respectively, are home to the steroidal pathways Δ^5 and Δ^4. Testosterone and its androgenic byproduct, dihydrotestosterone, exert biological effects directly by attaching to the androgen receptor and indirectly by aromatizing to estradiol, which enables activity via binding to the ER. Members of the steroid nuclear receptor superfamily, androgen and ERs have largely comparable structures with just the C-terminal ligand binding domain separating them from other members. The LH receptor is made up of a large extracellular domain that binds the LH molecule and the typical seven transmembrane-spanning helix sections found in G protein–coupled receptors. LH is a dimeric glycoprotein hormone made up of a subunit that is unique to LH and a subunit that is shared by other pituitary glycoprotein hormones. Most sex steroids bind to SHBG, which tightly binds and transports the majority of testosterone in the bloodstream.[4]

8.3.1.2 Secretion

In three stages of male development, testosterone is secreted at adult levels: briefly during the first trimester of intrauterine life (coinciding with the development of the masculine genital tract), early in the neonatal period as the perinatal androgen surge (of undetermined physiologic significance), and continuously after puberty to maintain virilization. The sudden increases in testosterone output from the testicles, which rise roughly 30-fold over levels found in prepubertal toddlers, women, or castrated men, are what cause the dramatic physical changes associated with male puberty. In males who are in good health but also have a chronic illness, there are steady decreases in circulating testosterone as well as increases in gonadotrophin and SHBG levels after middle age. However, these patterns are absent until late old age in these men.[35] There are also temporal trends, such as an increase in the incidence of obesity and variations in testosterone immunoassays caused by artifactual methods that differ from standard mass spectrometry results.[59] Ineffective hypothalamic control of testicular function, Leydig cell attrition, malfunction, and atherosclerosis of testicular arteries are all functional causes of these age-related alterations brought on by the accumulation of chronic illness states. This causes the aging HPT axis to gradually operate with multilevel functional abnormalities that, when combined, result in lower levels of circulating testosterone in men as they age.[62] Additionally, the mean circulating testosterone levels and the estimated testicular arteriovenous differences and testicular blood flow rate can both be used to estimate the metabolic clearance rate (from bolus injection or steady-state isotope infusion using high specific-activity tracers) and hormone production rates. Under the assumption of steady-state conditions, these techniques provide reliable estimates of a testosterone production rate of 3 to 10 mg/day utilizing tritiated or nonradioactive deuterated tracers with interconversion rates of around 4% to dihydrotestosterone (DHT) and 0.2% to estradiol (hours to days). These steady-state approaches are a simplification that ignores the effects of postural changes on hepatic blood flow and episodic fluctuations in circulating testosterone levels over shorter time frames (minutes to hours), which are influenced by pulsatile LH production. Circulating SHBG concentration, diurnal periodicity, and postural effects on hepatic blood flow are the main known factors of the testosterone metabolic clearance rate. Significant genetic influences on circulating testosterone levels have been reported, along with environmental implications via modifications in SHBG and other pathways.[52]

8.3.1.3 Transport

By attaching to circulating plasma proteins, testosterone circulates in the blood at levels higher than those at which it is soluble in water. The most significant is SHBG, a high-affinity but low-capacity binding protein. Albumin, corticosteroid-binding globulin, and α1 acid glycoprotein are examples of low-affinity binding proteins.[8] Testosterone has a strong affinity for circulating SHBG, a homodimer of two glycoprotein subunits with a combined amino acid count of 373 and three glycosylation sites, two of which are N-linked and one of which is O-linked.[29] Upon consecutive binding of an androgen, the two binding sites in the homodimer exhibit dynamic, cooperative binding affinities.[23] Acquired liver illness does not change the affinity of SHBG for binding testosterone, which is subject to genetic variations.[52] However, under physiological circumstances, between 60% and 70% of the testosterone in the blood is SHBG-bound, with the remaining 10% to 20% bound to lower affinity, high-capacity binding sites (albumin, α1 acid glycoprotein, corticosteroid-binding protein), and 1% to 2% remaining non-protein bound. According to the physico-chemical partitioning between the hydrophobic protein binding sites on circulating binding proteins, the hydrophilic aqueous extracellular fluid, and the lipophilic cellular plasma membranes, the transfer of hydrophobic steroids into tissues is therefore assumed to occur passively.

8.3.1.4 Measurement

In order to validate a clinical and pathological diagnosis of androgen deficit, monitoring blood testosterone concentration is a critical component of the clinical examination of androgen status. The amount of testosterone in the blood serves as a proxy for both the body's overall testosterone production rate and the tissues' apparent response to androgens. The emphasis on a single point measurement of blood testosterone concentration, however, ignores variations in the metabolic clearance rate over the entire body as well as other elements affecting net androgen effects at tissue levels. These parameters include pre-receptor, receptor, and post-receptor influences on testosterone activation, inactivation, and action in that tissue. They also include the effectiveness of blood testosterone transfer into nearby tissues during capillary transit. Additionally, dynamic circulating testosterone levels exhibit different circhoral and diurnal patterns. Although the buffering actions of the circulating steroid-binding proteins attenuate the pulsatility of blood testosterone concentrations, circhoral LH pulsatility entrains some pulsatility in blood testosterone levels. This is demonstrated by contrast with the startlingly pulsatile patterns of circulating testosterone in mice lacking the expression of the hepatic SHBG gene, which lacks the ability to produce circulating SHBG to stabilize fluctuations in testosterone levels.[12,17] Younger and healthier older men exhibit diurnal rhythms of morning peak testosterone levels and mid-afternoon nadir levels; however, some aging men lose these patterns.[28] As a result, it is customary to normalize testosterone values to blood samples taken in the morning on at least two distinct days. Utilizing tracer reference techniques such as equilibrium dialysis or ultrafiltration, assays to measure blood "free" testosterone levels directly in serum samples have been developed. Additionally, various formulas based on immunoassay measurements of total testosterone and SHBG have been calculated. Due to the arduous nature of measuring "free" or "bioavailable" testosterone, calculational equations with questionable validity have been extensively employed; nevertheless, large-scale evaluations have shown that these estimations for free or bioavailable testosterone are inaccurate. Generally speaking, the clinical applicability of various derived (free, bioavailable) measures of testosterone resulting from the unproven free hormone hypothesis is still being determined; as a result, they play a minor role in the clinical consensus guidelines for the diagnosis and treatment of androgen deficiency.

8.4 DRUG DEVELOPMENT FOR ANDROGENS ACROSS LIFE SPAN

The androgen receptor is necessary for the formation of a mature testis capable of supporting spermatogenesis and producing testosterone, which serve as the foundation for male fertility. These processes ultimately result in the differentiation of masculine sexuality and sexual maturation. One X chromosomal gene, which codes for a protein with 919 amino acids and is located at Xq11–12, defines the human androgen receptor. a traditional member of the large nuclear receptor superfamily, which also includes receptors for thyroid hormones, retinoic acid, vitamin D, and many orphan receptors (receptors for which the ligand was initially unknown) and the five classes of mammalian steroid hormones (androgen, estrogen, progesterone, glucocorticoid, and mineralocorticoid).[28] Although levels of expression and androgen sensitivity in nonreproductive tissues vary, androgen receptor expression is not restricted to reproductive organs and is widespread.

Depending on the dosage, kind of androgen, and treatment goals, androgen therapy can either be a physiologic replacement or a pharmacologic therapy. The goal of androgen replacement therapy is to raise tissue androgen exposure to levels that are comparable to those of eugonadal men in androgen-deficient men who have pathological hypogonadism (reproductive system disorders). Androgen replacement treatment strives to restore the whole spectrum of androgen effects while mimicking the efficacy and safety experience of eugonadal men of similar age. It uses the natural androgen testosterone and a dose that keeps blood testosterone levels within the eugonadal range. Because androgen deficiency, whether brought on by castration or a biological condition, has a modest impact on life duration, it is doubtful that testosterone replacement therapy can increase longevity.[37] Pharmacologic androgen therapy is an approach that uses androgens without limitations on type or amount in an effort to produce androgen effects on muscle, bone, brain, or other tissues. An androgen is used therapeutically to utilize the anabolic or other effects of androgens on muscle, bone, and other tissues as hormonal medications in a variety of nonreproductive illnesses, regardless of the androgen status in such pharmacological treatment. Both the use of testosterone, a natural androgen, and the use of physiological replacement doses or their equal are not restrictions on this type of pharmaceutical androgen therapy. Rather, it is evaluated similarly to any other hormonal or xenobiotic nonhormonal therapeutic medication for its efficacy, safety, and relative cost-effectiveness for that particular application. As more specialized treatments are discovered, many prior applications of pharmacologic androgen therapy are now regarded as second-line medicines.[38] While improved first-line drug treatments for endometriosis, osteoporosis, and advanced breast cancer have similarly reduced the use of androgen therapy to a last resort, newer mechanism-based agents in development for hereditary angioedema may replace 17-alkylated androgens. Erythropoietin has, however, largely replaced androgen therapy for anemia caused by marrow or renal failure.[68,39] Pharmacological androgen therapy, however, continues to be a viable, affordable option with a well-proven efficacy and safety profile in many clinical settings (Figure 8.3).

Androgen-deficient men with pathological reproductive system disorders (hypothalamus, pituitary, testes) that prevent the testes from producing enough testosterone to meet the body's normal needs are the only group of patients who have a clear clinical indication for testosterone replacement therapy. Finding well-defined abnormalities of the hypothalamus, pituitary, or testis with a known and clearly characterized pathological foundation is necessary to establish a pathological basis for

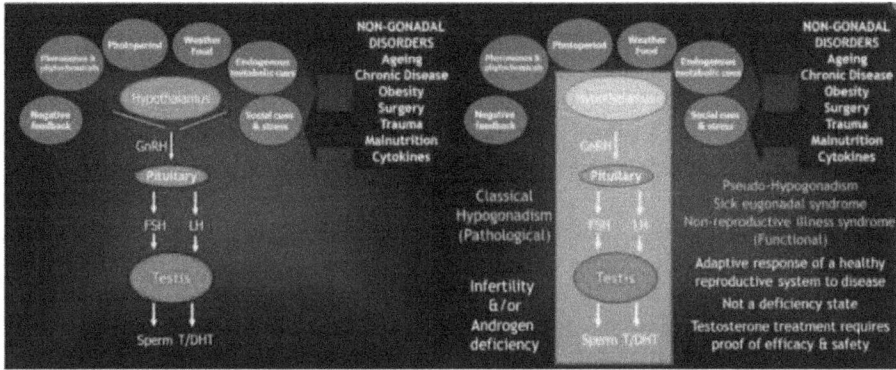

FIGURE 8.3 The hypothalamic–pituitary–testicular axis in health and intrinsic and extrinsic diseases.

testosterone replacement therapy. These conditions can and frequently do result in persistent testosterone deficiency, either as a result of conditions affecting the testis, where damaged Leydig cells are unable to produce enough testosterone, or as a result of conditions affecting the hypothalamus and/or pituitary, where impaired pituitary LH secretion eliminates the primary stimulator of Leydig cell testosterone synthesis. Furthermore, since 25%–35% of men who need androgen replacement therapy have Klinefelter's syndrome, it is possible to estimate the prevalence of male hypogonadism in the general population from the known prevalence of Klinefelter's syndrome in 33 prospective birth survey studies is 15.6 per 1000 male births.[27,28] The most prevalent hormonal deficiency disorder in males is androgen deficiency, with an estimated frequency of 5 per 1000 men in the general population. Although adult castration does not affect life expectancy and lifelong androgen shortage only mildly shortens it (two years), the hormonal imbalance results in avoidable morbidity and a poor quality of life.[27,28] Androgen deficiency is still vastly underdiagnosed due to its variable and frequently subtle clinical features, depriving sufferers of straightforward and efficient medical care with frequently striking benefits. In stark contrast to the typical expectation of reproductive health care for women, only 20% of men with Klinefelter's syndrome, which is characterized by the highly distinctive tiny (4 mL) testes, are diagnosed throughout their lifetime, meaning that the majority of men live without ever having their pelvis examined by a medical professional. Because all currently envisioned regimens using testosterone, either alone or in combination with a progestin or a GnRH antagonist, aim to suppress spermatogenesis (and thereby endogenous testosterone production), androgen replacement therapy can be considered a form of hormonal male contraception.

8.5 CONCLUSIONS

Because the endocrine system is crucial for cellular communication, metabolism, and growth, changes in hormone levels have an impact on the aging process. More specifically, there is a strong clinically significant correlation between age-related declines in muscle and bone mass and strength, declines in androgen and estrogen levels, and eventually human health span. To mitigate the dramatic and quick reductions in androgen and estrogen concentrations with aging and the role of these hormones in total human longevity, further research is required to determine the right roles, efficacies, and safe uses of hormone and exercise training therapies. In humans, genetic variables that induce organ development, particularly gonadal development and androgen-dependent programming, are tightly regulated in a tissue-specific, spatially and temporally connected manner. Endocrine, paracrine, and autocrine steroid production, as well as the recruitment of several additional regulators involved in the specificity of androgen action through change of the hormone–receptor complex, all contribute to the facilitation of modification. One way to measure this is as an "androgen sensitivity index." This may have a variety of therapeutic implications, including it is impossible to undo the effects of androgens during pregnancy or the absence of androgenization. This is visible in genital structures, but it is also conceivably implied in the development of other tissues, such as the brain. The supplementation of many substances may be helpful to elicit particular effects because any replacement of androgens should consider their variable effects on androgen action. Third, androgens have a specific influence and side effects, therefore the timing of treatment is crucial. In general, females secrete more glucocorticoids in response to different acute stressors, which is consistent with findings of sex differences in HPA axis regulation at all levels. There is also a ton of evidence that gonadal hormones play organizing and activating roles in sex variations in acute HPA axis activity. To reduce the chances of sex chromosomal effects that modify HPA activity both with and without gonadal steroids, more research is required. Finally, the neuroendocrine stress response to chronic stress differs significantly between the sexes. The HPA axis is dysregulated during chronic stress as opposed to acute stress, which may raise the risk of stress-related disorders in people. Therefore, future research on the roles of gonadal hormones and sex chromosomes in the sex differences in chronic stress-induced HPA dysregulation may have significant therapeutic implications.

REFERENCES

1. Acevedo-Rodriguez, A., Kauffman, A. S., Cherrington, B. D., Borges, C. S., Roepke, T. A., & Laconi, M. (2018). Emerging insights into hypothalamic-pituitary-gonadal axis regulation and interaction with stress signalling. *Journal of Neuroendocrinology*, *30*(10), e12590.
2. Aleksic, S., Desai, D., Ye, K., Duran, S., Gao, T., Crandall, J. P., ... Milman, S. (2021). The hypothalamic-pituitary-testicular axis in exceptionally old men. *Journal of the Endocrine Society*, *5*(Supplement_1), A727–A727.
3. Al-Hader, A. A., Lei, Z. M., & Rao, C. V. (1997). Neurons from fetal rat brains contain functional luteinizing hormone/chorionic gonadotropin receptors. *Biology of Reproduction*, *56*(5), 1071–1076.
4. Al-Hader, A. A., Lei, Z. M., & Rao, C. V. (1997). Novel expression of functional luteinizing hormone/chorionic gonadotropin receptors in cultured glial cells from neonatal rat brains. *Biology of Reproduction*, *56*(2), 501–507.

5. Arnold, A. P. (2009). The organizational–activational hypothesis as the foundation for a unified theory of sexual differentiation of all mammalian tissues. *Hormones and Behavior, 55*(5), 570–578.

6. Bangasser, D. A., & Valentino, R. J. (2014). Sex differences in stress-related psychiatric disorders: Neurobiological perspectives. *Frontiers in Neuroendocrinology, 35*(3), 303–319.

7. Blair, J. A., McGee, H., Bhatta, S., Palm, R., & Casadesus, G. (2015). Hypothalamic–pituitary–gonadal axis involvement in learning and memory and Alzheimer's disease: More than "just" estrogen. *Frontiers in Endocrinology, 6*, 45.

8. Bock, S. L., Chow, M. I., Forsgren, K. L., & Lema, S. C. (2021). Widespread alterations to hypothalamic-pituitary-gonadal (HPG) axis signaling underlie high temperature reproductive inhibition in the eurythermal sheepshead minnow (Cyprinodon variegatus). *Molecular and Cellular Endocrinology, 537*, 111447.

9. Brailoiu, E., Dun, S. L., Brailoiu, G. C., Mizuo, K., Sklar, L. A., Oprea, T. I., ... Dun, N. J. (2007). Distribution and characterization of estrogen receptor G protein-coupled receptor 30 in the rat central nervous system. *Journal of Endocrinology, 193*(2), 311–321.

10. Clements, J. A., Reyes, F. I., Winter, J. S. D., & Faiman, C. (1976). Studies on human sexual development. III. Fetal pituitary and serum, and amniotic fluid concentrations of LH, CG, and FSH. *The Journal of Clinical Endocrinology & Metabolism, 42*(1), 9–19.

11. Costantini, D., Marasco, V., & Møller, A. P. (2011). A meta-analysis of glucocorticoids as modulators of oxidative stress in vertebrates. *Journal of Comparative Physiology B, 181*(4), 447–456.

12. Coquelin, A., & Desjardins, C. (1982). Luteinizing hormone and testosterone secretion in young and old male mice. *American Journal of Physiology, 243*, E257–E263.

13. Dillon, E. L., Durham, W. J., Urban, R. J., & Sheffield-Moore, M. (2010). Hormone treatment and muscle anabolism during aging: Androgens. *Clinical Nutrition, 29*(6), 697–700.

14. Debiève, F., Beerlandt, S., Hubinont, C., & Thomas, K. (2000). Gonadotropins, prolactin, inhibin A, inhibin B, and activin A in human fetal serum from midpregnancy and term pregnancy. *The Journal of Clinical Endocrinology & Metabolism, 85*(1), 270–274.

15. De Kloet, E. R., Joëls, M., & Holsboer, F. (2005). Stress and the brain: From adaptation to disease. *Nature Reviews Neuroscience, 6*(6), 463–475.

16. Dieli-Conwright, C. M., Spektor, T. M., Rice, J. C., Sattler, F. R., & Schroeder, E. T. (2009). Hormone therapy attenuates exercise-induced skeletal muscle damage in postmenopausal women. *Journal of Applied Physiology, 107*(3), 853–858.

17. Ellis, G. B., & Desjardins, C. (1982). Male rats secrete luteinizing hormone and testosterone pisodically. *Endocrinology, 110*, 1618–1627.

18. Foradori, C. D., Weiser, M. J., & Handa, R. J. (2008). Non-genomic actions of androgens. *Frontiers in Neuroendocrinology, 29*(2), 169–181.

19. Figueiredo, H. F., Dolgas, C. M., & Herman, J. P. (2002). Stress activation of cortex and hippocampus is modulated by sex and stage of estrus. *Endocrinology, 143*(7), 2534–2540.

20. Green, M. R., & McCormick, C. M. (2016). Sex and stress steroids in adolescence: Gonadal regulation of the hypothalamic–pituitary–adrenal axis in the rat. *General and Comparative Endocrinology, 234*, 110–116.

21. Guimiot, F., Chevrier, L., Dreux, S., Chevenne, D., Caraty, A., Delezoide, A. L., & De Roux, N. (2012). Negative fetal FSH/LH regulation in late pregnancy is associated with declined kisspeptin/KISS1R expression in the tuberal hypothalamus. *The Journal of Clinical Endocrinology & Metabolism, 97*(12), E2221–E2229.

22. Greising, S. M., Baltgalvis, K. A., Lowe, D. A., & Warren, G. L. (2009). Hormone therapy and skeletal muscle strength: A meta-analysis. *The Journals of Gerontology. Series A, Biological Sciences, 64*(10), 1071–1081.

23. Goldman, A. L., Bhasin, S., Wu, F. C. W., Krishna, M., Matsumoto, A. M., & Jasuja, R. (2017). A reappraisal of testosterone's binding in circulation: Physiological and clinical implications. *Endocrine Reviews, 38*, 302–324.

24. Handa, R. J., & Weiser, M. J. (2014). Gonadal steroid hormones and the hypothalamo–pituitary–adrenal axis. *Frontiers in Neuroendocrinology, 35*(2), 197–220.

25. Heck, A. L., & Handa, R. J. (2019). Sex differences in the hypothalamic–pituitary–adrenal axis' response to stress: An important role for gonadal hormones. *Neuropsychopharmacology, 44*(1), 45–58.

26. Herman, J. P., McKlveen, J. M., Ghosal, S., Kopp, B., Wulsin, A., Makinson, R., ... Myers, B. (2016). Regulation of the hypothalamic-pituitary-adrenocortical stress response. *Comprehensive Physiology, 6*(2), 603.

27. Handelsman, D. J. (2007). Update in andrology. *Journal of Clinical Endocrinology and Metabolism, 92*, 4505–4511.

28. Handelsman, D. J. (2020). Androgen physiology, pharmacology, use and misuse. [Updated 2020 Oct 5]. *Endotext [Internet]. South Dartmouth (MA): MDText. com, Inc.*

29. Hammond, G. L., Wu, T. S., & Simard, M. (2012). Evolving utility of sex hormone-binding globulin measurements in clinical medicine. *Current Opinion in Endocrinology, Diabetes and Obesity, 19*, 183–189.

30. Hostetter, G., Gallo, R. V., & Brownfield, M. S. (1981). Presence of immunoreactive luteinizing hormone in the rat forebrain. *Neuroendocrinology, 33*(4), 241–245.

31. Hogervorst, E., Bandelow, S., Combrinck, M., & Smith, A. D. (2004). Low free testosterone is an independent risk factor for Alzheimer's disease. *Experimental Gerontology, 39*(11–12), 1633–1639.

32. Horstman, A. M., Dillon, E. L., Urban, R. J., & Sheffield-Moore, M. (2012). The role of androgens and estrogens on healthy aging and longevity. *Journals of Gerontology Series A: Biomedical Sciences and Medical Sciences, 67*(11), 1140–1152.

33. Jones, T. H. (2010). Testosterone deficiency: A risk factor for cardiovascular disease? *Trends in Endocrinology & Metabolism, 21*(8), 496–503.

34. Kaplan, S. L., & Grumbach, M. M. (1976). The ontogenesis of human foetal hormones. II. Luteinizing hormone (LH) and follicle stimulating hormone (FSH). *European Journal of Endocrinology, 81*(4), 808–829.

35. Kaufman, J. M., & Vermeulen, A. (2005). The decline of androgen levels in elderly men and its clinical and therapeutic implications. *Endocrine Reviews, 26*, 833–876.

36. Kuiri-Hänninen, T., Sankilampi, U., & Dunkel, L. (2014). Activation of the hypothalamic-pituitary-gonadal axis in infancy: Minipuberty. *Hormone Research in Paediatrics, 82*(2), 73–80.

37. Liu, P. Y., Death, A. K., & Handelsman, D. J. (2003). Androgens and cardiovascular disease. *Endocrine Reviews, 24*, 313–340.

38. Liu, P. Y., & Handelsman, D. J. (2004). Androgen therapy in non-gonadal disease. In E. Nieschlag & H. M. Behre (Eds.), *Testosterone: Action, Deficiency and Substitution* (3rd Ed., pp. 445–495). Berlin: Springer-Verlag.

39. Longhurst, H., & Cicardi, M. (2012). Hereditary angio-oedema. *Lancet, 379*, 474–481.

40. Lowe, D. A., Baltgalvis, K. A., & Greising, S. M. (2010). Mechanisms behind estrogen's beneficial effect on muscle strength in females. *Exercise and Sport Sciences Reviews, 38*(2), 61–67.

41. Menon, K. M. J., & Menon, B. (2012). Structure, function and regulation of gonadotropin receptors–a perspective. *Molecular and Cellular Endocrinology, 356*(1–2), 88–97.

42. Munck, A., Guyre, P. M., & Holbrook, N. J. (1984). Physiological functions of glucocorticoids in stress and their relation to pharmacological actions. *Endocrine Reviews, 5*(1), 25–44.
43. Michael, Y. L., Gold, R., & Manson, J. E. (2010). Hormone therapy and physical function change among older women in the Women's Health Initiative: A randomized controlled trial. *Menopause, 17*(2), 295–302.
44. Miller, W. L., & Auchus, R. J. (2011). The molecular biology, biochemistry, and physiology of human steroidogenesis and its disorders. *Endocrine Reviews, 32*, 81–151.
45. Miller, W. L., & Tee, M. K. (2015). The post-translational regulation of 17,20 lyase activity. *Molecular and Cellular Endocrinology, 408*, 99–106.
46. Miller, W. L. (2017). Disorders in the initial steps of steroid hormone synthesis. *The Journal of Steroid Biochemistry and Molecular Biology. 165*, 18–37.
47. Nieschlag, E., Nieschlag, S., & Behre, H. M. (1993). Lifespan and testosterone. *Nature, 366*(6452), 215.
48. Nieschlag, E. (2010). Male hormonal contraception. *Fertility Control, 198*, 197–223.
49. Palm, R., Chang, J., Blair, J., Garcia-Mesa, Y., Lee, H. G., Castellani, R. J., ... Casadesus, G. (2014). Down-regulation of serum gonadotropins but not estrogen replacement improves cognition in aged-ovariectomized 3xTg AD female mice. *Journal of Neurochemistry, 130*(1), 115–125.
50. Pawlak, M., Lefebvre, P., & Staels, B. (2012). General molecular biology and architecture of nuclear receptors. *Current Topics in Medicinal Chemistry, 12*(6), 486–504.
51. Peng, H. M., Im, S. C., Pearl, N. M., Turcu, A. F., Rege, J., Waskell, L., & Auchus, R. J. (2016). Cytochrome b5 activates the 17,20-lyase activity of human cytochrome P450 17A1 by increasing the coupling of NADPH consumption to androgen production. *Biochemistry, 55*, 4356–4365.
52. Perheentupa, A., Makinen, J., Laatikainen, T., Vierula, M., Skakkebaek, N. E., Andersson, A. M., & Toppari, J. (2013). A cohort effect on serum testosterone levels in Finnish men. *European Journal of Endocrinology, 168*, 227–233.
53. Pilavdzic, D., Kovacs, K., & Asa, S. L. (1997). Pituitary morphology in anencephalic human fetuses. *Neuroendocrinology, 65*(3), 164–172.
54. Rapp, S. R., Espeland, M. A., Shumaker, S. A., Henderson, V. W., Brunner, R. L., Manson, J. E., ... WHIMS Investigators. (2003). Effect of estrogen plus progestin on global cognitive function in postmenopausal women: The Women's Health Initiative Memory Study: A randomized controlled trial. *JAMA, 289*(20), 2663–2672.
55. Rybka, K. A., Sturm, K. L., De Guzman, R. M., Bah, S., Jacobskind, J. S., Rosinger, Z. J., ... Zuloaga, D. G. (2022). Androgen regulation of corticotropin releasing factor receptor 1 in the mouse brain. *Neuroscience, 491*, 185–199.
56. Ronkainen, P. H., Kovanen, V., & Alen, M. (2009). Postmenopausal hormone replacement therapy modifies skeletal muscle composition and function: A study with monozygotic twin pairs. *Journal of Applied Physiology, 107*(1), 25–33.
57. Seale, J. V., Wood, S. A., Atkinson, H. C., Harbuz, M. S., & Lightman, S. L. (2004). Gonadal steroid replacement reverses gonadectomy-induced changes in the corticosterone pulse profile and stress-induced hypothalamic-pituitary-adrenal axis activity of male and female rats. *Journal of Neuroendocrinology, 16*(12), 989–998.
58. Seale, J. V., Wood, S. A., Atkinson, H. C., Lightman, S. L., & Harbuz, M. S. (2005). Organizational role for testosterone and estrogen on adult hypothalamic-pituitary-adrenal axis activity in the male rat. *Endocrinology, 146*(4), 1973–1982.
59. Sikaris, K., McLachlan, R. I., Kazlauskas, R., de Kretser, D., Holden, C. A., & Handelsman, D. J. (2005). Reproductive hormone reference intervals for healthy fertile young men: Evaluation of automated platform assays. *Journal of Clinical Endocrinology and Metabolism, 90*, 5928–5936.

60. Trinh, N. H., Hoblyn, J., Mohanty, S., & Yaffe, K. (2003). Efficacy of cholinesterase inhibitors in the treatment of neuropsychiatric symptoms and functional impairment in Alzheimer disease: A meta-analysis. *JAMA, 289*(2), 210–216.

61. Troisi, R., Potischman, N., Roberts, J. M., Harger, G., Markovic, N., Cole, B., ... Hoover, R. N. (2003). Correlation of serum hormone concentrations in maternal and umbilical cord samples. *Cancer Epidemiology Biomarkers & Prevention, 12*(5), 452–456.

62. Veldhuis, J. D., Keenan, D. M., Liu, P. Y., Iranmanesh, A., Takahashi, P. Y., & Nehra, A. X. (2009). The aging male hypothalamic-pituitary-gonadal axis: Pulsatility and feedback. *Molecular and Cellular Endocrinology, 299*, 14–22.

63. Vasudevan, N., & Pfaff, D. W. (2008). Non-genomic actions of estrogens and their interaction with genomic actions in the brain. *Frontiers in Neuroendocrinology, 29*(2), 238–257.

64. Viau, V. (2002). Functional cross-talk between the hypothalamic-pituitary-gonadal and-adrenal axes. *Journal of Neuroendocrinology, 14*(6), 506–513.

65. Verdile, G., Laws, S. M., Henley, D., Ames, D., Bush, A. I., Ellis, K. A., ... Martins, R. N. (2014). Associations between gonadotropins, testosterone and β amyloid in men at risk of Alzheimer's disease. *Molecular Psychiatry, 19*(1), 69–75.

66. Yang, D., Zhang, W., Zhu, Y., Liu, P., Tao, B., Fu, Y., ... Yan, Z. (2019). Initiation of the hypothalamic–pituitary–gonadal axis in young girls undergoing central precocious puberty exerts remodeling effects on the prefrontal cortex. *Frontiers in Psychiatry, 10*, 332.

67. Zandi, P. P., Carlson, M. C., Plassman, B. L., Welsh-Bohmer, K. A., Mayer, L. S., Steffens, D. C., ... Cache County Memory Study Investigators. (2002). Hormone replacement therapy and incidence of Alzheimer disease in older women: The Cache County Study. *JAMA, 288*(17), 2123–2129.

68. Zuraw, B. L. (2008). Clinical practice. Hereditary angioedema. *New England Journal of Medicine, 359*, 1027–1036.

9 GH–IGF-1 Axis and Hypothalamic–Pituitary–Testicular Axis in Drug Development

Gabriel Gbenga Babaniyi, Ulelu Jessica Akor, and Ebunoluwa Elizabeth Babaniyi

9.1 INTRODUCTION

The study of endocrinology examines how hormones are made, where they are produced, and where and how they work and interact. But the study of endocrinology has grown to encompass the actions of growth factors that work through autocrine and paracrine mechanisms, the influence of neurons, especially those in the hypothalamus, that control endocrine function, and the reciprocal interactions of cytokines and other immune system components with the endocrine system.[4] The main roles of hormones include the control of energy synthesis, storage, and consumption; adaptability to novel surroundings or stressful situations; promotion of growth and development; and the maturation and operation of the reproductive system. Although hormones were initially thought of as the byproducts of ductless glands, we now recognize that many organs that were not previously thought of as "endocrine," such as the heart, kidneys, GI tract, adipocytes, and brain, synthesize and secrete hormones that are essential for a variety of physiological processes. Animal research implies that insulin-like growth factor 1 (IGF-1) may affect the function of the hypothalamic–pituitary–testicular (HPT) axis, particularly in childhood, but there is little evidence for this in human studies, according to Cannarella et al.[13] This problem might be resolved using the human IGF-1–deficient model known as Laron syndrome.

Furthermore, the male hypothalamic–pituitary–gonadal (HPG) axis is a meticulously controlled system whose function is to support spermatogenesis and androgen production. The gonadotropin-releasing hormone (GnRH)–gonadotrope secretory unit is hypothesized to be inhibited by testosterone, which is thought to feed back.[7] The stimulation of gonadotropin biosynthesis and secretion by GnRH is therefore dependent on the pulsatile character of GnRH delivery to the anterior pituitary, which is the mechanism by which GnRH is released from the hypothalamus.

DOI: 10.1201/9781003297826-9

Follicle-stimulating hormone (FSH) and luteinizing hormone (LH), which are gonadotropins, are glycoproteins made up of a common component and a hormone-specific β subunit that interact with one another noncovalently. GnRH increases the amounts of α, LH-β, and FSH-β subunit mRNAs as well as the transcriptional activity of the respective gene promoters, which in turn stimulates the production of gonadotropin subunits in vitro.[16,77,83] In contrast to its primarily indirect effect on FSH secretion, testosterone appears to exert a direct feedback control over LH secretion.

It has been hypothesized that the human HPT axis may be stimulated by IGF-1 acromegaly levels of this hormone that occur in pubertal-age healthy children.[14,12,77] This idea is supported by data from animal model studies and in vitro research, in particular, GnRH-secreting neurons in zebrafish chemomigrate in response to IGF-1 stimulation of GnRH production from GT1-7 cell lines.[83] The growth hormone receptor (GHR) and the insulin-like growth factor 1 receptor (IGF-1R) are both expressed in the Gn11 and GT1-7 cell lines. Both Gn11 cell migration and GnRH release from GT1-7 cells were induced by the presence of either growth hormone (GH) or IGF-1. In vitro models of developing (GnRH-secreting) neurons are represented by the Gn11 and GT1-7 cells, respectively. Accordingly, our results imply that GH and IGF-1 might stimulate GnRH neuron motility and secretion, and that their absence may negatively impact the GnRH neurons' ability to operate.[41]

IGF-1 appears to be important in testicular development and sex determination, which is interesting because it has been shown in mice models with a constitutive deletion for the IGF-1R. Through the same PI3K/AKT pathway, IGF-1R mediates the effects of FSH and mediates the proliferation and differentiation of Sertoli, germ, and Leydig cells in mammals.[12] Additionally, gonads have receptors for GH and IGF-1, which can control how active sex hormones are.[77] Contrary to popular belief, there is a stronger connection between the HPG and HPS (hypothalamic–pituitary–somatotropic) axes, which help to balance each other's functions. While total testosterone and GH secretions both gradually decline in late adulthood, GH secretion increases proportionally with sex hormone secretion during puberty.[17] The relationship between the two axes still needs to be fully understood. The cross talk is particularly complex because of the redundancy of reciprocal interactions at each regulation level, which alters over various developmental stages, and the mixture of endocrine and paracrine effects (Figure 9.1). Studies focused on the effects of GH and IGF-1 on gonadal development, steroidogenesis, and fertility yield conflicting results, although studies utilizing animal models offer some insights.

Similarly, applying this knowledge to people may emphasize the importance of IGF-1 in treating individuals with hypogonadotropic hypogonadism or delayed puberty. Given that the IGF-1R knockout is fatal to life, the paucity of human evidence is alarming. Laron dwarfism is the human phenotype that most closely resembles the animal model.[12] Resistance to GH brought on by mutations in the receptor characterizes the illness known as Laron syndrome. Due to this, a condition develops that is defined by elevated amounts of structurally normal GH and decreased levels of IGF-1. These individuals have the characteristic phenotype, which includes dwarfism, obesity, severe hypoglycemia, and a classic head shape with a small face and protruding forehead that results in a saddle nose. They have

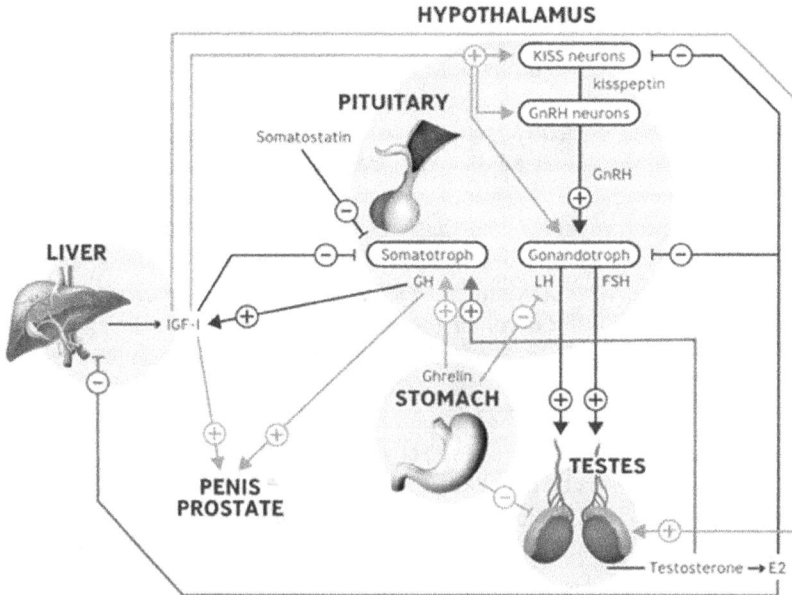

FIGURE 9.1 Cross talk between growth and gonadal hormones. The effects of growth hormones on gonadal hormones are indicated by light blue arrows. In order to encourage the liver to create IGF-1, pituitary somatotroph cells release GH. The primary antagonistic regulator of GH secretion is somatostatin. IGF-1 has a variety of effects. GH has several known effects, including (1) on the hypothalamus, which activates GnRH neurons and kisspeptin neurons for the development of puberty; (2) on the pituitary gland, which activates gonadotroph cells; (3) on the testicles; and (4) on the penis and prostate, probably influencing growth and development. GH can also directly act on the prostate and penis. The effects of gonadal hormones on growth hormones are indicated by green arrows. Testosterone released from the testes and E2 through aromatization are major facilitators of GH production from pituitary somatotroph cells. FSH and LH released from gonadotroph pituitary cells directly stimulate the testicle; IGF-1 synthesis in the liver can be slowed down by E2. The effects of ghrelin are indicated by orange arrows. Ghrelin can operate directly on the testes, suppressing both steroidogenesis and spermatogenesis. In addition, ghrelin can increase GH release from somatotroph cells and decrease LH release from gonadotroph cells.

thinning hair and a high-pitched voice. Poor genital development is another trait shared by male patients with Laron syndrome, which supports the link between IGF-1 and HPT axis function.[46] Since 1970, numerous studies have investigated these patients' andrological characteristics. Therefore, the goal of this systematic review is to emphasize the effects of low IGF-1 on the human HPT axis and assess the data gathered over the years on the GH–IGF-1 axis and the HPT axis as they relate to medication development. Furthermore, there is a close relationship between the HPS and HPG axes. These axes' interactions with one another are intricate and poorly understood. These interactions are distinguished by redundant reciprocal effects at each regulatory level and a combination of developmental/changing endocrine and paracrine effects.

9.1.1 How GH and IGF-1 Influence the HPG Axis

The hypothalamic GnRH neurons, kisspeptin neurons, and pituitary gonadotropin-secreting cells all respond centrally to GH and IGF-1. Kisspeptin neurons in the antero-ventral periventricular nucleus of rats that have received an injection of IGF-1, either centrally in the cerebrospinal fluid or peripherally, become activated. Additionally, both in rats and in cows, IGF-1 appears to promote LH release from pituitary cells.[35,36] In rodent models, it has been found that knocking out (KO) the genes for GHRs or IGF-1 or IGF-1Rs impairs sexual development and delays the start of puberty.[28] This phenotype resembles that of kisspeptin1R knockout mice, indicating that IGF-1R signaling is essential for the development of GnRH neurons and the synaptogenesis required for the onset of puberty.[69] Although systemic GH/IGF-1 hormone suppression does not prevent animals from becoming reproductively competent, gonadal development is significantly slowed.[77] This implies the existence of alternate or paracrine signals that maintain receptor signaling activity, albeit at a reduced intensity.

Additionally, Sertoli cells (SCs) and Leydig cells (LCs) of the testis both produce GH and IGF-1 (Figure 9.2). The SCs and LCs of the human testis exhibit the majority of the immunostaining for IGF-1. The germ cells (primary spermatocytes, secondary

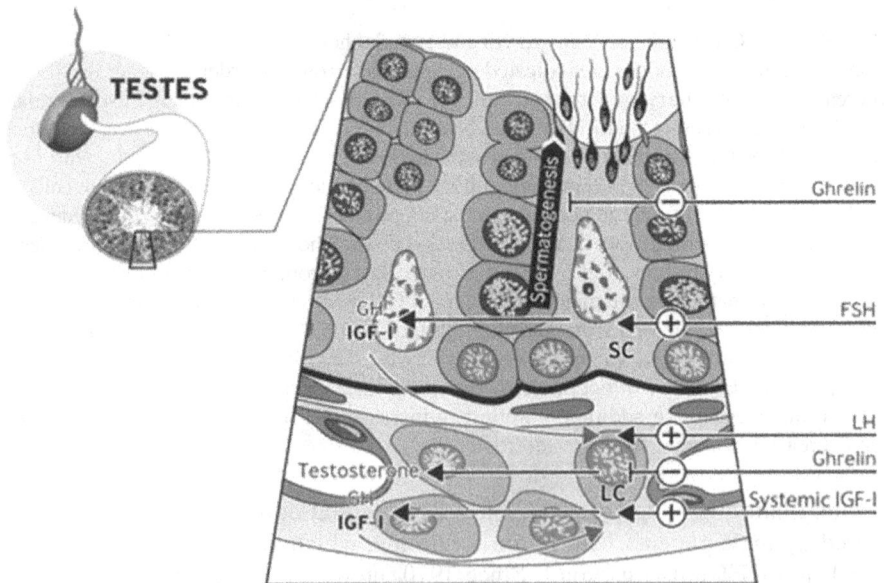

FIGURE 9.2 Cross talk between growth and gonadal hormones in the testis. Under the regulation of FSH and LH, Leydig cells (LCs) and Sertoli cells (SC) can both produce GH and even more IGF-1. Growth hormone release from LCs and SCs as well as spermatogenesis are both inhibited by ghrelin. Numerous paracrine and autocrine signals involved in spermatogenesis and steroidogenesis can be created by locally synthesized IGF-1 (green arrows). Alterations to steroidogenesis IGF-1 and GH both have the ability to promote the proliferation and differentiation of LC progenitors, while StAR and 3HSD gene expression are enhanced by IGF-1. The figure does not depict IGF-1 activity on spermatogenesis because it has not yet been fully verified.

spermatocytes, and early spermatids) as well as LCs and SCs all express GHR and IGF-1R.[79] In order to produce several paracrine and autocrine signals involved in spermatogenesis and steroidogenesis, testicular GH and, more significantly, locally generated IGF-1 play a crucial role. FSH and LH appear to be in charge of this ultra-short paracrine loop since they cause IGF-1 to be stimulated.[15] IGF-1 has also been shown to have a significant impact on steroidogenesis in numerous studies. IGF-1 administration alone has a minor impact on basal steroidogenesis in dwarf mice with growth hormone deficit (GHD), but it increases the number of hCG receptors on LCs, suggesting that IGF-1 may enhance gonadotropin-induced steroidogenesis.[48] Additionally, IGF-1 promotes the proliferation and differentiation of LC progenitors. Similar to this, GH stimulates 3-HSD gene expression in LCs and boosts steroido-genic acute regulatory protein (StAR).[80] IGF-1, meantime, might control spermato-genesis by an autocrine effect. Reduced fertility is evident in GHR-KO mice, which lends credence to this assertion. However, spermatogenesis is not completely sup-pressed, most likely because the seminal tubules produce IGF-1 independently of GH. In the same mouse model, IGF-1 therapy boosts sperm motility.

9.1.2 How Sex Hormones Can Shape the HPS Axis

The central neuroendocrine regulation of GH secretion and the peripheral modifi-cation of GH responsiveness can be used to describe the effects of sex steroids on the somatotropic axis. The hormones testosterone and estradiol (E2) play a key role in facilitating GH secretion. Due to an increase in the amplitude of GH secretion bursts during puberty, testosterone replacement therapy causes the pituitary gland to release more GH in hypogonadal patients.[64] The testosterone and its aromatiza-tion to E2 in these people is to blame for the impact. In addition, decreased GH and IGF-1 secretion in males with congenital aromatase insufficiency supports the role of estrogens. Nevertheless, sex-related variations in somatotropin-driven sex hor-mone release have been observed in animal models. Male mice exhibit more regular, high-amplitude GH secretory pulses, whereas female mice exhibit irregular, lower-amplitude secretory peaks with higher interpulse GH levels.[51] The primary negative regulator of GH secretion, somatostatin, which displays a similar sex-specific secre-tion pattern, appears to be the mediator of this sex-related effect.[63] Signal transduc-tion may be involved in the dimorphic effects of GH on growth, according to studies in rats. Despite the preservation of a male-like GH secretion pattern, the rhythmic GH release that is characteristic of men is more effective at activating the STAT5b signaling cascade, which when turned off in male STAT5b-KO rats, determines female-like growth.

GH secretion is also sexually dimorphic in humans; males have greater nocturnal pulses and somewhat smaller daily pulses than females, who exhibit more continu-ous production and numerous irregular pulses.[5] Given that sex hormone levels are incredibly low during puberty and that the HPS axis directs skeletal growth with-out clearly differentiating between boys and girls, sexual dimorphism in GH secre-tion is likely a factor in differences in body growth. Truncal growth is accelerated by sex hormones throughout puberty more so than appendicular growth, up until growth plate closure and growth arrest. Boys are taller than females and exhibit a longer growth period because of this mechanism, which is mostly mediated by E2.[68] The HPS axis appears to be influenced by the two sex hormones in adults as well. Ghrelin, a hormone that promotes GH production, is favorably modulated by testosterone to cause higher GH bursts. In addition, current research indicates that E2 is a crucial regulator of GH secretion in adult males.[65] Through high-affinity binding, the pituitary receptors ERα and ERβ can work in concert with the pituitary-specific transcription factor Pit1 to stimulate pituitary Gh gene transcription.

Similar to how sex hormones affect peripheral GH response, which is gender specific, sex hormones also play a significant role in this regulation. Boys and girls in the prepubertal stage have equivalent levels of GH and IGF-1.[65] Studies on adults have shown that men had lower levels of circulating GH than women, which can be explained, at least in part, by men having higher GH clearance than women due to androgenic effects.[68] In contrast, adult males have higher IGF-1 levels than females, even in the presence of GHD. This observation is mostly due to E2's ability to reduce the liver's sensitivity to GH's effect on IGF-1 release. This may be the reason why men with GHD are more likely than women to respond favorably to lower dosages of recombinant human growth hormone (rhGH), with higher increases in IGF-1 and bone mass.[5] This is similar to how normal or even acromegalic females typically exhibit lower IGF-1/GH ratios than males. The liver's stimulation of phospholipase C (PKC) and/or the overexpression of cytokine signaling-2 suppressors by estrogen together diminish Janus kinase 2 (JAK-2) phosphorylation, which in turn downregulates GH signal transduction in females.[77] The end outcome is an E2-dependent suppression of hepatocyte IGF-1 secretion.

9.2   HORMONES IN DRUG DEVELOPMENT

Due to the rational drug design using computational tools and bioinformatics approaches, drug discovery and development have accelerated. The process of developing a drug is difficult, expensive, and time-consuming. Pharmaceutical therapies, which fall between small molecules and biologics in the scientific hierarchy, are becoming more prevalent and significant in patient care. These medications, according to Ingallinera,[78] also include hormones, peptides (both natural and synthetic), and steroids. They are intricate, frequently present problems with solubility and stability, and mix chemical and microbiological activities. They cost a lot of money and have a high potency per dose. Therefore, there are major risks associated with the design and production of these complicated pharmaceuticals in terms of cost, safety, and product quality. Additionally, mistakes can jeopardize the ability to deliver outcomes to patients. Cross-contamination avoidance, single-use technology, and non-destructive testing techniques can all significantly reduce risks. The other inventive processes utilized by medicinal chemists for the desired modifications of leads for clinical therapeutic drugs include bioisosteric replacements and hybrid molecular approaches. It is known that testosterone and estrogen promote the growth of breast and prostate cancer. However, selective estrogen receptor modulators (SERMs), which are advantageous for estrogen-like activities, should induce inhibitory activity in the breast and uterine and agonist activity in other tissues. Therefore, the creation of ER selective ligands could be a useful strategy for treating breast cancer since ER subtypes α and β are hormone-dependent modulators of intracellular signaling and gene expression.[50] Inhibitors of aromatase and lyase as well as hormone receptor binders have been employed in hormonal therapy for these malignancies. The hormone therapy, however, causes some individuals to eventually develop resistance. In addition, the adverse consequences of the medication, such as reductions in libido, potency, and bone density, decreased patients' quality of life. When using antiestrogens for a long time, osteoporosis may become a problem. Tamoxifen, an estrogen receptor antagonist, has been shown to be effective in treating breast cancer, but there is some concern that this medication may also increase the growth of endometrium and uterine cancer.[44,50]

However, the target-based medication design strategy has been ineffective, as the majority of created pharmaceuticals have displayed negative side effects. Multidisciplinary techniques, the cornerstone of rational drug design, are required to meet this issue.[49] A medication target is essentially a biomolecule involved in metabolic or signaling pathways and unique to the illness process. But the biological impacts are brought about by:

1. Blocking the functions using tiny compounds that have a higher competitive binding affinity than their natural ligands for the active sites (within the biomolecules).
2. Preventing the interactions (between the biomolecules) at the bimolecular level.[30]

In a similar vein, the development of computer-aided techniques, molecular docking tools, and the availability of 3D crystal or solid-state nuclear magnetic resonance (NMR) structures of biomolecules have all greatly accelerated the process of finding new drugs.[54] Rational medication design strategies, however, primarily consist of the following:

1. Using the available 3D structural data, therapeutic compounds can be developed with the necessary qualities for target biomolecules (proteins or nucleic acids) in biological processes.
2. Analysis of global gene expression data from samples (untreated and treated with a drug) collected by applying cutting-edge computational technologies to identify previously unidentified targets (genes and proteins).

A lead molecule that exhibits adequate pharmacological action may have structural properties that affect its bioavailability, metabolism, and excretion from the body and are responsible for its adverse effects. Therefore, a different reasoning technique known as bioisosteric replacement is typically applied to achieve desired alterations in the leads to produce safer and therapeutically appropriate drug molecules. Because of this, the likelihood of successfully developing new chemical entities as pharmaceuticals has increased. Bioisosteres of functional groups are founded on an understanding of the physicochemical features of pharmacophore, including electro-negativity, steric size, and lipophilicity.[50] SERMs are structurally varied compounds that act as either agonists or antagonists when they come into contact with intracel-lular estrogen receptors in a variety of tissues. Therefore, a good SERM should have estrogen-like effects on the circulatory, skeletal, and central neurological systems as well as antagonistic activity in the breast and uterus and agonistic activity in other tissues.[55]

Likewise, rhGH therapy has been developed as a cure for a number of ailments linked to low stature, including Turner syndrome, GH deficiency, chronic renal fail-ure, short stature homeobox gene, and Noonan syndrome.[66] Although some studies have indicated that rhGH therapy did not connect with the early onset of puberty, there are worries that it can cause skeletal maturation and the onset of puberty too early.[37] Examining prepubertal rhGH treatment in mammals will help us better understand the mechanisms by which rhGH could cause early onset of puberty in males; changes in hypothalamic kisspeptin, GnRH, and IGF-1 levels; pituitary and circulating LH; spermatogenesis; testicular steroidogenesis; and IGF-1 in the cir-culation, liver, and testes. Ingallinera.[78] suggests using single-use equipment as a means of reducing the time-consuming process of thoroughly cleaning manufactur-ing facilities, mainly due to the growing use of disposable technology, which has also been enhanced to handle complicated formulations incorporating proteins, steroids, and hormones. So, although they are pricey, disposable bags are simple to use. To mix, contain, and store batches before and after filtering, single-use bags were cre-ated specifically for this purpose. Additionally, there are no risks associated with extractables and leachables from the material used to make the bags. Ingallinera.[78] added that the adulteration of a starting material, intermediate, or completed prod-uct with another starting material or product is referred to as cross-contamination. Cross-contamination can seriously jeopardize a drug product's quality and integrity if it is not properly controlled. Information that is essential for avoiding cross-con-tamination can be found in the initial safety assessment (ASI) of a medicine under development. The ASIs are used to create a toxicological report that identifies the acceptable residue limits (ARLs) and the allowable daily exposure (ADE).[47] This information assists the manufacturer in creating a cross-contamination prevention strategy by informing the cross-contamination risk assessment. Throughout the pro-duction process, all of this crucial information and the procedures designed to mini-mize cross-contamination must be computed, recorded, and measured.[50] Creating the preventive plan is a leadership responsibility when working with complicated formulations where cross-contamination poses a serious risk to quality, and opera-tional leaders need to be thoroughly familiar with the crucial specifics. Nevertheless, testing will be a part of every fill-finish process to guarantee accurate dosage quanti-ties and critical quality characteristics (CQAs), which is crucial when dealing with small amounts of highly potent medications. Underfilling has an impact on qual-ity and patient outcomes, whereas overfilling wastes valuable medication products. Randomly selecting finished goods for sampling is less accurate and wasteful.[19] Nondestructive testing can be used to test a complete batch, verify quality with accu-racy, and save time and money. The pharmaceutical business has access to a variety of nondestructive methods of evaluating finished goods, and the optimum inspection approach should be determined by the essential qualities of the final product (CQA). Testing might range from simple final product check weighing to intricate visual automated inspection systems to look for product particles, determine residual seal force (RSF), or assess the integrity of a prefilled syringe.[38,70]

9.3 HYPOTHALAMIC–PITUITARY–TESTICULAR AXIS IN DRUG DEVELOPMENT

Many medications have a negative impact on spermatogenesis. These effects may take place directly by impeding sperm production or testicular function, or they may take place inadvertently by affecting the HPT axis.[62,2] The recent drop in male fertility rates around the world has been attributed to lead exposure at work and environmental degradation. Lead may also influence the HPT axis, which regulates hormones, as well as the testes and sperm directly.[32] Normal testicular function in males depends on the flawless coordination of the HPG axis since human reproductive function changes significantly throughout life. Male fertility and typical testosterone production are included in this. Pulsatile release of the pituitary GnRH by the hypothalamus stimulates the production of LH, FSH, and other pituitary gonadotropins, which in turn support intragonadal testosterone synthesis and spermatogenesis.[21] However, chronic hormone replacement therapy using testosterone preparations is the preferred treatment if hypogonadism has been detected. However, suppression of the HPG axis via a negative feedback mechanism is unavoidable since exogenous testosterone formulations cannot imitate the natural endogenous pathway of the hypothalamic–pituitary hormonal axis.[62]

Low levels of GnRH also cause the pituitary gland to produce less LH and FSH, which in turn further reduces output. Low LH levels cause the Leydig cells in the testis to produce less testosterone. Prolactin can be suppressed and gonadotropin secretion frequently increased when dopaminergic medications like bromocriptine or cabergoline are administered in cases where prolactin levels are elevated. The glycoproteins LH and human chorionic gonadotropin (hCG) are heterodimeric and share a common component.[21] The transcription of the b subunit is the rate-limiting step in the synthesis of LH and hCG. They differ in stability, circulation half-life, and receptor affinities, but because of slight structural variations, they are both able to bind to and activate the same receptor in the gonads. Pharmacologic hCG operates as an LH analogue and is known to increase testosterone synthesis in Leydig cells, even though each hormone causes a specific set of actions to occur following receptor contact.[20,74] Often, hCG by itself can support spermatogenesis in people who have undergone a hypophysectomy or in those who have other pituitary disorders. As sperm generation takes several months, men must continue hCG subcutaneous or intramuscular injections, 1500 to 2000 IU three times a week, for at least six months.[85] Human menopausal gonadotropins or recombinant FSH can be added as an effective regimen to induce spermatogenesis in male patients with idiopathic hypogonadotropic hypogonadism after several months of hCG alone if sufficient spermatogenesis has not taken place. The therapeutic or negative effects of long-term hCG or recombinant

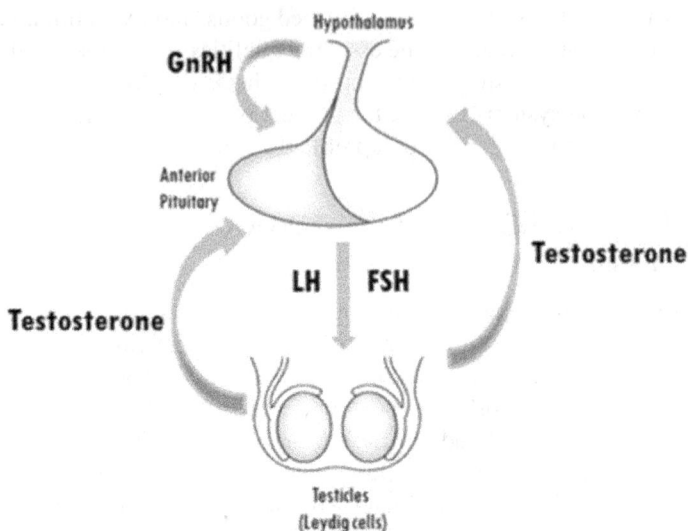

FIGURE 9.3 Hypothalamic–pituitary–gonadal axis.

FSH treatment for hypogonadism, however, are not well understood. Pulsatile sub-cutaneous or intravenous GnRH, administered using an infusion pump and tubing (similar to an insulin pump), may be utilized to promote proper pituitary gonado-tropin output in cases of hypothalamic illness. Naturally, this strategy would fail in treating pituitary disease, which also necessitates months of treatment.[43]

Thus, lead's effects on the HPT axis have been linked to dose-dependent changes in male endocrine systems following moderate lead exposure.[84] According to studies, lead's neurotoxic effects are mostly felt in the hypothalamus.[75] At modest levels of prolonged lead exposure, the impact may result from reduced GnRH mRNA expres-sion. By stopping prostaglandin E2 production or the release of prostaglandin E2 induced by norepinephrine, lead may also interfere with the release of hypothalamic GnRH.[45] By interfering with the calcium-dependent secondary messenger systems that control LH release from secretory granule storage, lead may have an effect on the hypothalamic–pituitary unit. This interferes with the hormonal feedback loop, which may account for the rise in stored β-LH (causing vacuolization of gonado-tropic cells). Lead's interaction with the metal-dependent testosterone receptor in the pituitary unit may also contribute to elevated LH mRNA and stored LH. Lead reduces testicular LH receptor levels and steroidogenesis at the pubertal stage.[67] Lead exposure during sexual development in animals resulted in degenerative alterations in the pituitary gland's gonadotropic cells, which explains why plasma levels of LH and testosterone are repressed into adulthood.[39]

Moderately exposed lead workers have routinely shown lower FSH levels, which could have an impact on spermatogenesis. On the other hand, elevated or stable FSH levels have also been noted.[60] This discrepancy in reporting may be due to variations in lead exposure levels and duration, as well as variations in the reproductive axis and testes' physiological conditions. Lead exposure during pubertal development may also affect the metabolic function of Sertoli cells, affecting spermatogenesis. Inhibin B overproduction has been linked to Sertoli cell malfunction from excessive lead exposure, which could explain the lower FSH levels previously reported.[56] In contrast, a lead exposure study in primates likewise found that Sertoli cell dysfunction was attributed to a reduced inhibin/FSH ratio. However, the majority of the research leads to reproductive axis malfunction rather than Sertoli cell dysfunction in adult lead-poisoning patients, as demonstrated by the lack of change in Sertoli cell morphology following lead exposure.[61]

9.3.1 EFFECTS OF DRUG DEVELOPMENT ON GH–IGF-1 AXIS

As the primary inducer of IGF-1 and IGF binding protein-3 (IGFBP-3) production from the liver, GH levels are lowered by liver failure and return to normal if hepatic function is restored.[82] GH, however, does not work alone in regulating the circulation's level of IGF-1. IGF-1 is released in response to insulin, thyroid hormone, androgens, androgens at low dosages and estrogens at high doses.[53] Serum concentrations are lowered by disorders that influence nutrition, such as celiac disease and anorexia, and malnutrition also has a severe inhibitory effect on IGF-1, IGFBP-3, and the acid-labile subunit.[73] Malnutrition may function at least in part by increasing fibroblast growth factor 21, which inhibits GH action and raises the levels of IGFBP-1 in the serum.[40,31] The physiological synergy of GH and IGF-1, also known as the dual-effector theory, can be disturbed by persistent inflammation, as demonstrated, for instance, in Crohn's disease or juvenile chronic arthritis. This is predicated on the idea that GH controls the expression of IGF-1 that is produced locally, which subsequently has an autocrine/paracrine effect. Pro-inflammatory cytokines, such as TNF-alpha, interfere with the effect of locally produced IGF-1 by reducing chondrocyte proliferation and differentiation in the growth plate as well as with circulating IGF-1 production, which results in hepatic GH resistance.[24]

Similar to this, IGF-1 assays that are available commercially and utilized in most hospital laboratories depend on an antibody's capacity to bind to IGF-1. As a result, there are significant differences between tests.[26] IGF-1 should have a high affinity for the antibody, which should have very little cross-reactivity with IGF-2. IGFBPs prevent the IGF-1 antibody from binding.[8,10,9] To combat this, excess IGF-2 is given to acidified serum samples, which is then neutralized. IGF-2 blocks the IGFBP binding site, freeing up the IGF-1 to attach to the antibody. There are several commercially available immunoassays for measuring IGFBP-3; these are unaffected by the presence of IGF-1 and do not call for an acidification step.[57] The body's capacity to create growth hormones is assessed using IGF-1. Growth hormone is crucial for the health of many different bodily tissues, including muscular tissue. Therefore, it has been demonstrated that many people with spinal cord injury (SCI) have lower levels of GH and IGF-1. The United States Food and Drug Administration (FDA) has approved the drug baclofen for the treatment of spasticity. It has been shown that people using long-term baclofen therapy had higher levels of growth hormone and IGF-1. IGF-1 levels are measured both before and after baclofen treatment. Therefore, it's crucial to establish the lowest baclofen dosage at which GH and IGF-1 levels improve.[11,86] All things considered, it makes sense to say that IGF-1's neuroprotective actions help mice with SCI recover functionally. The PI3K/Akt/mTOR signaling pathway may also be activated in the underlying process, which would then result in autophagy being inhibited. However, more research is needed to determine how IGF-1-regulated autophagy and the activation of certain PI3K subtypes are related. IGF-1, therefore, has a protective impact on neuropathy in studies and may be useful in the treatment of neuropathic ulcers. IGF-1 therapy for diabetes mellitus may provide advantages that haven't yet been fully understood.[86]

Additionally, there is likely a deficiency in the elderly that makes them more susceptible to the severity of the disease. As a man gets older, his GH level in the serum decreases. After the third decade of life, GH secretion gradually decreases by 15% for each additional decade of adulthood. Integrated assessments of GH secretion show that it peaks at puberty at about 150 micrograms per kilogram per day and thereafter by age 55 it declines to about 25 micrograms per kilogram per day.[29] Although the serum levels of adult men's and women's IGF-1 and GH have similar reference ranges, it has long been known that women secrete more GH than men. Additionally, GH plays a crucial role in controlling blood sugar levels, and adult patients with GHD have been found to have a compromised ability to use glucose, as well as insulin resistance and fasting hyperglycemia. Additionally, it has been observed that sex hormones affect the local synthesis of IGF-1 in target tissues, as well as the expression of the GH receptor in a variety of different tissues, in addition to influencing GH secretion.[42] The average range for GH levels is 0.4 to 10 nanograms per milliliter (ng/mL) for adult males, 1 to 14 ng/mL for adult females, and 10 to 50 ng/mL for youngsters.

Gradually, between the ages of 25 and 75, free testosterone concentrations decrease in males by roughly 50% as they age.[22,73] Lower levels of IGF-1 circulate as a result of the steady drop in testosterone levels that occurs with aging and the age-related decline in growth hormone production levels. The "push effect" of testosterone is a stimulatory effect that causes growth hormone to be secreted at the pituitary level. Contrarily, estrogen only stimulates pituitary GH release by inhibiting IGF-1 production in the liver, increasing GH secretion as a result; this is known as "a pull effect."[33] Compared to postmenopausal women or young men, young women have higher levels of spontaneous and induced GH secretion. It was discovered that the difference was closely tied to estrogen levels. Between the third and fifth decades, GH secretion drops more quickly in males than in women as they get older.[53] Although spontaneous GH secretion gradually declines with age, there is no dramatic decline during the menopausal years. Instead, age-related increases in body or abdominal fat account for the majority of the decrease.[6] However, GH is tethered to a high-affinity binding protein (GHBP) and circulates in the blood. GHBP, which is produced by proteolytic cleavage of the extracellular domain of the GHR, is primarily found in the liver. GHBP modifies GH activity and changes its pharmacokinetics and distribution. Women have considerably greater serum GHBP concentrations than men.[25]

9.3.2 EFFECT OF METABOLISM ON HYPOTHALAMIC– PITUITARY–TESTICULAR AXIS HEALTH

Although GnRH plays a part in the hypothalamic regulation of aging, the underlying mechanisms and their interactions with reproductive hormones are yet unknown. The case series and mechanistic investigations show that the HPT axis dysregulation in men can cause an energy deficit (acute over days or chronic over months), either from inadequate energy intake and/or excessive energy expenditure. Therefore, study of the HPT axis in men with unusual lifespans can provide insight into hypothalamic function in humans.[3] It is unclear to what extent the clinical effects of this may be separated from those of dietary deficiency, concurrent endocrine dysregulation, and accompanying comorbidities. Loss of GnRH pulsatility as a result of leptin's inability to trigger kisspeptin signaling is the main cause of HPT axis malfunction.[34] Furthermore, hypothalamic GnRH regulates the HPT axis, in which GnRH released from the hypothalamus stimulates the pituitary to create LH, which in turn stimulates the testes to produce testosterone (T). T inhibits the production of GnRH and LH via acting on the hypothalamus and pituitary through negative feedback, respectively.[18] Negative feedback is lost as T decreases, and GnRH and LH are elevated as a result. Due to its pulsatile secretion and low circulating levels, hypothalamic GnRH cannot be directly quantified in humans; however, its synthesis can be extrapolated from measurements of circulating LH and T. Hypothalamic dysfunction is indicated by low T levels that are not followed by compensatory production of GnRH and LH.[81] On the other hand, a compensatory increase in LH in response to age-related testicular failure suggests that hypothalamic function is still intact. In men with age-related testicular dysfunction, this compensatory hypothalamic–pituitary response may be sufficient to maintain normal T levels, resulting in compensated testicular dysfunction, or it may be inadequate, resulting in overt testicular dysfunction, similar to female menopause.[27] Furthermore, Debarba et al.[27] reported that 17-α-Estradiol (17aE2) treatment beginning at 4 months of age lengthens the male mouse life span and can lessen neuroinflammatory reactions in the hypothalamus of 12-month-old males. The longevity of male mice is increased by 17aE2, but female mice are unaffected, showing that life span regulation has a sexually dimorphic pattern.

9.4 SOLUTION TO THE EFFECTS

According to studies, the immune system is significantly influenced by the endocrine and neuroendocrine systems.[76] GH plays a critical function in the maturation of the immune system and may promote the growth of the thymus gland, which is in charge of producing T cells, the key component of cell-mediated immunity. Additionally, lymphoid tissues like the thymus, spleen, and immune cells create GH.[59,72] In addition, clinical research has indicated that GH plays a key role in immunological modulation, and several lymphocyte subpopulations express the GH receptor.[37] Immunoglobulin production is accelerated by GH-stimulated T and B cell proliferation. It also has the ability to control the cytokine response and accelerates the development of myeloid progenitor cells.[52] In 2012, a clinical investigation found that adult respiratory distress syndrome (ARDS) incidence and mortality were related to lower circulating levels of IGF-1. These findings indicate the IGF pathway's involvement in ARDS.[1] GH and IGF-1 may protect the host from deadly bacterial infection due to their immune-regulatory and anabolic actions. The hormones drive phagocyte migration, prepare phagocytes for the production of superoxide anions and cytokines, and boost opsonic action in addition to promoting myeloid cell maturation.[71] The negative effects of therapy can be more severe in older people and they are more sensitive to GH replacement. With proper dose titration, it is possible to prevent or alleviate the hormonal side effects of overreplacement that cause the acute side symptoms. Older, heavier, or female patients are more likely to experience problems.[58] Fluid retention, peripheral edema, arthralgia, and carpal tunnel syndrome are typical adverse effects of GH replacement. Although the onset of GH frequently results in a rise in glucose levels, these levels typically revert to normal with an improvement in body composition and decreased insulin resistance. Headache, tinnitus, and benign intracranial hypertension are other, less often reported side effects.[58,23] It would be important to investigate if raising growth hormone levels over the age-appropriate normal range has as many risks, acute and delayed, as benefits.

9.5 CONCLUSION

Complex formulations that lay somewhere between small molecules and biologics can provide a number of obstacles during development and production, including quality hazards, processes that squander expensive drug products, and patient and employee safety issues. Cross-contamination control, the utilization of single-use technology, and nondestructive testing of the finished product will result in higher-quality medications and improved patient outcomes. According to the evidence examined here, there is cross talk between the HPG and HPS axis. The expression of GH and IGF-1 receptors at every level of the HPG axis and on reproductive organs was established by molecular research. IGF-1 signaling, working directly and indirectly through kisspeptin neurons and LH-secreting cells, may be important for GnRH neuron maturation and timely pubertal start. Additionally, a paracrine network made up of locally generated GH and IGF-1 by the LC and SC operates within the testis to have quantifiable impacts on steroidogenesis and presumably less obvious effects on spermatogenesis.

Sex hormones then control HPS activity. The relationship between GH secretion and receptor sensitivity shows a distinct sex-related pattern. Additionally, it appears that E2 is the primary regulatory hormone at the peripheral level, where it inhibits the generation of IGF-1, and at the central level, where it exerts a stimulatory impact. Both testosterone and E2 appear to regulate GH secretion. The growing function of ghrelin, an orexigenic hormone and one of the primary triggers of HPS axis activation, which also decreases LH secretion, spermatogenesis, and steroidogenesis, adds to the intricacy of the interaction. Only until the transition age has passed do fertility and gonadal maturity attain their maximum potential, which is strongly dependent on metabolic balance. Also unclear are the somatotropic axis' actual effects in vivo on the reproductive system and sexual organs, but evidence from the literature suggests that the HPS axis must be active at physiological levels from the earliest stages of fetal development through childhood in order for the testicles to develop properly. Sexual differentiation depends heavily on insulin growth factors. Additionally, IGF-1 appears to be crucial for the maintenance of the proper testicular position throughout minipuberty and promotes linear growth in childhood.

IGF-1 also actively contributes to the activation of GnRH, the beginning of puberty, and the pubertal cycle. Patients with GHD and GHI (GH insufficiency) frequently experience poor genital development and delayed puberty. Prompt replacement therapy with rhGH/rhIGF-1 may help these individuals attain earlier pubertal onset, proper pubertal development, and larger testicular volumes and penile lengths than controls. Even though linear development is virtually over, IGF-1 levels throughout the transition age are still high, pointing to a role in the maturation of the reproductive tract. Although lower IGF-1 levels in adult males appear to be associated with inferior sperm parameters, there is yet no convincing evidence that medication can enhance semen properties and reproductive outcomes in either GHD or idiopathic infertility. There is unquestionably a need for studies on infertile males and long-term follow-up of GHD patients. Further research is needed to fully understand the significance of GH–IGF-1 interactions in sexual maturation and development during puberty and much more so at the transition age. However, it is always crucial to monitor gonadal growth in children with GHD in order to start treatment right away and ensure correct gonadal maturation. Additionally, research into how the HPS axis functions in kids with abnormalities of the urogenital system and gonadal development (micropenis, cryptorchidism, and hypospadias) may be crucial for therapeutic intervention. In conclusion, healthy puberty, complete gonadal development at the transition age, and adult fertility depend on accurate diagnosis and quick treatment. High-dose rhGH treatment in prepubescent male rats enhanced testicular IGF-1 levels, which may enhance LC production of testosterone and spermatogenesis. In terms of clinical use, reducing rhGH dosage to prevent precocious puberty can be explored to prevent the negative effects of rhGH in young patients.

REFERENCES

1. Ahasic, A. M., Zhai, R., Su, L., Zhao, Y., Aronis, K. N., Thompson, B. T., ... Christiani, D. C. (2012). IGF1 and IGFBP3 in the acute respiratory distress syndrome. *European Journal of Endocrinology/European Federation of Endocrine Societies*, *166*(1), 121.
2. Amory, J. K. (2007). Drug effects on spermatogenesis. *Drugs of Today*, *43*(10), 717–724.
3. Aleksic, S., Desai, D., Ye, K., Duran, S., Gao, T., Crandall, J., ... Milman, S. (2022). Integrity of hypothalamic–pituitary-testicular axis in exceptional longevity. *Aging Cell*, *21*(8), e13656.
4. Araujo, A. B., & Wittert, G. A. (2011). Endocrinology of the aging male. *Best Practice & Research Clinical Endocrinology & Metabolism*, *25*(2), 303–319.
5. Avtanski, D., Novaira, H. J., Wu, S., Romero, C. J., Kineman, R., Luque, R. M., ... Radovick, S. (2014). Both estrogen receptor α and β stimulate pituitary GH gene expression. *Molecular Endocrinology*, *28*(1), 40–52.
6. Baumann, G. (2001). Growth hormone binding protein 2001. *Journal of Pediatric Endocrinology and Metabolism*, *14*(4), 355–376.
7. Bleach, R., Sherlock, M., O'Reilly, M. W., & McIlroy, M. (2021). Growth hormone/insulin growth factor axis in sex steroid associated disorders and related cancers. *Frontiers in Cell and Developmental Biology*, *9*, 630503.

8. Blum, W. F., Ranke, M. B., & Bierich, J. R. (1988). A specific radioimmunoassay for insulin-like growth factor II: The interference of IGF binding proteins can be blocked by excess IGF-I. *European Journal of Endocrinology, 118*(3), 374–380.

9. Blum, W. F. (1994). Radioimmunoassays for IGFs and IGFBPs. *Growth Regulation, 4*(1).

10. Blum, W. F., Böttcher, C., & Wudy, S. A. (2011). Insulin-like growth factors and their binding proteins. In M B. Ranke & P. E. Mullis (Eds.), *Diagnostics of endocrine function in children and adolescents* (pp. 4157–4182). Basel: Karger.

11. Blum, W. F., Alherbish, A., Alsagheir, A., El Awwa, A., Kaplan, W., Koledova, E., & Savage, M. O. (2018). The growth hormone–insulin-like growth factor-I axis in the diagnosis and treatment of growth disorders. *Endocrine Connections, 7*(6), R212–R222.

12. Cannarella, R., Condorelli, R. A., La Vignera, S., & Calogero, A. E. (2018). Effects of the insulin-like growth factor system on testicular differentiation and function: A review of the literature. *Andrology, 6*(1), 3–9.

13. Cannarella, R., Crafa, A., La Vignera, S., Condorelli, R. A., & Calogero, A. E. (2021a). Role of the GH-IGF1 axis on the hypothalamus–pituitary–testicular axis function: Lessons from Laron syndrome. *Endocrine Connections, 10*(9), 1006–1017.

14. Cannarella, R., Paganoni, A. J., Cicolari, S., Oleari, R., Condorelli, R. A., La Vignera, S., ... Magni, P. (2021b). Anti-Müllerian hormone, growth hormone, and insulin-like growth factor 1 modulate the migratory and secretory patterns of GnRH neurons. *International Journal of Molecular Sciences, 22*(5), 2445.

15. Cailleau, J., Vermeire, S., & Verhoeven, G. (1990). Independent control of the production of insulin-like growth factor I and its binding protein by cultured testicular cells. *Molecular and Cellular Endocrinology, 69*(1), 79–89.

16. Caroppo, E. (2009). Male hypothalamic-pituitary-gonadal axis. In *Infertility in the male* (pp. 14–28). New York: Cambridge University.

17. Chandrashekar, V., Zaczek, D., & Bartke, A. (2004). The consequences of altered somatotropic system on reproduction. *Biology of Reproduction, 71*(1), 17–27.

18. Chellappa, K., Brinkman, J. A., Mukherjee, S., Morrison, M., Alotaibi, M. I., Carbajal, K. A., ... Lamming, D. W. (2019). Hypothalamic mTORC2 is essential for metabolic health and longevity. *Aging Cell, 18*(5), e13014.

19. Chen, L. Z., Sun, W. W., Bo, L., Wang, J. Q., Xiu, C., Tang, W. J., ... Liu, X. H. (2017). New arylpyrazoline-coumarins: Synthesis and anti-inflammatory activity. *European Journal of Medicinal Chemistry, 138*, 170–181.

20. Choi, J., & Smitz, J. (2014). Luteinizing hormone and human chorionic gonadotropin: Origins of difference. *Molecular and Cellular Endocrinology, 383*(1–2), 203–213.

21. Corradi, P. F., Corradi, R. B., & Greene, L. W. (2016). Physiology of the hypothalamic pituitary gonadal axis in the male. *Urologic Clinics, 43*(2), 151–162.

22. Chernecky, C. C., & Berger, B. J. (2013). *Laboratory tests and diagnostic procedures* (6th Ed., pp. 599–600). St Louis, MO: Elsevier Saunders. https://www.ucsfhealth.org/medical-tests/growth-hormone-test

23. Cianfarani, S. (2019). Risk of cancer in patients treated with recombinant human growth hormone in childhood. *Annals of Pediatric Endocrinology & Metabolism, 24*(2), 92.

24. Choukair, D., Hügel, U., Sander, A., Uhlmann, L., & Tönshoff, B. (2014). Inhibition of IGF-I–related intracellular signaling pathways by proinflammatory cytokines in growth plate chondrocytes. *Pediatric Research, 76*(3), 245–251.

25. Clasey, J. L., Weltman, A., Patrie, J., Weltman, J. Y., Pezzoli, S., Bouchard, C., ... Hartman, M. L. (2001). Abdominal visceral fat and fasting insulin are important predictors of 24-hour GH release independent of age, gender, and other physiological factors. *The Journal of Clinical Endocrinology & Metabolism, 86*(8), 3845–3852.

26. Clemmons, D. R. (2011). Consensus statement on the standardization and evaluation of growth hormone and insulin-like growth factor assays. *Clinical Chemistry, 57*(4), 555–559.

27. Debarba, L. K., Jayarathne, H. S., Miller, R. A., Garratt, M., & Sadagurski, M. (2022). 17-α-Estradiol has sex-specific effects on neuroinflammation that are partly reversed by gonadectomy. *The Journals of Gerontology: Series A, 77*(1), 66–74.

28. DiVall, S. A., Williams, T. R., Carver, S. E., Koch, L., Brüning, J. C., Kahn, C. R., ... Wolfe, A. (2010). Divergent roles of growth factors in the GnRH regulation of puberty in mice. *The Journal of Clinical Investigation, 120*(8), 2900–2909.

29. Elkarow, M. H., & Hamdy, A. (2020). A suggested role of human growth hormone in control of the COVID-19 pandemic. *Frontiers in Endocrinology, 11*, 569633.

30. Fuller, J. C., Burgoyne, N. J., & Jackson, R. M. (2009). Predicting druggable binding sites at the protein–protein interface. *Drug Discovery Today, 14*(3–4), 155–161.

31. Fazeli, P. K., & Klibanski, A. (2014). Determinants of GH resistance in malnutrition. *Journal of Endocrinology, 220*, R57–R65. https://doi.org/10.1530/JOE-13-0477

32. Gandhi, J., Hernandez, R. J., Chen, A., Smith, N. L., Sheynkin, Y. R., Joshi, G., & Khan, S. A. (2017). Impaired hypothalamic-pituitary-testicular axis activity, spermatogenesis, and sperm function promote infertility in males with lead poisoning. *Zygote, 25*(2), 103–110.

33. Garcia, J. M., Merriam, G. R., & Kargi, A. Y. (2019). Growth hormone in aging. In: Feingold KR, Anawalt B, Blackman MR, et al., editors. Endotext [Internet]. South Dartmouth (MA): MDText.com,Inc.; 2000-. Available from: https://www.ncbi.nlm.nih.gov/sites/books/NBK279163/.

34. Grossmann, M., & Wittert, G. A. (2021). Dysregulation of the hypothalamic–pituitary–testicular axis due to energy deficit. *The Journal of Clinical Endocrinology & Metabolism, 106*(12), e4861–e4871.

35. Hashizume, T., Kumahara, A., Fujino, M., & Okada, K. (2002). Insulin-like growth factor I enhances gonadotropin-releasing hormone-stimulated luteinizing hormone release from bovine anterior pituitary cells. *Animal Reproduction Science, 70*(1–2), 13–21.

36. Hiney, J. K., Srivastava, V. K., Pine, M. D., & Dees, W. L. (2009). Insulin-like growth factor-I activates KiSS-1 gene expression in the brain of the prepubertal female rat. *Endocrinology, 150*(1), 376–384.

37. Huh, K., Nah, W. H., & Xu, Y. (2021). Effects of recombinant human growth hormone on the onset of puberty, Leydig cell differentiation, spermatogenesis and hypothalamic KISS1 expression in immature male rats. *World Journal of Men's Health, 39*, 381–388.

38. Han, X., Luo, J., Wu, F., Hou, X., Yan, G., Zhou, M., Zhang, M., Pu, C., & Li, R. (2016). Synthesis and biological evaluation of novel 2, 3-dihydrochromeno [3, 4-d] imidazol-4 (1H)-one derivatives as potent anticancer cell proliferation and migration agents. *European Journal of Medicinal Chemistry, 114*, 232–243.

39. Hamadouche, N. A., Nesrine, S., & Abdelkeder, A. (2013). Lead toxicity and the hypothalamic-pituitary-testicular axis. *Notulae Scientia Biologicae, 5*(1), 1–6.

40. Hawkes, C. P., & Grimberg, A. (2015). Insulin-like growth factor-I is a marker for the nutritional state. *Pediatric Endocrinology Reviews: PER, 13*(2), 499.

41. Juul, A., & Skakkebæk, N. E. (2019). Why do normal children have acromegalic levels of IGF-I during puberty? *The Journal of Clinical Endocrinology & Metabolism, 104*(7), 2770–2776.

42. Johansson, A. G. (1999). Gender difference in growth hormone response in adults. *Journal of Endocrinological Investigation, 22*(5 Suppl), 58–60.

43. Kim, E. D., McCullough, A., & Kaminetsky, J. (2016). Oral enclomiphene citrate raises testosterone and preserves sperm counts in obese hypogonadal men, unlike topical testosterone: Restoration instead of replacement. *BJU International, 117*(4), 677–685.

44. Kudoh, M. (1996). Strategy of drug development for hormone-dependent tumor. *Gan to Kagaku ryoho. Cancer & Chemotherapy, 23*(6), 668–672.

45. Kasperczyk, A., Dobrakowski, M., Czuba, Z. P., Horak, S., & Kasperczyk, S. (2015). Environmental exposure to lead induces oxidative stress and modulates the function of the antioxidant defense system and the immune system in the semen of males with normal semen profile. *Toxicology and Applied Pharmacology, 284*, 339–344.

46. Laron, Z., & Kauli, R. (2016). Fifty seven years of follow-up of the Israeli cohort of Laron Syndrome patients—From discovery to treatment. *Growth Hormone & IGF Research, 28*, 53–56.

47. Li, X., Wu, C., Lin, X., Cai, X., Liu, L., Luo, G., You, Q., & Xiang, H. (2019). Synthesis and biological evaluation of 3-aryl-quinolin derivatives as anti-breast cancer agents targeting ERα and VEGFR2. *European Journal of Medicinal Chemistry, 161*, 445–455.

48. Maran, R. R. M., Sivakumar, R., Ravisankar, B., Valli, G., Ravichandran, K., Arunakaran, J., & Aruldhas, M. M. (2000). Growth hormone directly stimulates testosterone and oestradiol secretion by rat Leydig cells in vitro and modulates the effects of LH and T3. *Endocrine Journal, 47*(2), 111–118.

49. Mandal, S., Moudgil, M. N., & Mandal, S. K. (2009). Rational drug design. *European Journal of Pharmacology, 625*, 90–100.

50. Makar, S., Saha, T., Swetha, R., Gutti, G., Kumar, A., & Singh, S. K. (2020). Rational approaches of drug design for the development of selective estrogen receptor modulators (SERMs), implicated in breast cancer. *Bioorganic Chemistry, 94*, 103380.

51. Mauras, N., Rogol, A. D., & Veldhuis, J. D. (1990). Increased hGH production rate after low-dose estrogen therapy in prepubertal girls with Turner's syndrome. *Pediatric Research, 28*(6), 626–630.

52. Meazza, C., Pagani, S., Travaglino, P., & Bozzola, M. (2004). Effect of growth hormone (GH) on the immune system. *Pediatric Endocrinology Reviews, 1*, 490.

53. Meinhardt, U. J., & Ho, K. K. (2006). Modulation of growth hormone action by sex steroids. *Clinical Endocrinology, 65*(4), 413–422.

54. Muller, B. A. (2009). Imatinib and its successors-how modern chemistry has changed drug development. *Current Pharmaceutical Design, 15*, 120–133.

55. Maximov, P. Y., Lee, T. M., & Craig Jordan, V. (2013). The discovery and development of Selective Estrogen Receptor Modulators (SERMs) for clinical practice. *Current Clinical Pharmacology, 8*, 135–155.

56. Mahmoud, A., Kiss, P., Vanhoorne, M., De Bacquer, D., & Comhaire, F. (2005). Is inhibin B involved in the toxic effect of lead on male reproduction? *International Journal of Andrology, 28*, 150–155.

57. Mohamed-Ali, V., & Pinkney, J. (2002). Therapeutic potential of insulin-like growth factor-1 in patients with diabetes mellitus. *Treatments in Endocrinology, 1*(6), 399–410.

58. Molitch, M. E., Clemmons, D. R., Malozowski, S., Merriam, G. R., & Vance, M. L. (2011). Evaluation and treatment of adult growth hormone deficiency: An Endocrine Society clinical practice guideline. *The Journal of Clinical Endocrinology & Metabolism, 96*(6), 1587–1609.

59. Napolitano, L. A., Schmidt, D., Gotway, M. B., Ameli, N., Filbert, E. L., Ng, M. M., ... McCune, J. M. (2008). Growth hormone enhances thymic function in HIV-1–infected adults. *The Journal of Clinical Investigation, 118*(3), 1085–1098.

60. Ng, T. P., Goh, H. H., Ng, Y. L., Ong, H. Y., Ong, C. N., Chia, K. S., Chia, S. E., & Jeyaratnam, J. (1991). Male endocrine functions in workers with moderate exposure to lead. *British Journal of Industrial Medicine, 48*, 485–491.

61. Nathan, E., Huang, H. F., Pogach, L., Giglio, W., Bogden, J. D., & Seebode, J. (1992). Lead acetate does not impair secretion of Sertoli cell function marker proteins in the adult Sprague Dawley rat. *Archives of Environmental Health, 47*, 370–375.
62. Osuntokun, O. S., Olayiwola, G., Atere, T. G., Adekomi, D. A., Adedokun, K. I., & Oladokun, O. O. (2020). Hypothalamic–pituitary–testicular axis derangement following chronic phenytoin–levetiracetam adjunctive treatment in male Wistar rats. *Andrologia, 52*(11), e13788.
63. Painson, J. C., & Tannenbaum, G. S. (1991). Sexual dimorphism of somatostatin and growth hormone-releasing factor signaling in the control of pulsatile growth hormone secretion in the rat. *Endocrinology, 128*(6), 2858–2866.
64. Rochira, V., Zirilli, L., Maffei, L., Premrou, V., Aranda, C., Baldi, M., ... Lanfranco, F. (2010). Tall stature without growth hormone: Four male patients with aromatase deficiency. *The Journal of Clinical Endocrinology & Metabolism, 95*(4), 1626–1633.
65. Roelfsema, F., Yang, R. J., Takahashi, P. Y., Erickson, D., Bowers, C. Y., & Veldhuis, J. D. (2018). Aromatized estrogens amplify nocturnal growth hormone secretion in testosterone-replaced older hypogonadal men. *The Journal of Clinical Endocrinology & Metabolism, 103*(12), 4419–4427.
66. Romano, A. A., Dana, K., Bakker, B., Davis, D. A., Hunold, J. J., Jacobs, J., & Lippe, B. (2009). Growth response, near-adult height, and patterns of growth and puberty in patients with Noonan syndrome treated with growth hormone. *The Journal of Clinical Endocrinology & Metabolism, 94*(7), 2338–2344.
67. Ronis, M. J., Badger, T. M., Shema, S. J., Roberson, P. K., & Shaikh, F. (1996). Reproductive toxicity and growth effects in rats exposed to lead at different periods during development. *Toxicology and Applied Pharmacology, 136*, 361–371.
68. Russell, N., & Grossmann, M. (2019). Mechanisms in endocrinology: Estradiol as a male hormone. *European Journal of Endocrinology, 181*(1), R23–R43.
69. Qiu, X., Dowling, A. R., Marino, J. S., Faulkner, L. D., Bryant, B., Brüning, J. C., ... Hill, J. W. (2013). Delayed puberty but normal fertility in mice with selective deletion of insulin receptors from Kiss1 cells. *Endocrinology, 154*(3), 1337–1348.
70. Saha, T., Makar, S., Swetha, R., Gutti, G., & Singh, S. K. (2019). Estrogen signaling: An emanating therapeutic target for breast cancer treatment. *European Journal of Medicinal Chemistry, 177*, 116–143.
71. Saito, H., Inoue, T., Fukatsu, K., Ming-Tsan, L., Inaba, T., Fukushima, R., & Muto, T. (1996). Growth hormone and the immune response to bacterial infection. *Hormone Research in Paediatrics, 45*(1–2), 50–54.
72. Savino, W., Postel-Vinay, M. C., Smaniotto, S., & Dardenne, M. (2002). The thymus gland: A target organ for growth hormone. *Scandinavian Journal of Immunology, 55*(5), 442–452.
73. Stanworth, R. D., & Jones, T. H. (2008). Testosterone for the aging male; current evidence and recommended practice. *Clinical Interventions in Aging, 3*(1), 25.
74. Shores, M. M., & Matsumoto, A. M. (2014). Testosterone, aging and survival: Biomarker or deficiency. *Current Opinion in Endocrinology, Diabetes, and Obesity, 21*(3), 209.
75. Sokol, R. Z. (1987). Hormonal effects of lead acetate in the male rat: Mechanism of action. *Biology of Reproduction, 37*, 1135–1138.
76. Tang, M. W., Garcia, S., Gerlag, D. M., Tak, P. P., & Reedquist, K. A. (2017). Insight into the endocrine system and the immune system: A review of the inflammatory role of prolactin in rheumatoid arthritis and psoriatic arthritis. *Frontiers in Immunology, 8*, 720.

77. Tenuta, M., Carlomagno, F., Cangiano, B., Kanakis, G., Pozza, C., Sbardella, E., ... Gianfrilli, D. (2021). Somatotropic-testicular axis: A crosstalk between GH/IGF-I and gonadal hormones during development, transition, and adult age. *Andrology, 9*(1), 168–184.

78. Ingallinera, T. S. (2020). Complex drug development and manufacturing—Steroids, peptides, and hormones. *Pharmaceutics International, Inc.* https://www.pharm-int .com/2020/12/28/complex-drug-development-and-manufacturing-steroids-peptides -and-hormones/

79. Vannelli, B. G., Barni, T., Orlando, C., Natali, A., Serio, M., & Balboni, G. C. (1988). Insulin-like growth factor-1 (IGF-I) and IGF-I receptor in human testis: An immuno-histochemical study. *Fertility and Sterility, 49*(4), 666–669.

80. Wang, G. M., O'Shaughnessy, P. J., Chubb, C., Robaire, B., & Hardy, M. P. (2003). Effects of insulin-like growth factor I on steroidogenic enzyme expression levels in mouse Leydig cells. *Endocrinology, 144*(11), 5058–5064.

81. Wang, Z., Wu, W., Kim, M. S., & Cai, D. (2021). GnRH pulse frequency and irregular-ity play a role in male aging. *Nature Aging, 1*(10), 904–918.

82. Weber, M. M., Auernhammer, C. J., Lee, P. D., Engelhardt, D., & Zachoval, R. (2002). Insulin-like growth factors and insulin-like growth factor binding proteins in adult patients with severe liver disease before and after orthotopic liver transplantation. *Hormone Research in Paediatrics, 57*(3–4), 105–112.

83. Xu, Y., Han, C. Y., Park, M. J., & Gye, M. C. (2022). Increased testicular insulin-like growth factor 1 is associated with gonadal activation by recombinant growth hormone in immature rats. *Reproductive Biology and Endocrinology, 20*(1), 1–15.

84. Yoshida, K., Sako, N., Baba, T., Kashiwabara, S., Okabe, M., Noguchi, J., & Hagiwara, H. (2016). Abnormal spermatogenesis and male infertility in testicular zinc finger pro-tein Zfp318-knockout mice. *Development, Growth & Differentiation, 58*, 600–608.

85. Zhang, M., Tong, G., Liu, Y., Mu, Y., Weng, J., Xue, Y., ... HHIS Study Group. (2015). Sequential versus continual purified urinary FSH/hCG in men with idiopathic hypo-gonadotropic hypogonadism. *The Journal of Clinical Endocrinology & Metabolism, 100*(6), 2449–2455.

86. Zhang, D., Yuan, Y., Zhu, J., Zhu, D., Li, C., Cui, W., ... Liu, B. (2021). Insulin-like growth factor 1 promotes neurological functional recovery after spinal cord injury through inhibition of autophagy via the PI3K/Akt/mTOR signaling pathway. *Experimental and Therapeutic Medicine, 22*(5), 1–9.

10 Reproductive Endocrinology Drug Development
Hormones, Metabolism, and Fertility in Female Reproductive Health

Gabriel Gbenga Babaniyi, Babatunde Hadiyatullahi Ajao, Ulelu Jessica Akor, and Elizabeth Babaniyi

10.1 INTRODUCTION

Mechanisms have been created in female mammals to integrate environmental, dietary, and hormonal inputs to ensure reproduction under favorable energy conditions and to prevent it in the event of food scarcity. In situations with insufficient nutrition, this metabolic technique might be advantageous, but it is currently having an impact on the health of women. In combination with lower energy expenditure, the unlimited availability of calories alters numerous metabolic pathways and impairs the well-calibrated relationship between energy metabolism and reproduction, which in turn affects female fertility. Being underweight, overweight, obese, or engaging in vigorous physical activity are all factors that change the profiles of particular hormones, such as insulin and adipokines, which reduce women's fertility.[19] Over the past few decades, the prevalence of infertility regarding female reproductive health has been rising. Frequently, the clinical picture shows that the root cause of infertility may be endocrine in origin.[10] It is estimated that 186 million people worldwide suffer from infertility, which is defined as being unable to conceive after a year of unprotected sex.

Clinical reproductive endocrinology is the study of disorders and hormonal secretory conditions of the endocrine glands involved in reproduction and the reproductive hormones that are produced as a result. The hormones and methods of control that govern sexual development, sexual function, and reproduction are described by reproductive endocrinology.[11] Women's reproductive health issues may be treated using a medication that works by the body's natural "kisspeptin"

DOI: 10.1201/9781003297826-10

hormone system. The naturally occurring version of kisspeptin known as kiss-peptin-54 (KP54) has been studied for a number of years to treat reproductive diseases, but in a recent study, MVT-602 triggered more strong signaling of the kisspeptin system over a longer length of time than KP54.[27] Follicle-stimulating hormone and luteinizing hormone, which are two naturally occurring hormones that stimulate ovulation, are two examples of how fertility drugs typically work, according to Mayo Clinic Staff.[35] They are also employed by women who ovulate in an effort to stimulate the production of a better egg or additional egg or eggs. Also linked to female infertility is bisphenol-A (BPA), according to reports. A possible effect of BPA on spontaneous fecundity and natural conception has been hypothesized, according to Pivonello et al.,[39] who noted that BPA has been found to be more frequently detected in infertile women. More specifically, peak serum estradiol levels during gonadotropin stimulation, the number of retrieved oocytes, the number of normally fertilized oocytes, and implantation have all been found to be negatively correlated with BPA exposure. In addition, BPA's harmful effects are more severe during perinatal exposure because it alters the hypothalamic–pituitary–ovarian axis in pups and adults, resulting in early maturity of the axis through disruption to gonadotropin-releasing hormone pulsatility, gonadotropin signaling, and sex steroid hormone synthesis.

10.1.1 FEMALE REPRODUCTIVE FUNCTION AND ENDOCRINOLOGY

The ovaries and other sexual organs undergo similar physical changes during the normal reproductive years of the female, which are characterized by monthly rhythmical changes in the rates of female hormone release. There are three hierarchies in the female hormonal system, and they are as follows:

1. Gonadotropin-releasing hormone: Gonadotropin-releasing hormone (GnRH) release by the hypothalamus is the first step in the regulation of sexual behavior in both males and females. The release of gonadotropic hormones, including luteinizing hormone and follicle-stimulating hormone, is stimulated by GnRH.[50]
2. Gonadotropic hormones: Follicle-stimulating hormone (FSH) and luteinizing hormone (LH), which are gonadotropic hormones, are released by the anterior pituitary gland (Figure 10.1). These hormones regulate the changes to the ovary during the female sexual cycle. The ovaries are dormant in the absence of these hormones, which is the situation throughout childhood when essentially no pituitary gonadotropic hormones are released.[17,26] Normal monthly sexual cycles start between the ages of 11 and 15 years old after the pituitary starts to emit progressively more FSH and LH starting at age 9 to 12 years. Menarche, or the beginning of the first menstrual cycle, occurs during this time of transition known as puberty. In response to GnRH, the pituitary secretes FSH, which circulates in the blood to the ovary and promotes follicle growth. The preovulatory follicle's main hormone output is estradiol. The developing follicle(s) causes the concentration

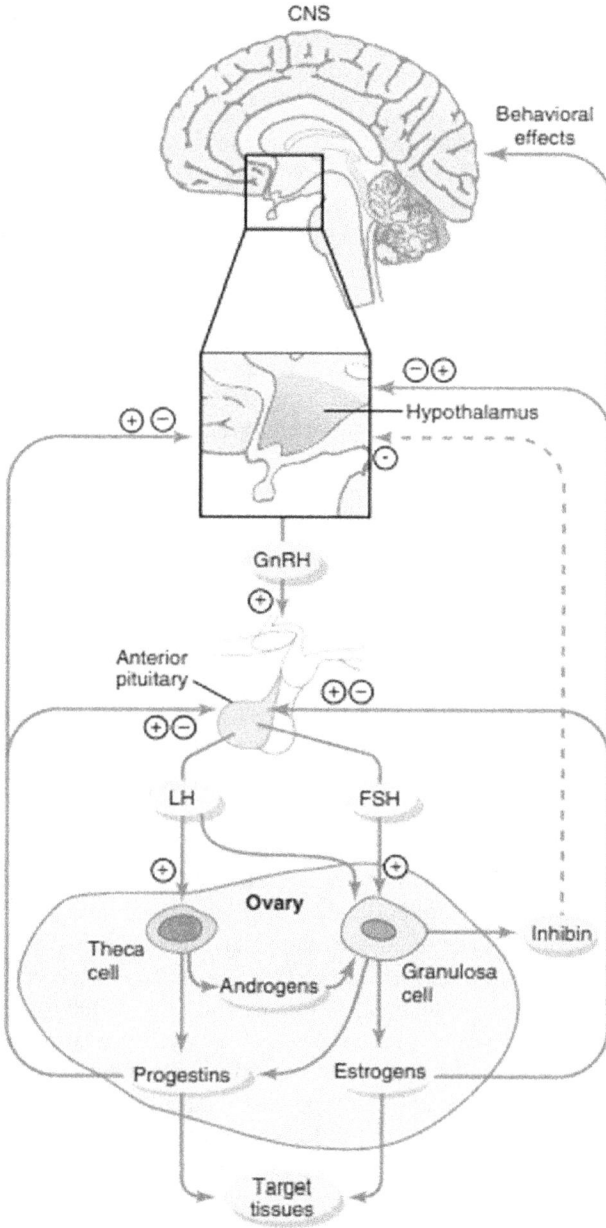

FIGURE 10.1   Gonadotropin hormones.

of estradiol to gradually rise (Graafian follicle). An LH surge from the pituitary is activated whenever a certain estradiol concentration is attained. Progesterone secretion increases while estrogen secretion is decreased further by LH. In the end, this creates an inflammatory reaction that ruptures the follicle and ends in ovulation. The follicular phase is the first stage of the female reproductive cycle. High estradiol levels are a defining feature, and it concludes with ovulation.[32]

The second phase of the ovarian cycle, known as the luteal phase, starts after ovulation. The follicle changes into the corpus luteum (CL) once the egg has been discharged. The CL is a transient endocrine structure that secretes a lot of progesterone to help the uterine lining form. Progesterone limits the production of GnRH during this time, which prevents the pituitary from producing LH and FSH. This is accomplished by sending a negative feedback signal to the brain. If an implanted embryo sends a signal to the CL, the CL's structure is preserved and it continues to release progesterone. The corpus albicans is the tissue that remains after the CL experiences luteolysis (luteal regression), which occurs in the absence of this signal. Progesterone levels drop at this time, and the endometrial lining either sheds as a result of menstruation or is reabsorbed.[26,32]

3. Progestin and estrogen: Only the ovaries secrete large amounts of estrogen in a normal, non-pregnant female, however, the adrenal cortices also secrete minuscule amounts of the hormone. Huge amounts of estrogen are also released by the placenta during pregnancy.[50]

BPA may impact female fertility and may play a role in the pathophysiology of female infertility, according to mounting evidence. According to Zegers-Hochschild et al.,[53] infertility is the inability of a woman to become pregnant after 12 months of regular unprotected intercourse and affects 25% of couples in developing nations. Couple infertility is therefore dependent on female factors in about 37% of cases, male factors in about 29%, and combined male and female infertility in about 18% of cases. The remaining 16% of cases are caused by genetic factors (1%), unidentified factors (15%), or other factors (16%), and are therefore classified as idiopathic infertility. The rise in environmental pollutants recorded globally has also been linked to an increase in the occurrence of couples, especially female infertility.[38]

The hypothalamic–pituitary–ovarian (HPO) axis's optimal operation is also directly tied to female reproduction in humans and rats. Following sexual maturation, the HPO axis integrates ovarian activity, especially ovarian steroidogenesis and folliculogenesis, with the last ovulation and primes the reproductive system to support a future pregnancy.[21] Similarly, humans and rodents share the same HPO axis-mediated regulation of the reproductive system. This includes the regulatory hypothalamic system, which releases GnRH in rhythmic pulses; the pituitary gland, which secretes FSH and LH; and the ovary itself, which releases sex hormones that regulate the function of the reproductive system. These include estrogens, particularly E2, and progesterone (P), particularly ovarian and uterine function in the classical cycles.[6,5] But how precisely ovarian and uterine cycles function varies greatly between animals. Some female primates, like female humans, have a menstrual cycle, in which menstruation takes place in the absence of pregnancy and the females are capable of being sexually receptive at any point throughout the cycle. The ovarian and uterine cycles can be used to characterize the menstrual cycle. The term "ovarian cycle" refers to a sequence of alterations that occur in the ovary during folliculogenesis when a recruited primordial follicle matures into a specialized Graafian follicle that can either be fertilized or perish due to atresia. The follicular phase, ovulation, and luteal phase make up the ovarian cycle.[6,5] Menstruation, proliferative, and secretory phases make up the three phases of the uterine cycle, which describe a succession of alterations in the endometrial lining of the uterus. The main functional unit of the female reproductive system is represented by the follicles, which are found in the cortex of the ovary.

For humans, the formation of primordial follicles marks the beginning of follicular development. The granulosa cells, which are somatic cells enclosing the oocyte within the follicle, and the theca cells, which are endocrine cells encircling the follicle, make up the follicle.[6] However, at the endocrine level, the electrical GnRH neuronal activity in the brain secretes the GnRH in rhythmic pulses to the anterior pituitary. The hypothalamic structure known as the GnRH pulse generator releases GnRH produced in specific neurons.[47] In contrast, the majority of GnRH neurons in humans are found in the mediobasal hypothalamus. GnRH neurons, which lack the estrogen receptor (ER), receive E2 signals from other neurons in the hypothalamus that do express the ER, such as the kisspeptin (Kiss1) neurons. As a result, two significant populations of Kiss1 neurons have been found in humans: one in the preoptic area (POA) and the other in the arcuate nucleus (ARC). Nearby GnRH neurons receive projections from Kiss1 neurons, causing the latter to produce GnRH.[31] Pulsatile releases of FSH and LH, which operate on the ovary and uterus to regulate ovarian and uterine cycles, are brought about by secreted pulses of GnRH into the portal blood arteries.[47] LH and FSH concentrations change over the course of the menstrual cycle. FSH predominates over LH in the early follicular and luteal phases, while LH predominates over FSH in the late follicular phase.[47] Under the stimulation of FSH, the activated primordial follicles with a single layer of granulosa cells surrounding the primordial oocytes develop into primary, secondary, and eventually antral follicles during the follicular phase of the ovarian cycle and the proliferative phase of the uterine cycle. Only a small percentage of antral follicles progress to the preovulatory stage, whereas the majority have atretic degeneration. Theca cells of the antral follicle are stimulated by LH to transform cholesterol into androgens, boosting the synthesis of endogenous intraovarian androgens, particularly testosterone. Simultaneously, FSH promotes aromatase production and activity in granulosa cells, causing androgens to be converted into estrogens, primarily E2. In order to further regulate follicular maturation, increase the development and differentiation of granulosa cells, and regulate the HPO through a negative feedback mechanism, the antral follicle releases E2 to its maximum circulating level in the preovulatory stage.[3,2] The innermost layer of the uterus, the endometrium, and its mucous membrane thicken as a result of increased E2 synthesis, which also activates Kiss-1 neurons and raises the frequency and amplitude of GnRH pulses. LH synthesis is induced by rapid GnRH pulse frequency, resulting in the LH surge.[47]

The dominant preovulatory follicle ovulates during ovulation, releasing the mature egg for fertilization. This is brought on by the surge in LH. The remaining theca and granulosa cells convert in the luteal phase following ovulation to create the corpus luteum, which generates P and E2.[6] Luteinization of the granulosa cells causes an increase in P production, which works to stabilize the endometrium at the ideal thickness to support implantation, to become receptive to the fertilized egg and prepare the endometrium for the potential of egg implantation, to thrive for the duration of the pregnancy, and to slow GnRH pulse frequency, which in turn causes a decrease in LH production and an increase in FSH production to stimulate the next round of ovulation. In the absence of fertilization, the corpus luteum begins to degrade, which lowers the levels of E2 and P and causes monthly discharges because the endometrium sheds and collapses. The uterine lining thickens in response to FSH-dependent estrogen stimulation, and the cycle restarts.[6,48]

Similar to rodent females, non-primate females also exhibit an estrus cycle during which the endometrium is reabsorbed. In the event that conception does not take place during the cycle, there will be recurrent times when the females are fertile and sexually responsive (estrus), which will be interrupted by periods when the females are neither fertile nor sexually receptive (anestrus).[43] In sexually mature females, estrus cycles begin after puberty and often last until death. In rodents, estrus cycles last the entire year.[43] However, in neonatal life, when primordial follicles form, rodent follicle development begins. Furthermore, the POA and rostral hypothalamus of rodents contain GnRH cell bodies, and the rostral periventricular region of the third ventricle contains Kiss1 neurons (RP3V). In mice, RP3V is made up of Kiss1 cells that are grouped in the anteroventral periventricular nucleus (AVPV) and extend caudally into the nearby periventricular preoptic zone (PeN).[31] In close proximity to GnRH neurons, Kiss1 neurons send projections to the RP3V, causing the latter to produce GnRH. Numerous data suggest that RP3V-AVPV Kiss1 neurons control the production of GnRH/LH surges. Meanwhile, the ARC Kiss1 neuronal population controls the production of GnRH pulses.[31,51] Similar to how humans' reproductive cycles are regulated by the hypothalamus in rodents. But unlike in humans, the reproductive processes of rat females are characterized by cyclical anatomical changes in the female reproductive system and cyclical sexual receptivity.[43] Estrus is the name for the cycle of receptivity, or "hot." According to Sato et al.,[43] the complete estrus cycle, which lasts four to five days, is composed of the following four stages:

1. Diestrus is characterized by the presence of tiny follicles in the ovary and big corpora lutea from the preceding ovulation. Low motility and atrophic uterus are both present. E2 levels start to rise at this time, although FSH and LH levels are low.
2. Proestrus is a period of rapid ovarian follicle growth and hypertrophy and strong contractility in the uterus. This stage corresponds to the preovulatory day, which is marked by elevated E2 and P levels and the onset of ovulation following increases in LH and FSH.
3. Estrus is a phase of the menstrual cycle when the uterus reaches its peak endometrial development and more than 15 eggs are ovulated. E2 levels are high in the morning and drop in the afternoon.
4. The uterus shrinks in size and vascularity during the metestrus as endometrium degenerates and is replaced, and many corpora lutea only release P for a brief period of time. There are low amounts of LH, FSH, and E2.

10.1.2   FUNCTIONS OF PROGESTERONE IN FEMALE REPRODUCTION

The most significant progestin in the body is progesterone, which is an ovarian sex hormone. Because it encourages secretory changes in the uterine endometrium during the second part of the monthly female reproductive cycle, progesterone is crucial for female reproduction because it prepares the uterus for implantation of the fertilized ovum (Table 10.1).

10.1.3   PHYSIOLOGICAL ANATOMY OF THE FEMALE REPRODUCTIVE SYSTEM

The vulva and vagina make up the lower tract of the female reproductive system, and the uterus and cervix, as well as the accompanying uterine (fallopian) tubes and ovaries, make up the upper tract.[41] During fetal development, a germinal epithelium that is embryologically descended from the epithelium of the germinal ridges covers the outer surface of the ovary. Primordial ova migrate into the ovarian cortex's substance when the female fetus grows and differentiates from this germinal epithelium. Then, a layer of spindle cells from the ovarian stroma (the ovary's supporting

---

TABLE 10.1
Roles of estrogen and progesterone

Estrogen	Progesterone
The primary role of estrogens is to promote cellular proliferation and growth in tissues relevant to reproduction, including cells in the sex organs.	Breast lobules and alveoli develop more quickly due to progesterone, which also causes the alveolar cells to multiply, expand, and have a secretory character. Progesterone does not, however, make the alveoli secrete milk.
Estrogens significantly enhance the growth of the endometrial glands and the endometrial stroma, which will later help to feed the implanted ovum.	The mucosal lining of the fallopian tubes secretes more fluid when progesterone is present. These fluids are essential for the fertilized ovum, dividing the ovum's nourishment as it travels through the fallopian tube before implantation.
Estrogens cause the glandular tissues of this lining to proliferate; especially, they cause the number of ciliated epithelial cells that line the fallopian tubes to increase.	Progesterone lessens the frequency and force of uterine contractions, which helps to prevent the implanted ovum from being expelled.
Breast stromal tissues expand, an extensive ductile system grows, and fat is deposited as a result of estrogen use.	
Estrogens cause the stratified vaginal epithelium, which is significantly more resilient to injury and infection than the prepubertal cuboidal cell epithelium, to transform from a cuboidal type.	
Estrogens increase the size of the uterus, vagina, fallopian tubes, and ovaries by several times.	

tissue) gathers around each ovum and gives them the epithelioid properties that give them the name granulosa cells. A primordial follicle is an ovum that is surrounded by a single layer of granulosa cells. At this point, the ovum is still developing and needs to undergo two more cell divisions before a sperm can fertilize it. The ovum is known as a primary oocyte at this point. Between the ages of 13 and 46, which are the entire reproductive years of adulthood, 400 to 500 primordial follicles mature enough to discharge one egg per month, while the other follicles degenerate (become atretic). Only a few primordial follicles are left in the ovaries when a woman reaches menopause, and even these quickly deteriorate.[24]

10.2 HORMONES IN DRUG DEVELOPMENT

In female animals, metabolism and reproduction are closely related and mutually regulated processes. Energy metabolism is continuously regulated during the reproductive stage of life due to the physiological activity of the gonads and their cyclical synthesis of sex hormones. The energetic costs of puberty, pregnancy, and lactation depend on women's capacity to conserve oxidizable fuels, which means that energy metabolism in female mammals is focused on reproductive needs.[46] Even more so, menarche and reproductive health are linked to physical activity (PA). Subfecundity and infertility are all associated with PA frequency, duration, and intensity. Particularly, in obese women, modest exercise and weight loss enhance metabolic function and hormonal profile, frequently increasing fertility. Contrarily, women who exercise until they are completely exhausted have a 2.3–3-fold higher chance of infertility. It was once thought that ovarian dysfunction in athletes might be related to body fat mass, however, it is now becoming apparent that the effects of physical activity on reproduction are unrelated to body fat accumulation. Even without changes in body weight and fat mass, the menstrual cycle resumes in female athletes when energy expenditure decreases. It is conceivable that disrupting the menstrual cycle is caused by a negative energy balance brought on by intense activity without accompanying increases in calorie intake.[22]

In addition, kisspeptin-54 (KP54), a naturally occurring type of kisspeptin, has been studied for many years as a potential treatment for reproductive diseases. However, MVT-602 has been discovered to elicit more robust kisspeptin system signaling over a longer time span than KP54. According to the research, MVT-602 may be used to successfully treat a variety of reproductive conditions that affect fertility, including hypothalamic amenorrhea (HA), which causes women to stop menstruating, and polycystic ovary syndrome (PCOS), a common condition that affects how a woman's ovaries function.[27] Women all across the world frequently struggle with reproductive health difficulties. These illnesses' effects on infertility might be quite upsetting. There is a need for more effective treatments, despite the fact that treatments for infertility and other reproductive problems have come a long way. But prior research has demonstrated that kisspeptin can be utilized to induce ovulation in women receiving in vitro fertilization (IVF) treatment. However, there are some restrictions when employing the naturally occurring kisspeptin hormone because its potency wears out after a few hours.[39] In light of this, a preliminary investigation has revealed that MVT-602 may be able to activate kisspeptin for a longer amount of time without causing any negative side effects. As a result, MVT-602 may be able to treat a larger variety of reproductive diseases.[19]

Similar to this, women with PCOS and diabetes have been found to have an increased risk of infertility due to lower insulin sensitivity. According to Douglas et al.,[18] the quantity and type of carbohydrates consumed may have an impact on reproductive processes. The literature contains a great deal of contradictory information, making it difficult to properly understand the existence and mechanism of the association between carbohydrates and reproduction in healthy premenopausal women. The quantity and quality of dietary carbohydrates have also been linked in certain studies to the ovulatory infertility of nulliparous women. The mechanism could mostly be attributed to decreased insulin sensitivity, which results in elevated levels of free IGF-I and testosterone and reproduces some clinical characteristics of PCOS.[12] In a long-term study of female respondents, a low-fat, high-carbohydrate diet was found to significantly lower blood levels of E2 and P4 and to significantly increase blood levels of FSH and the ratio of FSH:E2, regardless of age or weight. This suggests that carbohydrates have an impact on the hypothalamic–pituitary–gonadal (HPG) axis. The prolonged menstrual periods and lower E2 levels seen in these women's blood are partially a reflection of the alterations in the years before menopause. Additionally, other research did not discover a connection between dietary intake of these macronutrients and plasma levels of sex steroids.[13,12] These differences could be attributed to the diverse protocols used (carbohydrate intake and sources, duration of the treatment, and sample size). Insulin and its signaling pathway may play a major role in mediating the consequences of increased carbohydrate intake by influencing the HPG axis. As a result, extremely low levels of leptin, which indicate a lack of energy, would hinder reproduction at the HPG level, but high levels of leptin, like those associated with obesity, could have an immediate inhibitory effect on the gonads.

10.2.1 Female Infertility Clinical Presentations

10.2.1.1 Amenorrhea

Women with ovulatory dysfunction do not experience regular menstrual cycles, which typically last 26 to 35 days, or the premenstrual symptoms they are expected to experience, such as breast soreness, lower abdomen bloating, and moodiness. The absence of menstruation, or amenorrhea, is abnormal unless it's brought on by prepuberty, pregnancy, lactation, or menopause. Anatomic abnormalities, genetic flaws, ovarian failure, hypothalamus dysfunction, pituitary dysfunction, and other endocrine abnormalities are some of the pathological reasons for amenorrhea.[10] Amenorrhea, the lack of menstrual periods that is typically caused by the failure of normal cycle estrogen production as demonstrated by low estrogen levels, is a symptom of female infertility. Pregnancy, uterine or endometrial abnormalities (congenital malformations and intrauterine adhesions), ovarian failure (hyper- and hypogonadotropic hypogonadism, menopause, and hyperprolactinemia), chronic anovulatory syndromes, and hyperandrogenism are also causes of amenorrhea (ovarian or adrenal). Excessive activity, obesity, injuries, infections, malignancies, stress, and hypo- and hyperthyroidism are other causes of amenorrhea. A woman's age and the severity of her symptoms will determine the clinical evaluation of amenorrhea. Menopause examination is part of the initial assessment for older women.[9] To rule out pregnancy as the reason for amenorrhea in younger women of childbearing age, a serum human chorionic gonadotropin (hCG) test should be done. To determine whether hyperprolactinemia is the root of the amenorrhea, serum prolactin testing is done. Serum LH and FSH are included in further evaluation. Hypogonadotropic hypogonadism is indicated by decreased LH and FSH levels along with decreased sex steroid levels; the pituitary or hypothalamus is the site of the abnormality. The most likely cause of amenorrhea when LH is unusually increased in relation to FSH is polycystic ovarian syndrome. FSH, which is typically >40 mIU/mL in women, is consistent with menopause brought on by primary ovarian failure. While androgen levels only marginally decline, estrogen levels are significantly reduced.[8]

Hirsutism results from female hyperandrogenemia. Hirsutism is a term used to describe an abnormal androgen effect that is characterized by excessive female hair growth in areas of the skin that are androgen-responsive and typically associated with masculine distribution. Local androgen metabolism at the hair follicle is what is responsible for this excessive hair growth. The source of this commonly familial hyperandrogenemia is the ovaries, adrenals, or peripheral organs. Conditions associated with elevated androgen levels include Polycystic Ovary Syndrome (PCOS), Cushing's syndrome, androgen-secreting tumors originating from either the adrenal or ovarian glands, the use of anabolic steroids, increased peripheral androgen sensitivity, enhanced peripheral androgen production, as well as congenital adrenal hyperplasia (CAH), encompassing defects in androgen synthesis such as 21-hydroxylase deficiency, 11-β-hydroxylase deficiency, and 3-β-hydroxysteroid dehydrogenase deficiency.[7] Tests to identify the source of androgens include those that measure total and free testosterone, dehydroisoandrosterone sulfate (DHEAS), LH, FSH, sex hormone–binding globulin (SHBG), 17-hydroxyprogesterone, dihydrotestosterone, androstenediol, and androstenedione. As the source of the excess androgens, elevated DHEAS levels, >7200 ng/mL cut-off, implicate the adrenals (>99% of adrenal origin), whereas elevated testosterone, >200 ng/mL cut-off, implicate the ovaries (20% of ovarian origin). A tumor is thought to be the source of the androgen if virilization is also present.[25]

10.2.1.2　Adrenogenital Syndromes

Adrenogenital disorders result in either the lack or deficiency of one of the enzymes necessary for the synthesis of the adrenal steroid hormones. They are inherited as autosomal recessive characteristics. Which adrenal hormone class is (are) decreased depends on which enzyme is lacking. Cortisol production is reduced and adrenocorticotropic hormone (ACTH) is elevated in adrenogenital disorders. ACTH stimulation results in congenital adrenal hyperplasia (CAH) and hormone synthesis without the need for the insufficient enzyme.[54] Depending on the extent of the enzyme shortage, the clinical appearance might range from mild to life-threatening in severity. Increased androgen levels result from 21-hydroxylase and 11-β-hydroxylase deficiencies. The elevated levels of circulating testosterone cause ambiguous genitalia in genetic females with a 21-hydroxylase impairment. After puberty, females with minor deficiencies develop hirsutism. Low levels of estrogens and the majority of androgens result from a 3-β-hydroxysteroid dehydrogenase deficit.[48]

10.2.1.3 Polycystic Ovarian Disease

Polycystic ovarian syndrome (PCOS), also known as Stein-Leventhal syndrome, is a condition in which the adrenal glands or the ovaries produce too much androgen, causing the organs to swell and contain numerous cysts. Menstrual abnormalities, obesity, and hyperandrogenemia are all symptoms of this condition in women. The LH:FSH ratio is more than 3.0 despite the reproductive axis being intact due to altered gonadotropin production by the pituitary.[37]

Research generally demonstrates that any infection, including human papillomavirus (HPV), makes it more challenging for a woman to become pregnant and maintain her pregnancy. But it's crucial to keep in mind that the majority of HPV infections go away on their own. Scarring and obstructions in the fallopian tubes are listed by the American College of Obstetricians and Gynecologists (ACOG) as possible risk factors for infertility. While sexually transmitted infections (STIs) like HPV can occasionally cause this kind of harm, the ACOG does not specifically mention HPV as a cause of infertility. According to Stinson,[44] women who have HPV may encounter the following issues:

- Difficulties conceiving since HPV may make it more difficult for the embryo to attach to the uterine or womb wall. Additionally, HPV infections might harm the embryo.
- Risk of spontaneous preterm birth and pregnancy loss are linked to HPV, however, the severity of these hazards varies depending on the type of HPV a person has contracted. Studies reveal a strong connection between cervical HPV infections and miscarriage.

It is vital to remember that the body's immune system clears most HPV infections without any additional treatment.

10.2.2 CLINICAL USE OF ESTROGEN AND PROGESTERONE

Advances in oocyte and embryo cryopreservation for assisted reproduction prompted new approaches to ovarian stimulation. Attention has been paid to progesterone and its derivatives to block the LH surge, as oocyte vitrification removes possible harmful effects of progestins on endometrial receptivity. The following have been highlighted by D'Antonio et al.[14] and La Marca and Capuzzo[30] as the clinical use of estrogen and progesterone:

ESTROGEN

1. Estrogens are used to treat young females with hypogonadism.
2. Women with estrogen shortage brought on by early ovarian failure, menopause, or surgical removal of the ovaries are treated with estrogen as part of hormone replacement therapy. Hot flashes and atrophic alterations in the urogenital tract are improved with HRT.
3. Osteoporosis and bone loss can both be prevented by estrogen.
4. They are elements of hormonal birth control.

PROGESTERONE

1. Progestins can be used alone or in conjunction with estrogen as contraceptives.
2. In hormone replacement therapy, they are combined with an estrogen to prevent estrogen-induced endometrial cancer.
3. In assisted reproductive technology, progesterone is used to encourage and maintain pregnancy.

10.2.3 Testosterone and Related Androgens

The testicles, adrenal glands, and, to a lesser extent, the ovary all produce testosterone and related androgens. Progesterone and dehydroepiandrosterone (DHEA) are used to make testosterone. The transport protein SHBG and testosterone are partially bonded together in the plasma. Dihydrotestosterone (DHT), the hormone that is active in those tissues, is created when the hormone is transformed in a number of organs, including the prostate. Oral testosterone has a low impact due to quick hepatic metabolism. It can be administered intravenously in the form of transdermal patches or long-acting esters. Oral alternatives are also offered.[14] More so, testosterone enters cells and binds to cytosolic receptors like other steroid hormones do. Upon entering the nucleus, the hormone-receptor complex modifies the expression of the target genes.[14]

10.2.4 Uses of Testosterone and Related Androgens

1. When a man's androgen output is insufficient, androgenic drugs are employed. (Hypogonadism can result from pituitary or hypothalamic malfunction as well as testicular dysfunction [primary hypogonadism, secondary hypogonadism]. Androgen treatment is advised in each case.)
2. Anabolic effects: Senile osteoporosis and chronic wasting brought on by cancer or HIV can be treated with anabolic steroids. They may also be used as a further kind of treatment for severe burns to hasten healing after surgery or to treat chronic illnesses that are incapacitating.
3. Anabolic steroids are used by sportsmen and bodybuilders to increase lean body mass, muscle strength, and endurance.
4. DHEA, which is a precursor to testosterone and estrogen, has been promoted as a hormone that fights aging and improves performance.
5. Endometriosis (ectopic development of the endometrium) and fibrocystic breast disease are treated with moderate androgen danazol.[42]

10.3 DRUG DEVELOPMENT IN FEMALE REPRODUCTIVE FERTILITY

A wide range of underlying conditions, including ovulation problems, damage to the fallopian tubes (tubal infertility), cervical conditions (benign polyps or tumors and cervical stenosis), and hormonal imbalances, can result in female infertility.

PCOS, endometriosis, premature ovarian failure (POF), hypothalamus dysfunction, hyperprolactinemia (excess prolactin), uterine fibroids, and pelvic inflammatory disease (PID) are some of these hormonal diseases.[34] The most significant risk factors include smoking, heavy drinking, chemotherapy or radiation therapy, long-term use of high-dosage NSAIDs, antipsychotic medications, usage of recreational substances (including cocaine and marijuana), obesity, advancing age, and sexually treated diseases/illnesses. In the meanwhile, two broad categories can be used to describe the effects of infertility on women. Infertility-related physical problems fall under the first group, and psychosocial disorders fall under the second. Menstrual irregularities and weight gain are among the physical signs of infertility. Interpersonal relationship issues, lower self-esteem, feelings of shame, social isolation, risk of mental health harm, sadness, anxiety, despair, guilt, and worthlessness are among the psychosocial illnesses brought on by infertility.[1,28]

But evidence-based herbal therapy could be a viable option for treating female infertility. Some plants and/or their secondary metabolites controlled the steroid and folliculogenesis processes. Some plants and/or their secondary metabolites are used to treat female reproductive problems like polycystic ovary syndrome, premature ovarian failure, endometriosis, hyperprolactinemia, and hypothalamus dysfunction.[1,28] But numerous studies have demonstrated the value of micronutrients in treating female infertility both on their own and in conjunction with other therapies. Antioxidants, B vitamins, vitamin D, and fatty acids (saturated fatty acids, monounsaturated fatty acids [MUFS], polyunsaturated fatty acids [PUFAs], docosapentaenoic acid, eicosapentaenoic acid, linoleic acid, omega-3, and omega-6) are some of the micronutrients that make up this group.[45,36] The propensity for women to utilize herbal medications is rising as a result of the harmful effects of chemical treatments on reproductive health, expensive drug costs, and cutting-edge fertility treatment techniques. Because it contains a variety of chemicals with phytoestrogenic, antioxidant, and nutritional benefits, herbal medicine is seen to be a good alternative to pharmaceutical medications. One of the helpful and healthful methods to lessen the symptoms of menopause in women who are estrogen deficient is to utilize phytoestrogens that mimic estrogen.[4,16]

The use of ovulation-inducing medications like clomiphene and gonadotrophins, assisted reproductive technologies like in vitro fertilization and intrauterine insemination, egg and sperm donation, ovulation-inducing medications like gonadotrophins, induction of ovulation, and micronutrients, as well as other new therapies, have made it possible for women to conceive and have children today.[33] A variety of reproductive problems in women that impair fertility have been discovered to be successfully treated with MVT-60, a drug that targets the body's natural kisspeptin hormone system to boost the reproductive hormones that control fertility, sexual development, and menstruation.

10.4 EFFECTS OF DRUG DEVELOPMENT ON REPRODUCTIVE ENDOCRINOLOGY HORMONES AND METABOLISM

Most side effects from fertility medicines are moderate and include injection site discomfort, infection, blood blisters, swelling, or bruising (Table 10.2). Ovarian hyperstimulation, a syndrome that causes ovaries to enlarge and become sensitive,

TABLE 10.2

Side effects of estrogen and progesterone

Estrogen	Progesterone
For healthy female reproductive development, estrogen is necessary. It is in charge of the development of secondary sexual traits, the growth spurt related to puberty, and the expansion of the genital structures (vagina, uterus, and uterine tubes) during childhood.	Headache, depression, weight gain, and changes in libido are the main side effects of progestin use.
Estrogen alters serum protein concentrations and slows bone resorption.	There are some progestins that exhibit androgenic activity, such as the 19-nortestosterone derivatives, which can raise the ratio of low-density lipid to high-density lipid cholesterol and result in acne and hirsutism. Women with acne could prefer less androgenic progestins such as norgestimate and drospirenone.
Blood coagulability is improved, plasma triglyceride levels are raised, low-density lipoprotein (LDL) cholesterol is decreased, and high-density lipoprotein (HDL) cholesterol is increased.	Because injectable medroxyprogesterone acetate has been linked to an increased risk of osteoporosis, there have been suggestions to limit its use.
Continuous estrogen medication, especially when combined with a progestin, prevents the anterior pituitary from secreting gonadotropins.	

Source: D'Antonio et al.[14]

is also a possibility. Multiple births are also more likely while using medicines like clomid.[29] Other side effects include headache, nausea, bloating, heat flashes, and impaired vision. Additionally, clomid can alter cervical mucous, which may make it more difficult to determine a woman's reproductive status and may prevent sperm from entering the uterus. Even though much of the evidence comes from retrospective research, the harmful consequences of smoking on female fertility have garnered a lot of attention in recent years. However, the information that is now available shows a significant link between smoking—both actively and passively—and decreased female fertility, as well as between in utero exposure and several unfavorable pregnancy outcomes and decreased fertility of female descendants in adulthood.[16]

Furthermore, progesterone is quickly absorbed when taken orally. Its half-life in plasma is brief, and the liver almost entirely breaks it down, less quickly than natural progestins are digested. The action of medroxyprogesterone acetate lasts for three months and is injected intramuscularly or subcutaneously. The duration of the other progestins is one to three days.[42]

10.4.1 EFFECT OF TESTOSTERONE AND RELATED ANDROGENS

1. Androgens can make women more masculine by causing acne, facial hair growth, voice deepening, male pattern baldness, and excessive muscular gain. Also possible are irregular menstrual cycles. Due to the risk of the fetus becoming virilized, pregnant women should avoid using testosterone.
2. In men, an excess of androgens can lead to gynecomastia, impotence, priapism, and reduced spermatogenesis. Female-specific cosmetic changes like those mentioned for females may also take place. Additionally, androgens can promote prostate development.
3. Androgens can lead to aberrant sexual maturation in youngsters as well as growth problems brought on by the epiphyseal plates closing too soon.
4. The use of anabolic steroids (such as DHEA) by athletes might result in the early closure of the epiphyses of long bones, which slows growth and disrupts development. These young athletes may experience reduced testicular size, liver problems, and increased aggression as a result of the high quantities they consume.[42]

10.5 SUGGESTED SOLUTIONS TO FERTILITY CHALLENGES

FSH and LH, two of the body's naturally occurring hormones, are the basis for how fertility medicines stimulate ovulation, which occurs when the ovaries make and release an egg. Additionally, fertility drugs or hormone injections may be the next step in the conception process if assistance is needed to produce healthier eggs or more of them.[20] As a result, some drugs and injections can assist ovulation when a person is having trouble getting pregnant owing to ovulation problems, bringing their body a little bit closer to their goal. There are four broad categories of medications that can be taken during fertility treatment, according to Gurevich:[23]

1. Medications designed to increase ovulation (fertility drugs).
2. Medications designed to stop or regulate menstruation (used during IVF).
3. Prescription drugs for an underlying illness that affects fertility.
4. Drugs designed to address different elements of fertility.

However, drugs can be used either on their own or in conjunction with surgical procedures, IVF treatment, or intrauterine insemination. Women are still more likely than males to seek fertility treatment medicines, despite the fact that infertility affects both genders virtually equally. This is because medicine cannot usually be used to address the majority of male infertility issues. Men may, however, occasionally also take hormones or other medications as part of fertility treatment. Commonly prescribed fertility drugs include:

- Clomiphene promotes the monthly release of an egg (ovulation) in women who do not ovulate regularly or who are incapable of ovulating at all.
- Tamoxifen is a possible clomiphene substitute when ovulation issues arise.

- Women with PCOS may benefit especially from metformin.
- Gonadotrophins can aid in promoting ovulation in females and possibly enhance male fertility.
- Dopamine agonists and gonadotrophin-releasing hormone are two other medications used to help women ovulate.

The adverse effects of these medications include nausea, vomiting, migraines, and hot flashes. Headaches, nausea, bloating, breast tenderness, mood fluctuations, and discomfort at the injection site are among the most frequent side effects of gonadotropins. When compared to oral medications like clomid, gonadotropins have a much higher risk of causing the conception of twins, triplets, or higher-order multiples.[15] Additionally, there is a considerably larger chance of getting ovarian hyperstimulation syndrome. While injectable fertility medicines may be recommended to men with hypogonadotropic hypogonadism in order to increase testosterone levels and enhance the health of their sperm, gonadotropins are generally used in women. Similarly, some drugs used for reproductive treatment stop ovulation.[52] Drugs are administered during IVF to delay ovulation until the eggs may be surgically removed. The eggs cannot be discovered or used for IVF after they have been ovulated into the body. To time cycles with a potential egg donor or gestational carrier, ovulation may also be repressed. Thomas[49] stated that ovarian swelling is a typical adverse reaction to the medications used to stimulate ovulation during IVF and intracytoplasmic sperm injection. Bloating, stomach discomfort, and nausea are examples of symptoms. Codeine and paracetamol are two safe prescription painkillers that should help with pain relief. Because they can harm the kidneys, anti-inflammatories like ibuprofen and aspirin should be avoided. Last but not least, occasionally an undiagnosed medical problem is affecting fertility. It needs to be treated first in these situations. To increase fertility, the underlying problem may not even need to be addressed. After therapy, spontaneous conception is easily possible.[40] Other times, though, a combination of remedies is necessary. There may be a need for therapy for other medical conditions in addition to fertility medications or surgical procedures. Various research indicates that regular exercise and a healthy diet, especially the daily intake of various nutrient groups, could greatly improve reproductive outcomes. The holy grail of treating female infertility remains the discovery of a fertility diet.

10.6 CONCLUSION

Although various research points to the potential for physical activity and a healthy diet, particularly the daily intake of various nutrient groups, to considerably enhance reproductive results, discovering a fertility diet remains the holy grail of treating female infertility. The key contributing factors to infertility include a lack of understanding of the function and methods of action of numerous nutrients, as well as other elements like lifestyle, physical activity, genetics, and cultural backgrounds. Though, as Hippocrates said in the 4th century BC, "if we could give every individual the right amount of nourishment and exercise, not too little and not too much, we would have found the safest way to health," nutrition and lifestyle changes are still among the most valuable and promising interventions in preserving human health and women's fertility. They also represent the most captivating challenge that we have to take up.

Unfortunately, we are still far from illuminating this field of study, mostly due to the dearth of studies that are available in the literature. Partially, it is still challenging to find and convince healthy volunteers to take part in long-term studies based on dietary and lifestyle changes. Additionally, the various protocols used throughout clinical trials frequently produced underpowered and nonrandomized outcomes, which produced contradictory findings. One major issue is the dearth of longitudinal research on the effects of nutrition on reproduction that might also assess lifestyle, physical activity, genetic, and cultural variations. Additionally, because there is no standard technique for analysis (various studies often utilize different methods, parameters, and outcomes), it is impossible to integrate the highly heterogeneous data that is currently accessible, which is a major barrier to producing definitive results. In conclusion, it has been discovered that the start of PCOS-like anomalies occurs after causing a corresponding reduction of sex hormone secretion that affects ovarian morphology and functions, particularly folliculogenesis. The several limitations of the reported studies prevent drawing final conclusions.

REFERENCES

1. Akbaribazm, M., Goodarzi, N., & Rahimi, M. (2021). Female infertility and herbal medicine: An overview of the new findings. *Food Science & Nutrition*, *9*(10), 5869–5882.
2. Alviggi, C., Mollo, A., Clarizia, R., & De Placido, G. (2006). Exploiting LH in ovarian stimulation. *Reproductive Biomedicine Online*, *12*(2), 221–233.
3. Alviggi, C., Clarizia, R., Mollo, A., Ranieri, A., & De Placido, G. (2011). Who needs LH in ovarian stimulation? *Reproductive BioMedicine Online*, *22*, S33–S41.
4. Ascenzi, P., Bocedi, A., & Marino, M. (2006). Structure–function relationship of estrogen receptor α and β: Impact on human health. *Molecular Aspects of Medicine*, *27*(4), 299–402.
5. Bates, G. W., & Bowling, M. (2013). Physiology of the female reproductive axis. *Periodontology 2000*, *61*(1), 89–102.
6. Buffet, N. C., & Bouchard, P. (2001). The neuroendocrine regulation of the human ovarian cycle. *Chronobiology International*, *18*(6), 893–919.
7. Burtis, C. A. (Ed.). (1999). *Tietz textbook of clinical chemistry*. Saunders.
8. Cook, J. D. (2000). Laboratory management of infertility. *AACC Diagnostic Endocrinology, Immunology and Metabolism*, *18*, 13–31.
9. Cook, J. D., & Noel, S. (2002). *Special topics in endocrinology: Thyroid, infertility and malignancies*. ASCP.
10. Cook, J. D. (2004). Reproductive endocrinology in infertility. *Laboratory Medicine*, *35*(9), 558–569.
11. Corenblum, B., & Boyd, J. (2017). Endocrinology and disorders of the reproductive system. In *Endocrine biomarkers* (pp. 351–397). Elsevier.
12. Cui, X., Rosner, B., Willett, W. C., & Hankinson, S. E. (2010). Dietary fat, fiber, and carbohydrate intake and endogenous hormone levels in premenopausal women. *Hormones and Cancer*, *1*(5), 265–276.

13. Chavarro, J. E., Rich-Edwards, J. W., Rosner, B. A., & Willett, W. C. (2009). A prospective study of dietary carbohydrate quantity and quality in relation to risk of ovulatory infertility. *European Journal of Clinical Nutrition, 63*(1), 78–86.

14. D'Antonio, F., Berghella, V., Di Mascio, D., Saccone, G., Sileo, F., Flacco, M. E., ... Khalil, A. (2021). Role of progesterone, cerclage and pessary in preventing preterm birth in twin pregnancies: A systematic review and network meta-analysis. *European Journal of Obstetrics & Gynecology and Reproductive Biology, 261,* 166–177.

15. Diamond, M. P., Mitwally, M., Casper, R., Ager, J., Legro, R. S., Brzyski, R., ... Zhang, H. (2011). Estimating rates of multiple gestation pregnancies: Sample size calculation from the assessment of multiple intrauterine gestations from ovarian stimulation (AMIGOS) trial. *Contemporary Clinical Trials, 32*(6), 902–908.

16. de Angelis, C., Nardone, A., Garifalos, F., Pivonello, C., Sansone, A., Conforti, A., Di Dato, C., Sirico, F., Alviggi, C., Isidori, A., Colao, A., & Pivonello, R. (2020). Smoke, alcohol and drug addiction and female fertility. *Reproductive Biology and Endocrinology: RB&E, 18*(1), 21. https://doi.org/10.1186/s12958-020-0567-7

17. Dobrzyn, K., Smolinska, N., Kiezun, M., Szeszko, K., Rytelewska, E., Kisielewska, K., ... Kaminski, T. (2018). Adiponectin: A new regulator of female reproductive system. *International Journal of Endocrinology*, vol. 2018, Article ID 7965071, 12 pages, 2018. https://doi.org/10.1155/2018/7965071.

18. Douglas, C. C., Gower, B. A., Darnell, B. E., Ovalle, F., Oster, R. A., & Azziz, R. (2006). Role of diet in the treatment of polycystic ovary syndrome. *Fertility and Sterility, 85*(3), 679–688.

19. Fontana, R., & Della Torre, S. (2016). The deep correlation between energy metabolism and reproduction: A view on the effects of nutrition for women fertility. *Nutrients, 8*(2), 87.

20. Geddes, J. K. (2021, April 5). *Common fertility treatment drugs to help women get pregnant.* What to Expect; www.whattoexpect.com. https://www.whattoexpect.com/getting-pregnant/fertility-tests-and-treatments/fertility-drugs/

21. Gregoraszczuk, E. L., & Ptak, A. (2013). Endocrine-disrupting chemicals: Some actions of POPs on female reproduction. *International Journal of Endocrinology, 2013*.

22. Gudmundsdottir, S. L., Flanders, W. D., & Augestad, L. B. (2014). Menstrual cycle abnormalities in healthy women with low physical activity: The North-Trøndelag population-based health study. *Journal of Physical Activity and Health, 11*(6), 1133–1140.

23. Gurevich, R. (2020, September 23). *Overview of common fertility treatment drugs.* Verywell Family; www.verywellfamily.com. https://www.verywellfamily.com/fertility-drugs-1960184

24. Hall, J. E., & Guyton, A. C. (2011). Fisiología médica. *Guyton y Hall, 120,* 1003–1017.

25. Hershman, J. M. (1977). *Endocrine pathophysiology: A patient oriented approach.* Lea & Febiger.

26. Hewitt, S. C., Winuthayanon, W., & Korach, K. S. (2016). What's new in estrogen receptor action in the female reproductive tract. *Journal of Molecular Endocrinology, 56*(2), R55–R71.

27. Imperial College London. (2020, November 16). New drug can improve fertility in women with reproductive health problems. *ScienceDaily.* Retrieved August 12, 2022 from www.sciencedaily.com/releases/2020/11/201116161207.htm

28. Inhorn, M. C., & Patrizio, P. (2015). Infertility around the globe: New thinking on gender, reproductive technologies and global movements in the 21st century. *Human Reproduction Update, 21*(4), 411–426.

29. Johnson, T. C. (2021, June 8). *An overview of fertility drugs.* WebMD; www.webmd .com. https://www.webmd.com/infertility-and-reproduction/guide/fertility-drugs

30. La Marca, A., & Capuzzo, M. (2019). Use of progestins to inhibit spontaneous ovulation during ovarian stimulation: The beginning of a new era?. *Reproductive Biomedicine Online, 39*(2), 321–331.

31. Lehman, M. N., Hileman, S. M., & Goodman, R. L. (2013). Neuroanatomy of the kisspeptin signaling system in mammals: Comparative and developmental aspects. *Kisspeptin Signaling in Reproductive Biology, 784,* 27–62.

32. Lorenzen, M., Boisen, I. M., Mortensen, L. J., Lanske, B., Juul, A., & Jensen, M. B. (2017). Reproductive endocrinology of vitamin D. *Molecular and Cellular Endocrinology, 453,* 103–112.

33. Mascarenhas, M., Sunkara, S. K., Antonisamy, B., & Kamath, M. S. (2017). Higher risk of preterm birth and low birth weight following oocyte donation: A systematic review and meta-analysis. *European Journal of Obstetrics & Gynecology and Reproductive Biology, 218,* 60–67.

34. Mustafa, M., Sharifa, A. M., Hadi, J., IIIzam, E., & Aliya, S. (2019). Male and female infertility: Causes, and management. *IOSR Journal of Dental and Medical Sciences, 18,* 27–32.

35. Mayo Clinic Staff. (2021, August 27). *Female infertility – Diagnosis and treatment – Mayo Clinic.* Mayo Clinic; www.mayoclinic.org. https://www.mayoclinic.org/diseases -conditions/female-infertility/diagnosis-treatment/drc-20354313

36. Naseri, L., Khazaei, M., Ghanbari, E., & Bazm, M. A. (2019). Rumex alveollatus hydroalcoholic extract protects CCL4-induced hepatotoxicity in mice. *Comparative Clinical Pathology, 28*(2), 557–565.

37. Pasquali, R., Casanueva, F., Haluzik, M., Van Hulsteijn, L., Ledoux, S., Monteiro, M. P., ... Dekkers, O. M. (2020). European Society of Endocrinology Clinical Practice Guideline: Endocrine work-up in obesity. *European Journal of Endocrinology, 182*(1), G1–G32.

38. Petraglia, F., Serour, G. I., & Chapron, C. (2013). The changing prevalence of infertility. *International Journal of Gynecology & Obstetrics, 123,* S4–S8.

39. Pivonello, C., Muscogiuri, G., Nardone, A., Garifalos, F., Provvisiero, D. P., Verde, N., ... Pivonello, R. (2020). Bisphenol A: An emerging threat to female fertility. *Reproductive Biology and Endocrinology, 18*(1), 1–33.

40. Quaas, A., & Dokras, A. (2008). Diagnosis and treatment of unexplained infertility. *Reviews in Obstetrics and Gynecology, 1*(2), 69.

41. Sairbanu, S., & Mohammed, R. (2020). Reproductive Endocrine Physiology. In *Subfertility: Recent Advances in Management and Prevention*, Rehman, R., & Sheikh, A. (Eds.). Elsevier Health Sciences, 65–76.

42. Richard, D. Y., Boulay, F., Wang, J. M., Dahlgren, C., Gerard, C., Parmentier, M., ... Murphy, P. M. (2009). International Union of Basic and Clinical Pharmacology. LXXIII. Nomenclature for the formyl peptide receptor (FPR) family. *Pharmacological Reviews, 61*(2), 119–161.

43. Sato, J., Nasu, M., & Tsuchitani, M. (2016). Comparative histopathology of the estrous or menstrual cycle in laboratory animals. *Journal of Toxicologic Pathology, 29*(3), 155–162.

44. Stinson, A. (2018, October 30). *What to know about HPV and fertility.* Medical News Today; www.medicalnewstoday.com. https://www.medicalnewstoday.com/articles /323512#hpv-and-mens-fertility

45. Silva, T., Jesus, M., Cagigal, C., & Silva, C. (2019). Food with influence in the sexual and reproductive health. *Current Pharmaceutical Biotechnology, 20*(2), 114–122.

46. Torre, S. D., Benedusi, V., Fontana, R., & Maggi, A. (2014). Energy metabolism and fertility—A balance preserved for female health. *Nature Reviews Endocrinology*, *10*(1), 13–23.

47. Tsutsumi, R., & Webster, N. J. (2009). GnRH pulsatility, the pituitary response and reproductive dysfunction. *Endocrine Journal*, *56*(6), 729–737.

48. T'Sjoen, G., Arcelus, J., Gooren, L., Klink, D. T., & Tangpricha, V. (2019). Endocrinology of transgender medicine. *Endocrine Reviews*, *40*(1), 97–117.

49. Thomas, C. (2021). *How can I offset the side effects of fertility drugs?* BabyCentre UK; www.babycentre.co.uk. Retrieved August 22, 2022, from https://www.babycentre.co .uk/x553909/how-can-i-offset-the-side-effects-of-fertility-drugs

50. Victoria, M., Labrosse, J., Krief, F., Cédrin-Durnerin, I., Comtet, M., & Grynberg, M. (2019). Anti Müllerian hormone: More than a biomarker of female reproductive function. *Journal of Gynecology Obstetrics and Human Reproduction*, *48*(1), 19–24.

51. Wang, X., Chang, F., Bai, Y., Chen, F., Zhang, J., & Chen, L. (2014). Bisphenol A enhances kisspeptin neurons in anteroventral periventricular nucleus of female mice. *Journal of Endocrinology*, *221*(2), 201–213.

52. Yang, S., Chen, X. N., Qiao, J., Liu, P., Li, R., Chen, G. A., & Ma, C. H. (2012). Comparison of GnRH antagonist fixed protocol and GnRH agonists long protocol in infertile patients with normal ovarian reserve function in their first in vitro fertilization-embryo transfer cycle. *Zhonghua fu Chan ke za zhi*, *47*(4), 245–249.

53. Zegers-Hochschild, F., Adamson, G. D., de Mouzon, J., Ishihara, O., Mansour, R., Nygren, K., ... Vanderpoel, S. (2009). International committee for monitoring assisted reproductive technology (ICMART) and the world health organization (WHO) revised glossary of ART terminology. *Fertility and Sterility*, *92*(5), 1520–1524.

54. Zimmermann, M. B., & Andersson, M. (2021). Global Endocrinology: Global perspectives in endocrinology: Coverage of iodized salt programs and iodine status in 2020. *European Journal of Endocrinology*, *185*(1), R13–R21.

11 Novel Drugs
Clinical Trials and Approval Process

J. Sarada, Y. Aparna, and S. Anju

11.1 INTRODUCTION

Clinical application of any new or novel drug/device needs to be evaluated thoroughly before it is commercialized for public usage. A drug, a therapeutic compound other than food recommended for the prevention, diagnosis, treatment, or relief of disease symptoms, needs proper testing in a systematic manner. Every novel drug undergoes various levels of testing to determine its safety, efficacy for treating the condition it is intended for, and the correct dosage and administration route before it reaches a patient. This process may span 10 to 15 years, and several pharmaceutical regulatory bodies play vital roles in approval.

The evaluation process investigates the efficacy and safety of a drug by testing it in humans in clinical trials. The National Institutes of Health (NIH) has defined clinical trials as "a research study in which one or more human subjects are prospectively assigned to one or more interventions to evaluate the effects of those interventions on health-related biomedical or behavioral outcomes" (1). Clinical trials help in deciding the correct medical approach that works best for certain types of diseases or for a specific group of people. Each trial focuses on a specific scientific question, finding better ways to prevent, screen, diagnose, and/or treat various diseases. Trials can also look for comparisons between new and existing treatments. Therefore clinical trials are an essential component in advancing medical knowledge (2).

Clinical trials help researchers in finding different:

- Interventions for treating certain diseases or conditions.
- Methods to prevent the development or recurrence of certain diseases or conditions, including vaccines and lifestyle changes.
- Evaluation of different methods designed to identify or diagnose certain diseases or conditions.

Clinical trials are conducted by a research team consisting of doctors, nurses, pharmacists, social workers, and other health care professionals for carrying out the trial protocol and recording the data (3). Usually, clinical trials are sponsored or funded by pharmaceutical companies (4). Academic medical centers, voluntary specialty

DOI: 10.1201/9781003297826-11

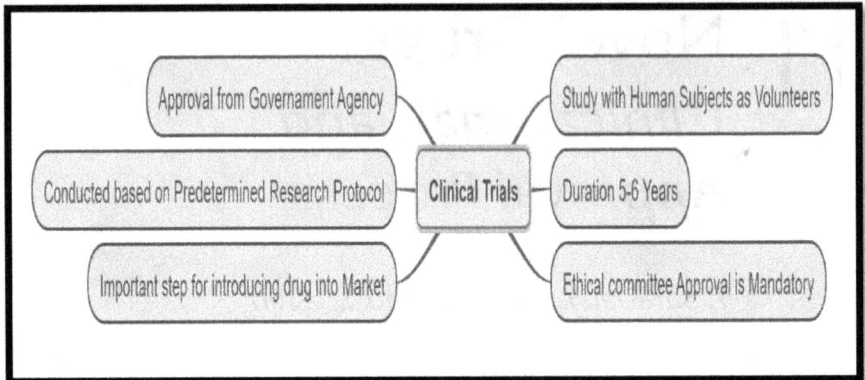

FIGURE 11.1   Features of a clinical study.

groups, governmental agencies, and other health care providers can also sponsor clinical trials. The implementation of clinical trials involves a rigorous approach based on scientific, statistical, ethical, and legal considerations (Figure 11.1). Thus, it is crucial for health care providers to understand the base on which well-performed clinical trials relay in order to maintain a partnership with patients and industry in pursuit of efficient therapies (5).

All clinical trials may not be successful and every investigation has its own set of potential benefits and risks. Therefore, participants/volunteers of clinical trials should be informed about the risks and protection given to them as human subjects in the form of consent before participating in the study. Patients need to be well informed that clinical trials are not fail-proof, and that funding, bias, trial errors, and other factors can affect results (6). Additionally, clinical studies are conducted only after US Food and Drug Administration (FDA) approval, and any new side effects and/or complications, especially unprecedented long-term risks, can always happen.

In a typical clinical trial, a research plan or protocol is made explaining the purpose of the study, the procedure or methods that will be followed, and their necessity. Every study requires certain specifications to be met and specific groups of participants such as only males or females, age range, diseased individuals, or healthy individuals. All participants should be provided with details of the trial like purpose of the study, number of participants, period of the study, eligibility criteria, schedule of tests, procedures, drugs and/or dosages, and type of information to be collected (7). Each clinical trial has its own specification or eligibility criteria that need to be mentioned in the protocol and specify whether participants must be healthy or diagnosed with certain diseases or conditions. Exclusion criteria like age, gender, type and stage or progression of certain diseases or conditions, prior treatment history, and other medical conditions might disqualify an individual from participating in the clinical trial (8).

Some trials may provide participants with prospective medical benefits, while others may not. At times, trials also require participants to go through additional procedures, tests, and assessments based on the particular study protocol that should be included in the informed consent document prior to the beginning of the research.

After completion of the clinical trial, researchers carefully examine the collected data before determining whether further testing will be needed. Following phase I and phase II trials, researchers have to decide whether to stop testing if the new drug, device, or other treatment being tested is found to be unsafe or ineffective. After phase III trials, researchers make conclusions regarding the medical importance of the new treatment approach to certain diseases or conditions.

11.2 TYPES OF CLINICAL TRIALS

Depending on what researchers focus on in clinical trials, the trials can be differentiated into seven types (Figure 11.2) (9).

1. **Preventive trials**

Preventive trials are conducted to test new medications/supplements like vitamins, preventive doses of vaccines, and/or lifestyle changes that might lower a person's risk of certain diseases. These studies include healthy people and individuals who previously had certain conditions like cancer and the most susceptible group of individuals.

2. **Screening trials**

Screening trials aim to find the best methods to diagnose certain diseases or conditions prior to patients experiencing symptoms. Screening trials are often used to decrease a person's risk of serious harm or death by earlier detection of illnesses.

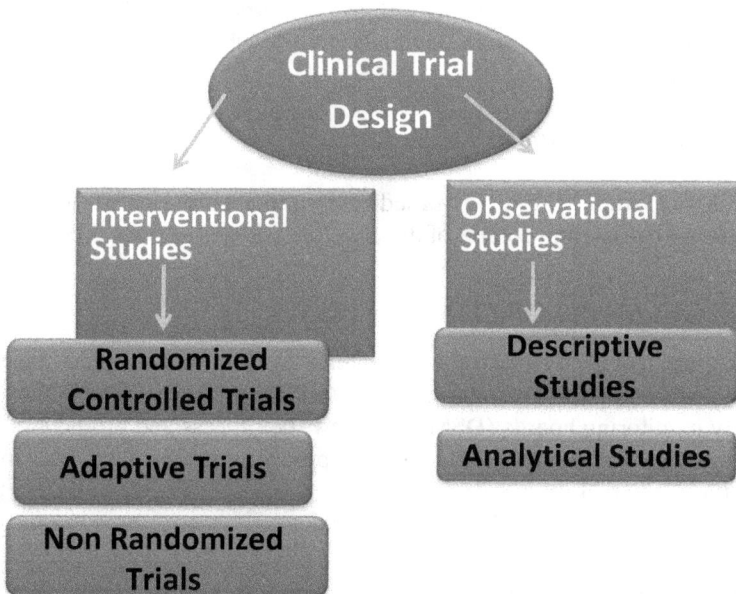

FIGURE 11.2 Methods for clinical studies.

3. **Diagnostic trials**

Diagnostic trials deal with novel or innovative scientific tests or procedures to identify certain diseases or conditions more accurately. These trials include participants
who exhibit the signs and symptoms required for investigation.

4. **Treatment (intervention) trials**

Treatment trials include an intervention like medication, psychotherapy, a new
device, a new approach to surgery, or another type of therapy or treatment. They
focus on finding new treatments by collecting clinical data and ensure the safety of
participants while evaluating the drug or device.

5. **Genetic studies**

Genetic studies aim to improve predictive markers of certain diseases or conditions
by identifying and understanding the role of responsible genes in certain illnesses.
Research conducted during these studies examines how a person's genes put them
at risk of developing certain disorders. This is important in determining various
treatments.

6. **Quality-of-life studies**

Quality-of-life studies aim to determine the best methods of managing side effects
of various diseases or conditions and treatments, for example, nausea, vomiting, and
depression associated with cancer as well as chemotherapy used in treating cancer.
They evaluate a person's comfort and quality of life when they are suffering from a
chronic illness.

7. **Epidemiological studies**

Epidemiological studies are survey-based analyses that help scientists identify prevalence patterns, causes, and control of different disorders in various groups of people.

11.3   REGULATION OF CLINICAL TRIALS

To ensure the drug evaluation process adheres to local and national standards of
safety and ethics, regulatory bodies like institutional review boards (IRBs) and data
and safety monitoring boards (DSMBs) review the process and protocol of clinical
trials. These agencies review, monitor, and approve biomedical research involving
human subjects (10, 11).

General criteria for research approval include:

- Risks to subjects are minimal.
- Reasonable in relation to benefits.

- Selection of subjects is equitable.
- Informed consent forms.
- Sufficient procedures for data monitoring to maintain subjects' safety.
- Adequate mechanisms for subject confidentiality.
- Rights and welfare of vulnerable populations are protected.

In compliance with the guidelines of the Code of Federal Regulations (CFR), one non-scientist member and one independent of the IRB are authorized to approve, modify, or reject a research activity. Depending on the perceived risk involved in a study, the IRB conducts a number of reviews from exempting for "minimal risk" studies (not greater than those encountered in daily life or routine clinical examinations or tests) to lengthy full-board reviews for higher-risk studies.

DSMBs, also referred to as data safety committees or data monitoring committees, are often required by IRBs for study approval. Their responsibilities are safeguarding the interests of study subjects, preserving the integrity and credibility of the trial, and ensuring reliable trial results are made available to the medical community (12).

DSMBs are usually organized by the trial sponsor and principal investigator, and are often composed of biostatisticians, ethicists, and physicians from relevant specialties, among others. The complexity and expense of monitoring human research have prompted the establishment of contract research organizations (CROs) to supervise clinical trials (13). They are commonly commercial or academic organizations hired by the study sponsor "to perform one or more of a sponsor's trial-related duties and functions," such as organizing and managing a DSMB, or managing and auditing trial data to maintain data quality.

The drug development and approval process has been defined and regulated by the FDA where safety and efficacy of the drug is the primary focus (Figure 11.3). The Center for Drug Evaluation and Research (CDER) works to evaluate new drugs before they enter the market for sale (14). CDER's evaluation checks dishonest practices and claims about drugs and provides the information to doctors and patients/ consumers for proper use of medicines. It also ensures that both brand-name and generic drugs' health benefits are more than their side effects. Initially, the drug company or sponsor conducts a series of laboratory and animal-based tests to establish drug mechanisms of action and their safety in humans. Next, clinical trials will be taken up to determine whether the drug is safe against the targeted disease or application in therapy and its health benefits.

FDA approval for a drug is based on the review by CDER. The drug approval process is carried out within a framework of guidelines:

- *Understand the target for the new drug and alternative treatments available.* The FDA reviews the disease for which the drug is developed and evaluates the current treatment in order to assess the possible risks of the drug and its benefits. If a new drug is proposed for therapy for a life-threatening disease in which there is no treatment, the drug is recommended if the benefits outweigh the risks.

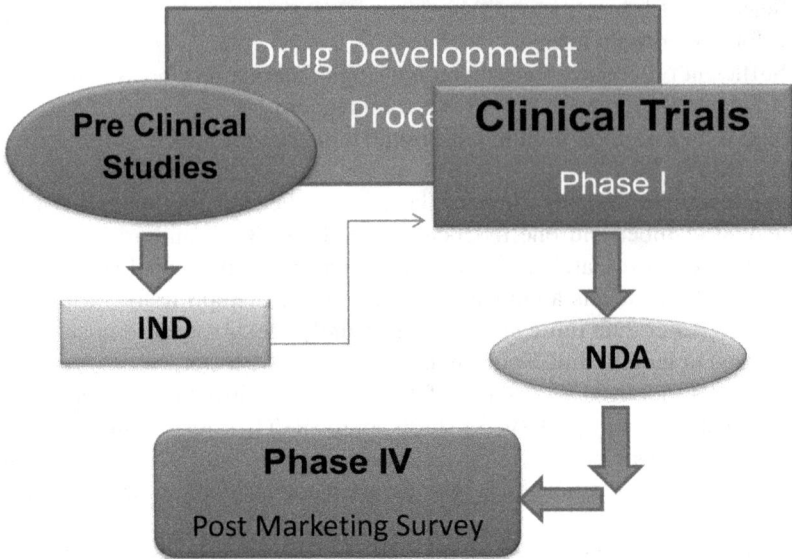

FIGURE 11.3 Drug development process.

- *Assessment of benefits and risks.* The FDA assesses the clinical benefits along with risks from the clinical information submitted by the drug manufacturer, considering any uncertainties that may arise from incomplete data. The FDA looks into submitting results of two well-designed clinical trials, and the first trial results are neither by chance nor biased. In cases of rare disease where multiple trials may not be possible, convincing proof from one clinical trial may be considered. Clinical proof states that the clinical benefits of new drugs should always outweigh any possible risks and uncertainties.
- *Strategies for managing risks.* This includes an FDA-approved drug label, with a clear description of the benefits and risks of the new drug. Detection and management of risks need to be specified. Risk Evaluation and Mitigation Strategy (REMS) help could be obtained by the drug manufacturer in case more effort is needed to manage risks. Although risk-benefit assessments and decisions are straightforward at times, they may be difficult to interpret or predict. The FDA and the drug manufacturer may reach different conclusions or there may be differences of opinion among the FDA's review team. Therefore, the FDA often uses the best scientific and technological information available for making decisions in a deliberative process.
- *Accelerated approval* is used exclusively for novel therapies to treat life-threatening diseases with therapeutic benefits. This approval is especially useful when the drug is for long-term use and its effect can be measured only over a period of time. In case a drug enters the market for sale under this category, then the drug producer needs to conduct postmarketing clinical trials to verify and describe the drug's benefit. The FDA may withdraw

the given approval if further trials fail to verify the predicted benefit. Many drugs have entered the market through this approval process, for example, antiretroviral drugs for HIV/AIDS and anticancer therapeutics, and subsequently changed the treatment process.

11.4 DRUG DEVELOPMENT DESIGNATIONS

The FDA also encourages the development of drugs that are the first available for an illness or possess significant benefits over current drugs. These approaches are for specific needs and, if applicable, a new drug application may receive more than one designation.

- *Fast track* is a process that facilitates the development and review process of drugs that are developed to treat serious conditions. This approach provides a way to bridge the gap for an unmet medical need if data on animal or human trials are available. This process helps to introduce new drugs into market at a very early stage.
- *Breakthrough therapy* designation expedites the development and review of drugs that are intended to treat a serious condition, and preliminary clinical evidence indicates that the drug may demonstrate substantial improvement over available therapy. A drug with breakthrough therapy designation is also eligible for the fast track process. The drug company must request a breakthrough therapy designation.
- *Priority review* means that the FDA aims to take action on an application within six months, compared to the ten-month standard review. A priority review designation directs attention and resources to evaluate drugs that would significantly improve the treatment, diagnosis, or prevention of serious conditions.

After a drug proves to be promising in preclinical studies, an investigational new drug (IND) application could be filed by the drug sponsor or sponsor-investigator. The drug is put under clinical trial phases I–III after approval. During these trials, if the drug is reported to be safe and efficacious on the targeted population, then the drug's sponsors submit a new drug application (NDA) to the FDA. After an extensive review by the FDA, it determines whether the therapeutic status can be granted and permitted for marketing. After final approval, the drug can continue to be studied in phase IV trials, in which safety and effectiveness for the indicated population are monitored (Figure 11.3).

Therefore, the evaluation process for any drug is made in a very systematic manner by approved agencies/authorities in a phase-wise manner.

11.5 PRECLINICAL TRIALS

Preclinical trials include animal studies to investigate a drug's safety dose for human therapy. This data on preclinical investigations is essential for IND approval for

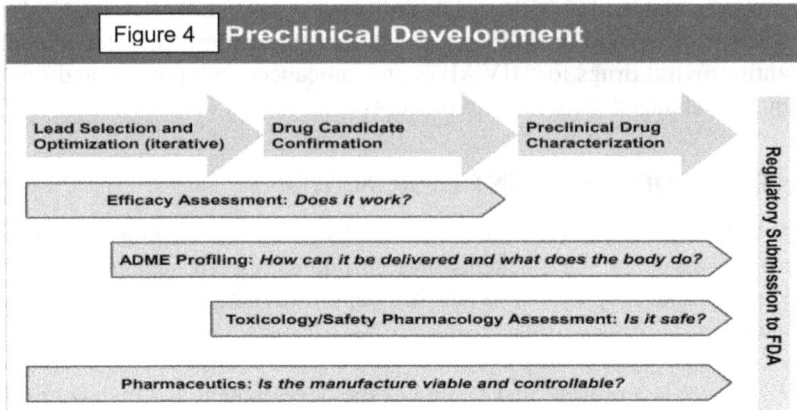

FIGURE 11.4 Preclinical development. (Adapted from TetraQ.)

further testing in humans. As the FDA emphasizes the *safety of the drug*, the initial phases of a clinical trial are made to test the safety and maximum tolerated dose (MTD) of a drug, along with the pharmacokinetics and pharmacodynamics of the drug (Figure 11.4).

11.6   CLINICAL TRIALS PROCESS

See Table 11.1.

11.6.1   PHASE I TRIALS

Phase I trials are usually performed in a small number of "healthy" and/or "diseased" volunteers. The MTD can be determined using various statistical designs (15). Dose escalation is based on very strict criteria, and subjects are closely followed for evidence of drug toxicity over a sufficient period. Improvements to the process of informed consent could help dispel some of these misconceptions while still maintaining adequate enrollment numbers.

11.6.2   PHASE II TRIALS

Also referred to as *therapeutic exploratory* trials, phase II trials are usually larger than phase I studies and are conducted with a small number of volunteers who have the disease of interest. They are designed to test safety, pharmacokinetics, and pharmacodynamics, but may also be designed to answer questions essential to the planning of phase III trials, including determination of optimal doses, dose frequencies, administration routes, and endpoints (16). In addition, they may offer preliminary evidence of drug efficacy by

TABLE 11.1
Clinical trial process

Phase	Length/period	Number of people	Purpose		
Phase I	1 month	10–20	How safe is the drug?	How does it get metabolized in body?	What are the side effects?
Phase II	3–12 months	50–75	Is it safe?	How well is it working?	What is the dosage?
Phase III	6–12 months	100–300	Is it safe?	How well it is working?	Does the benefit outweigh the risk?
FDA approval	Application submitted	Application reviewed	Application approved	Available for public	
Phase IV	3–12 months	100–300	Does it appear to be safe?	Are there any rare side effects?	Cost-effective ness and comparison with similar drugs

1. comparing the study drug with "historical controls" from published case series or trials that established the efficacy of standard therapies,
2. examining different dosing arms within the trial, or
3. randomizing subjects to different arms (such as a control arm).

However, the small number of participants and primary safety concerns within a phase II trial usually limit its power to establish efficacy and thereby supports the necessity of a subsequent phase III trial. Sponsor(s), investigator(s), and the FDA meet at the conclusion of the initial trials to review the preliminary clinical data, IND, and ascertain the viability of progressing further.

11.6.3 PHASE III TRIALS

Phase III trials are also referred to as *therapeutic confirmatory, comparative efficacy*, or *pivotal trials*. To confirm efficacy and figure out the incidence of common adverse reactions, this phase of drug assessment is organized in a more diverse target population. Phase III trials are usually conducted with 100–300 subjects, and these trials have the statistical power to establish an adverse event rate of no less than 1 in 100 persons. This is one of the reasons why the FDA requires more than one phase III trial to establish drug safety and efficacy.

Comparative efficacy trials are the most common type, also known as *superiority* or *placebo-controlled trials*, comparing the intervention of interest with either a standard therapy or a placebo. An equivalence trial or *positive-control study* is designed to confirm whether the experimental treatment is similar to the comparator as prespecified by the investigator. Hence, in such trials, a placebo is not included in this study design. The intervention will be deemed equivalent to the comparator when differences between the intervention and the comparator remain within the prespecified margin. A *non-inferiority study* is a variant of the equivalency trial in which the goal of the study is to exclude the possibility that experimental intervention is less effective than the standard treatment by some prespecified magnitude.

The balance in treatment allocation for comparison of treatment efficacy is the hallmark of phase III trial design. This clinical trial tries to eliminate the imbalance of confounders and/or biases between treatment groups through randomization.

In a *simple randomization model*, each subject to a trial arm is randomly allocated regardless of those already assigned. This strategy is less ideal because of imbalances in treatment assignments or distribution of covariates. *Block randomization* can be used to improve a simple randomized model, where a constraint can be placed on randomization forcing the number of subjects randomly assigned per arm to be equal and balanced after a specified block size. Another trial design is *stratification*, which is used in combination with randomization to further balance study arms based on prespecified characteristics instead of size in the case of blocking. Stratification facilitates analysis by ensuring that specific prognostic factors of clinical importance are properly balanced in the arms of a clinical trial. To minimize assessment bias of subjective outcomes, phase III trial design insists that the interventions be *blinded* or masked.

Specific blinding strategies to remove information bias include the subject only as *single blinding*, both the subject and investigator as *double blinding*, or *triple blinding* if the data analyst, subject, and investigator are involved. However, methods of drug delivery cannot be blinded.

The development of established drug toxicities may lead to improper unmasking and pose ethical and safety issues. Additional strategies can be applied to enhance study efficiency, like assigning each subject to serve as their own control, i.e., using a crossover study or evaluating more than one treatment simultaneously as the factorial design. The most common approach is the *intention-to-treat analysis*, where subjects are assessed based on the intervention arm in which they were randomized, irrespective of the treatment they receive. A complementary or secondary analysis is an *as-treated* or *per-protocol* analysis, in which subjects are evaluated based on the treatment they actually received, irrespective of whether they were randomized to that treatment arm. For the primary analysis of random trials, intention-to-treat analyses are preferable because they eliminate selection bias by preserving randomization. However, an interventional trial as-treated or per-protocol approach may eliminate any benefit of random treatment selection. This study appears to be similar to an interventional cohort study with the potential for treatment selection bias. An intention-to-treat analysis may fail to show a difference in outcomes if adherence to the treatment is poor and contamination in the control group is high. This is in contrast to a per-protocol analysis, which takes into account such protocol violations. The Consolidated Standards of Reporting Trials (CONSORT) guideline was established to improve the quality of trial reporting and assist with evaluating the conduct and validity of trials and their results (17, 18).

11.6.4 PHASE IV TRIALS

Phase IV trials, commonly known as therapeutic use or postmarketing trials, are observational studies performed on FDA-approved drugs. They aim to:

1. Identify less common adverse reactions.
2. Evaluate cost.
3. Evaluate drug effectiveness in diseases, populations, or doses similar to or markedly different from the original study population.

Premarketing or phase III studies are limited, as statistics show that approximately 20% of drugs get new black box warnings at postmarketing, and 4% of new drugs are finally withdrawn for safety reasons (19). This helps in understanding societal decisions because one needs to look into delays in accessing new drugs and delays in information regarding rare adverse reactions. Over the past decade, there has been a steady rise in voluntarily and spontaneously reported serious adverse drug reactions submitted directly to the FDA by physicians and consumers, or indirectly via drug manufacturers. The most common criticisms during postmarketing surveillance are:

1. The reliance on voluntary reporting of adverse events.
2. The trust in drug manufacturers to collect, evaluate, and report drug safety data that may risk their financial interests.
3. The dependence on one government body to approve a drug and then actively seek evidence that might lead to its withdrawal.

Proposed solutions include the establishment of a national health data network to oversee postmarketing surveillance independent of the FDA approval process, a preplanned meta-analysis of a series of related trials to assess less common adverse events, and large-scale simple randomized controlled trials with few eligibility and treatment criteria.

Clinical trials are one of the powerful approaches to making progress in medical research. Modern clinical trials are based on numerous ethical principles and practices that guide the investigator in performing human research without violating rules. The general procedure for a new drug to be established as a therapeutic agent starts with the establishment of the maximum tolerated dose in humans in phase I, followed by pharmacodynamics and pharmacokinetic studies, and understanding of its therapeutic benefit in phase II. Comparison of drug efficacy with an established therapeutic agent in a larger population of volunteers is carried out in phase III, and finally postmarket evaluation for adverse reactions and effectiveness after administration to the general public is investigated in phase IV.

REFERENCES

1. https://grants.nih.gov/policy/clinical-trials/definition.htm.
2. https://www.fda.gov/drugs.
3. https://www.fda.gov/patients/drug-development-process/step-1-discovery-and-development.
4. https://www.hopkinsmedicine.org/research/understanding-clinical-trials/clinical-research-team.html.
5. Umscheid CA, Margolis DJ, Grossman CE. Key concepts of clinical trials: a narrative review. *Postgraduate Medicine*. 2011;123(5):194–204. doi:10.3810/pgm.2011.09.2475.
6. Department of Health and Human Services, editor. Code of Federal Regulations–The common rule: Protection of human subjects. 45, p. 2009. https://www.hhs.gov/ohrp/regulations-and-policy/regulations/index.html
7. Ridpath JR, Wiese CJ, Greene SM. Looking at research consent forms through a participant-centered lens: The PRISM readability toolkit. *American Journal of Health Promotion*. 2009;23(6):371–375.
8. Dixon JR Jr. The International Conference on Harmonization Good Clinical Practice guideline. *Qual Assur*. 1998 Apr-Jun;6(2):65–74. doi: 10.1080/105294199277860. PMID: 10386329.
9. https://www.fda.gov/patients/clinical-trials-what-patients-need-know/what-are-different-types-clinical-research.
10. Ellenberg S, Fleming TR, DeMets DL. *Data Monitoring Committees in Clinical Trials: A Practical Perspective*. West Sussex: John Wiley & Sons, 2002, 50.
11. Guidance for Industry. E6. Good clinical practice–consolidated guidance. Bethesda, MD: US Department of Health and Human Services, 1996.

12. https://www.fda.gov/science-research/clinical-trials-and-human-subject-protection/regulations-good-clinical-practice-and-clinical-trials.
13. https://www.technologynetworks.com/drug-discovery/articles/exploring-the-drug-development-process.
14. https://www.fda.gov/about-fda/fda-organization/center-drug-evaluation-and-research-cder.
15. Mapstone J, Elbourne D, Roberts I. Strategies to improve recruitment to research studies. *Cochrane Database of Systematic Reviews.* 2007 Apr 18;(2):MR000013. doi: 10.1002/14651858.MR000013.pub3. Update in: Cochrane Database Syst Rev. 2010;(1):MR000013. PMID: 17443634.
16. Treweek S, Pitkethly M, Cook J, Fraser C, Mitchell E, Sullivan F, Jackson C, Taskila TK, Gardner H. Strategies to improve recruitment to randomised controlled trials. *Cochrane Database of Systematic Reviews* 2018 Feb 22;2(2):MR000013. doi: 10.1002/14651858.MR000013.pub6. PMID: 29468635; PMCID: PMC7078793.
17. Moher D, Schulz KF, Altman D, CONSORT Group (Consolidated Standards of Reporting Trials). The CONSORT statement: Revised recommendations for improving the quality of reports of parallel-group randomized trials. *JAMA.* 2001;285(15):1987–1991.
18. Schulz KF, Altman DG, Moher D. CONSORT 2010 statement: Updated guidelines for reporting parallel group randomised trials. *BMJ.* 2010;340:c332.
19. Fontanarosa PB, Rennie D, DeAngelis CD. Post marketing surveillance–lack of vigilance, lack of trust. *JAMA.* 2004;292(21):2647–2650.

12 Quorum Quenching–Based Drug Development
Challenges and Futurity

Y. Aparna, S. Anju, and J. Sarada

12.1 INTRODUCTION

Quorum sensing is a mechanism in which bacteria communicate with each other by secreting signaling molecules termed acyl-homoserine lactones, or AHLs. This mechanism is very well noted in many pathogens, as it increases virulence gene expression, biofilm formation, and development of antibiotic resistance. The emergence of multidrug-resistant bacteria and the threat they pose to humans has posed a major challenge to the treatment of various diseases, especially with nosocomial infections. The increasing awareness of quorum-sensing mechanisms and their ability to increase virulence gene expression paved the way for the search for quorum-sensing inhibitory molecules, otherwise termed quorum-quenching agents. The emergence of multidrug-resistant bacteria has become a major health concern worldwide and there is a need for novel strategies to combat the multidrug resistance.

Quorum-sensing signals are broadly classified as autoinducers (AI-2), N-acyl-homoserine lactones (AHLs) (Kalia, 2012) oligopeptides, methyl dodecanoic acid, hydroxy palmitic acid methyl ester, diffusible signal factor, and Cis-11 methyl dodecanoic acid. Oligopeptides are involved in communication in gram-positive bacteria while AHLs are signaling molecules in gram-negative bacteria (Dong and Zhang, 2005; Sifri, 2008, Dougald, 2007). These quorum-sensing molecules enable pathogenic bacteria to resist antibiotics and biofilm development. To combat these quorum-sensing mechanisms, a search has started for quorum-quenching agents to prevent infections.

Recent research on hospital surveillance studies referred to microbes with antimicrobial resistance as "ESKAPE" pathogens. The term refers to six potent pathogens: *Enterococcus faecium*, *Staphylococcus aureus*, *Klebsiella pneumoniae*, *Acinetobacter baumannii*, *Pseudomonas aeruginosa*, and *Enterobacter* spp. These ESKAPE organisms escape antibacterial treatments and are considered multidrug-resistant bacteria (Tommasi et al., 2015; Micoli et al., 2018; Boucher et al., 2009).

DOI: 10.1201/9781003297826-12

Quorum quenching (QQ) agents are novel alternatives for antimicrobial approaches (Qin et al., 2018). QQ prevents or controls pathogenic microorganisms by interfering with their quorum sensing (QS) signaling molecules. Many recent research reviews state that more than 60 infections caused by bacteria are known to cause biofilms, which is a QS-related phenomenon.

Biofilm is an extracellular mucopolysaccharide produced by many pathogenic bacteria. It prevents the action of antibiotics and is also involved in the evasion of host immune responses. This phenomenon was well established in *Pseudomonas aeruginosa*, an opportunistic pathogen that causes nosocomial infection. Research by Bauer et al. (2002) demonstrated that QS-controlled biofilm production can be inhibited by interfering with autoinducer signal molecules.

Many approaches and methods have been developed in recent years to block signaling molecules. They include denaturing signaling molecules either by biological or chemical degradation, blocking a receptor level, inhibiting the transport of signal molecules, and competitive inhibition of signal molecules and receptors. Several natural and synthetic compounds have been identified in recent years that act as antagonists to QS circuits.

Many reports state that combating the antibiotic resistance is focused on the inhibition of QS signals. They have become the novel areas for many new therapeutic approaches (Shaaban et al., 2019, Sai Priya et al., 2020).

Based on the molecular weight, QQ substances are classified into two types: small molecule quorum-sensing inhibitors (QSIs) and macromolecular QQ substances. It was noted that both QSIs and the macromolecular QQ system inhibit the QS mechanism in different ways. Also, many research studies stated that many pathogens contain multiple QS systems. Such pathogens pose a threat to controlling them (Fong et al., 2018),

12.2 CLASSIFICATION OF AHL-DEGRADING ENZYMES

AHL-degrading enzymes are of two types: (1) natural QQ molecules and (2) synthetic QQ molecules.

12.2.1 NATURAL QQ AGENTS AS TARGETS FOR DRUG DEVELOPMENT

AHL-degrading degrading enzymes exist in nature and are produced by bacteria, Archaebacteria, plants, and other eukaryotes. Plants produce QQ compounds to reduce the pathogenicity of invading microorganisms. The first natural product found to exhibit QQ activity was isolated from *Delisea pulchra*, which produces brominated furanones. These furanones are known to inhibit AHLs and autoinducer peptides (AIPs) (Defoirdt et al., 2007). Coumarins are another group of compounds that exhibit QQ activity by inhibiting biofilm-producing bacteria, plant pathogens, and infections in aquaculture (Reen et al., 2018). Witch hazel tannin inhibits the QS system in methicillin-resistant *Staphylococcus aureus* and *Staphylococcus epidermidis* (Kiran et al., 2008). Flavonoids from *Combretum albiflorum* are known to inhibit pyocyanin, elastase, and biofilm formation in *Pseudomonas aeruginosa* (Vandeputte et al., 2010). Table 12.1 is a list of some noteworthy QQ agents.

TABLE 12.1

Quorum quenching agents from prokaryotes

Organism	Target	Reference
Delftia tsuruhatensis SJO1	AHL degradation, anti-biofilm potential	Singh et al., 2017
Vibrio alginolyticus	Inhibits *Pseudomonas aeruginosa* PAO1 mobility, elastase, rhamnolipid production, and biofilm production	Song et al., 2018
Bacillus cereus D28	QS signaling of *Chromobacterium violaceum*, *Vibrio harveyi*, and *Vibrio fischeri*	Teasdale et al., 2011
Halobacillus salinus C42	QS circuits of *Vibrio harveyi*	Teasdale et al., 2011
Delisea pulchra	LuxR and Lux S	Defoirdt et al., 2007
Lyngbya majuscula	Las R	Kwan et al., 2011
Aspergillus spp.	Lux R	Dobretsov, 2011
Candida albicans	PqsA	Ramage et al., 2002
Penicillium spp.	Las R and RhlR	Xavier and Bassler, 2005
Allium sativum	LuxR family	Von Bodman et al., 2008
Curcuma longa	CviR	Packiavathy et al., 2014
Hamamelis virginiana	RNAIII	Giacometti et al., 2005

12.2.2 Synthetic QQ Agents as Drug Targets

It is important to understand the roles of QQ agents in controlling bacterial infections and competitive signal molecules that are synthesized to mimic the structure of natural QS molecules. Synthesized AI-2 homologues play a potential role in inhibiting biofilm formation. thereby inhibiting pathogenesis in *Vibrio harveyi*. They are also known to inhibit methylthioadenosine (MTA) nucleoside activity, which is involved in the synthesis of AI-2 peptides in bacterial pathogens. Boronic acid compounds and DPD homologues also act as antagonists to AI-2.

AIPs are QS signaling molecules in gram-positive bacteria like *S. aureus*. To control these signaling molecules, many synthetic analogues are synthesized. For example, RNAIII-inhibiting peptide (RIP), a linear peptide, is used for reducing the virulence of *S. aureus*. It showed good therapeutic impact in controlling *S. aureus* infections. They are also demonstrated to inhibit biofilm production in various gram-positive and gram-negative organisms. Another example is synthetic AIPs that contain only sulfur ring structure, which are used to control QS mechanisms in gram-positive bacteria (Zhang et al., 2019).

12.3 QQ MOLECULES FROM PROKARYOTES

Depending on the AHL-degrading mechanism and mode of action, AHL-degrading molecules are classified into three types. They are AHL lactonases, AHL acylases, and AHL oxidoreductases.

12.3.1   AHL Lactonases

AHL lactonases are metallo-β-lactamase members that can hydrolyze the ester bonds of a lactone ring. They are known to have very broad specificity. They are coded by aiiA, an autoinducer inactivation gene. This was identified in *Bacillus* spp., *Pseudomonas aeruginosa*, and *Burkholderia thailandensis*. They decreased the AHL accumulation in the aforementioned bacteria and changed their QS-dependent AHL accumulation. Some AHL lactonases also could alter the expression of virulence factors in pathogens like *Pseudomonas aeruginosa* and *Pectobacterium carotovorum* by altering the swarming motility, protease, biofilm production, and pyocyanin production, which is a QS-dependent virulence gene expression (Dong et al., 2007). Though AHL lactonase enzymes can cleave the lactone ring, the product formed is unstable and restores the AHL molecule under acidic conditions (Schipper et al., 2009).

Different types of lactonases have been identified, including phosphotriesterase-like lactonases, metallo-β-lactamase–like lactones, α/β-hydrolase fold lactones, and paraoxonases. These lactonases are well distributed in bacteria, archaea, and eukaryotes (Sikdar and Elias, 2020) (Table 12.2).

12.3.2   AHL Acylases

Acylases are the enzymes that hydrolyze amide bonds in AHLs (Table 12.3). They come under the superfamily Ntn-hydrolases, i.e., N-terminal nucleophile hydrolases. They have a specific α β/β α-fold. PvdQ from *Pseudomonas aeruginosa* is a well-studied QQ acylase. They cleave AHLs with an acyl side chain length of more than ten carbons (Wahjudi et al., 2011). They are also termed amidases.

12.3.3   AHL OXIDOREDUCTASES

AHL oxidoreductases modify AHLs by oxidizing or reducing the acyl side chain without degrading the AHLs. These changes result in the alteration of AHL signals by modifying the QS responses. For example, BpiB09 reductase from *Acidobacterium* spp. reduces 3-oxo-AHLs to 3-hydroxy-AHLs in *P. aeruginosa* altering motility, pyocyanin secretion, and biofilm production (Chen et al., 2013; La Sarre and Federle, 2013).

TABLE 12.2
AHL lactonases from different bacteria

Gene	Organism	Activity
AiiA	*Bacillus* sp. 240B1	Degrades AHL signals in *Erwinia carotovora*
MomL	*Muricauda olearia* Th120	Inhibits virulence factor production in *P. aeruginosa*
BpiB01	*Nitrobacter* sp. strain Nb-311A	Inhibits biofilm production
BpiB04	*Pseudomonas fluorescence*	AHL degradation
BpiB07	*Xanthomonas campestris*	Inhibits biofilm production

TABLE 12.3
AHL acylases

Molecule	Organism	Reference
AhlM	*Streptomyces* spp. M664	Park et al., 2005
PvdQ, QuiP	*P. aeruginosa* PAO1	Sio et al., 2006; Huang et al., 2003
AiiC	*Anabaena* spp. PCC7120	Romero et al., 2008
AiiD	*Ralstonia* spp. XJ12B	Lin et al., 2003

12.4 QQ AGENTS FROM EUKARYOTES FOR DRUG DEVELOPMENT

Many QQ agents are derived from eukaryotic organisms like plants, animals, algae, and fungi. These compounds are known to interfere with bacterial QS signaling circuits. They are found to have wider applications in medicine for the treatment of various ailments, as they are efficient and biocompatible. Higher organisms are known to evolve many defense mechanisms. Some of these mechanisms include the production of antibodies, antimicrobial peptides, and lysozymes. QQ enzymes are identified in various animal models like zebrafish, mice, rats, and higher organisms (Zhang et al., 2004).

Endophytic microorganisms of plant origin produce secondary metabolites like camptothecin, paclitaxel, hypericin, azadirachtin, podophyllotoxin, and deoxypodophyllotoxin. They also are known to exhibit QQ, antimicrobial, and anticancer properties (Kusari et al., 2014). Endophytic bacteria like *Brevibacteria borstelensis* and *Bacillus megaterium* from the plant *Cannabis sativa* are known to exhibit QQ activity (Kusari et al., 2014). Strains of endophytic bacteria *Microbacterium testaceum* from the *Phaseolus vulgaris* plant exhibited QQ activity on bioluminescence in *E. coli* pSB403 and violacein production from *C. violaceum CV026* (Lopes et al., 2015)

The secondary metabolite derived from garlic, ajoene (4,5,9-trithiadodeca 1,6,11 triene 9 oxide), is rich in sulfur, which is known to control QS circuits and virulence factors in *P. aeruginosa*. Ajoene acts as a broad-spectrum QQ inhibitor by enzymatic degradation of amide bonds and lactone rings (Jakobsen et al., 2017).

Gingerol and curcumin act as QQ agents in reducing infections caused by *P. aeruginosa* by inhibiting virulence factors like biofilm production, pyocyanin, and exopolysaccharide production (Shukla et al., 2021).

Fragin, a member of the diazeniumdiolate class of natural compounds, is known to have antibacterial, antifungal, and antitumor properties because of the presence of a metallophore that exhibits metal chelation capability. This is also known to regulate AHL-dependent QS systems (Jenul et al., 2018).

Furanones derived from the macroalga *Delisea pulchra* are used in the treatment of QS-mediated infections. These furanones block QS circuits in various pathogens by competitively inhibiting AHLs (Givskov, 1996). They were tested in mice models to understand bacteriostatic action against *P. aeruginosa*, which causes lung infections (Hentzer, 2003).

Secondary metabolites from fungi like patulin and penicillanic acid from penicillium species act as QQ agents. Marine-derived fungi secrete a secondary metabolite called equisetin that inhibits virulence genes in *Pseudomonas aeruginosa* (Rasmussen et al., 2005; Zhang et al., 2018).

Mammalian enzymes like paraxonases and lactonases show hydrolytic activities on lactones and esters. They mimic the drug metabolism and hence can act as detoxifying nerve agents. They are able to destroy AHLs.

12.5   ANTIBODIES AS QQ AGENTS

Studies by Sandra De Lamo Marin's group demonstrated for the first time that antibodies exhibit QQ activity. They were able to inhibit QS systems in *P. aeruginosa*. The monoclonal antibodies developed, such as XYD-11G2 and RS2-IG9, were efficient in destroying the 3OC12 HSL in *P. aeruginosa*. Studies have demonstrated that antibody-based QQ therapy can be a novel approach to inhibit QS in pathogenic bacteria, thereby reducing virulence (Marin et al., 2007).

12.6   ANTIBIOTICS AS QQ AGENTS

Antibiotics act not only as bacteriostatic and bactericidal agents but also exhibit QQ activity. Antibiotics like ciprofloxacin, azithromycin, ceftazidime, and erythromycin inhibited virulence gene expression like phospholipase C, elastase, leucocidin, protease, and DNase in *P. aeruginosa* (Mookherjee et al., 2018). Previous studies have revealed that subinhibitory concentrations of tobramycin could block rhII and rhIR genes by reducing C4HSL generation in certain bacteria. They are known to interfere with bacterial signaling mechanisms. Reduction in protease activity was noted with antibiotics like ciprofloxacin, ceftazidime, and azithromycin (Skindersoe et al., 2008).

12.7   NANOPARTICLES AS QQ AGENTS

In recent years, nanoparticles have gained significance due to their antimicrobial activity. They are the most promising compounds to combat antimicrobial resistance to antibiotics and to fight against multidrug-resistant bacteria. Studies are in progress to explore the toxicity index and pharmacokinetic features to develop alternate methods to combat antibiotic resistance. Chitosan nanoparticles are demonstrated to have QQ properties by decreasing the expression of lasR and rhlR genes, biofilm production, increasing permeability into the cell membrane, and pyocyanin inhibition in *P. aeruginosa* PAO1 strains (Muslim et al., 2017).

12.8   TARGET SPECIFICITY OF QQ AGENTS

QQ agents exhibit different modes of action. Understanding the mechanism of action may help in the development of new-generation drugs with target specificity that may help in combating antibiotic resistance. Different modes of action of QQ agents are presented in Figure 12.1.

Compound	Activity
Sinefungin	Precursor synthesis
Solenopsin A	QS signal/sensor complex formation
Halogenated furanone	QS sensor turnover
AiiA Lactonase, PvdQ acylase	QS signal diffusion
J8-C8	QS signal synthesis
RS2-1G9 Sequestring antibody	QS signal diffusion

Action on AHL

Compound	Activity
Phospho-AI-2 LsrK	QS Signal transport
Ribosyl-cysteine compounds	QS Signal synthesis
Immucillin A analog	Precursor synthesis
Cinnemaldehyde derivatives	QS signal/Sensor complex formation

Action on AI-2 ← MODE OF ACTION OF QQ AGENTS → Action on PQS

Compound	Activity
Hod dioxygenase	QS Signal diffusion
Haloginated anthranilic acid	QS Signal synthesis
Farnesol	QS signal/sensor complex formation
PqsD inhibitor	Precursor synthesis

Action on AIP

Compound	Activity
Ambuic acid	QS Signal synthesis
Savirin	QS signal/sensor complex formation
AP4-24H11 sequestring antibody	QS signal diffusion

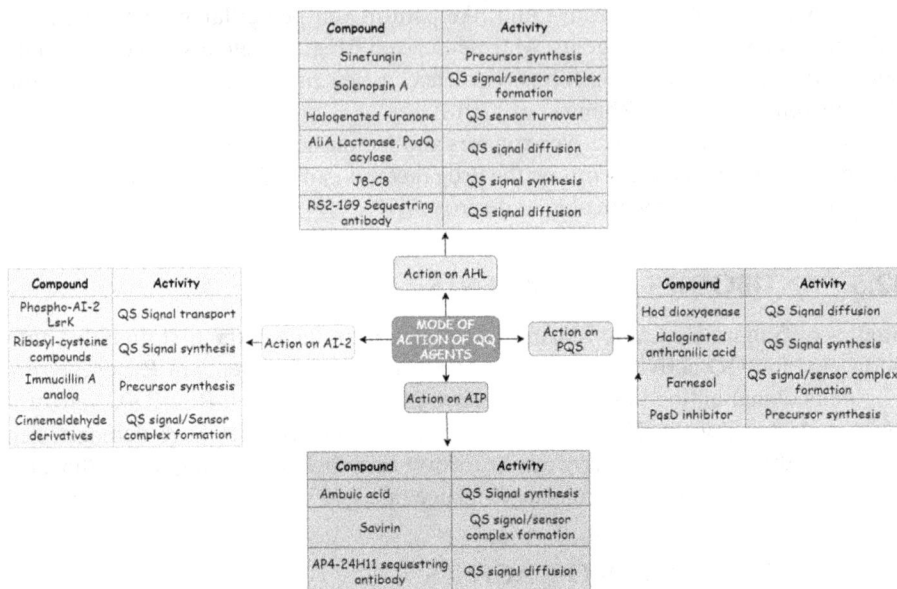

FIGURE 12.1   Target specificity of different QQ agents.

12.9   CHALLENGES AND FUTURE APPROACHES

The main challenge is the presence of an extremely diverse group of signaling molecule distribution in varied species. Studies by Kalia et al. (2014) and Maeda et al. (2012) hypothesized that bacteria may become resistant to QSIs and QQ compounds, and novel strategies are required to increase the range of QSIs and QQ compounds to avoid resistance. Most research on QSIs has been studied in vitro by using strains that are basically domesticated. It is a very big challenge to understand how most virulent bacteria respond in in vivo conditions. Also, knowledge of screening QSI compounds is in the beginning stages and needs to be standardized. Knowledge of the specificity of various QSIs is also a major drawback in understanding how different bacterial systems respond.

A lack of suitable animal models to check the mode of action of QQ-based drugs, host cytotoxicity, and stability of drugs is a major concern that needs to be addressed. It is very important to understand and analyze the chemical and kinetic behavior of QQ-based drugs and their role in modulating immune responses. The major challenge lies in understanding the signaling mechanisms in polymicrobial communities and their spatial conformation with respect to QQ, and therapy is still an unanswered question. The ecological behavior of microbes and their evolutionary sharing is a big challenge in developing QQ-based drugs and checking their efficacy in controlling QS circuits.

Commercial production of QQ metabolites for large-scale production is still in its early stages. The biggest challenge lies in understanding the human–microbiome interactions with respect to QS and QQ abilities exhibited by bacteria and human systems, respectively.

12.10 FUTURE PERSPECTIVES

Recombination QQ enzymes are used in destroying biofilm production by *A. baumannii* (Chow et al., 2014). These may open a new area in the treatment of various infectious diseases. The search for novel QQ or QSI agents may help in reducing virulence by targeting the QS network and may help in eliminating bacterial resistance to antibiotics giving a scope for treatment of diseases. Computer-aided drug development, high-throughput omics, and system biology platforms may play a crucial role in the future by modifying the inhibitors for targeting a broad range of QS signaling molecules for target specificity and inhibitory activity.

ACKNOWLEDGMENTS

The authors thank the principal and management of Bhavan's Vivekananda College of Science, Humanities and Commerce for their constant support and encouragement.

REFERENCES

Bauer, W. D., and Robinson, J. B. 2002. Disruption of bacterial quorum sensing by other organisms. *Current Opinion in Biotechnology* 13, 234–237. https://doi.org/10.1016/S0958-1669(02)00310-5

Boucher, H. W., Talbot, G. H., Bradley, J. S., Edwards, J. E., Gilbert, D., Rice, L. B. Scheld, M., Spellberg, B., and Bartlett, J. 2009. Bad bugs, no drugs: No ESKAPE! An update from the Infectious Diseases Society of America. *Clinical Infectious Diseases* 48, 1–12. https://doi.org/10.1086/595011

Chen, F., Gao, Y., Chen, X., Yu, Z., and Li, X. 2013. Quorum quenching enzymes and their application in degrading signal molecules to block quorum sensing-dependent infection. *International Journal of Molecular Sciences* 14(9), 17477–17500. https://doi.org/10.3390/ijms140917477

Chow, J. Y., Yang, Y., Tay, S. B., Chua, K. L., and Yew, W. S. 2014. Disruption of biofilm formation by the human pathogen Acinetobacter baumannii using engineered quorum-quenching lactonases. *Antimicrobial Agents and Chemotherapy* 58, 1802–1805. https://doi.org/10.1128/AAC.02410-13

Defoirdt, T., Miyamoto, C. M., Wood, T. K., Meighen, E. A., Sorgeloos, P., Verstraete, W., and Bossier, P. 2007. The natural furanone (5Z)-4-bromo-5-(bromomethylene)-3-butyl-2 (5H)-furanone disrupts quorum sensing-regulated gene expression in Vibrio harveyi by decreasing the DNA-binding activity of the transcriptional regulator protein LuxR. *Environmental Microbiology* 9, 2486–2495.

Dobretsov, S., Teplitski, M., Bayer, M., Gunasekera, S., Proksch, P., and Paul, V. J. 2011. Inhibition of marine biofouling by bacterial quorum sensing inhibitors. *Biofouling* 27, 893–905.

Dong, Y.-H., and Zhang, L.-H. 2005. Quorum sensing and quorum-quenching enzymes. *Journal of Microbiology* 43(1), 101–109.

Dong, Y.-H., Wang, L.-H., and Zhang, L.-H. 2007. Quorum-quenching microbial infections: Mechanisms and implications. *Philosophical Transactions of the Royal Society B* 362, 1201–1211.

Fong, J., Zhang, C., Yang, R., Boo, Z. Z., Tan, S. K., Nielsen, T. E., Givskov, M., Liu, X. W., Bin, W., Su, H., and Yang, L. 2018. Combination therapy strategy of quorum quenching enzyme and quorum sensing inhibitor in suppressing multiple quorum sensing pathways of *Pseudomonas aeruginosa*. *Scientific Reports* 8, 1155.

Giacometti, A., Cirioni, O., Ghiselli, R., Dell'Acqua, G., Orlando, F., D'Amato, G., Mocchegiani, F., Silvestri, C., DelPrete, S. M., Rocchi, M., Balaban, N., Saba, V., and Scalise, G. 2005. RNAIII-inhibiting peptide improves efficacy of clinically used antibiotics in a murine model of Staphylococcal sepsis. *Peptides* 26, 169–175. https://doi.org/10.1016/j.peptides.2004

Givskov, M., De Nys, R., Manefield, M., Gram, L., Maximilien, R., Eberl, L., Molin, S., Steinberg, P. D., and Kjelleberg, S. 1996. Eukaryotic interference with homoserine lactone-mediated prokaryotic signalling. *Journal of Bacteriology* 178, 6618–6622.

Hentzer, M., Wu, H., Andersen, J. B., Riedel, K., Rasmussen, T. B., Bagge, N., ... Givskov, M. 2003. Attenuation of *Pseudomonas aeruginosa* virulence by quorum sensing inhibitors. *The EMBO Journal* 22(15), 3803–3815.

Huang, J. J., Han, J.-I., Zhang, L.-H., and Leadbetter, J. R. 2003. Utilization of acyl-homoserine lactone quorum signals for growth by a soil pseudomonad and *Pseudomonas aeruginosa* PAO1. *Applied and Environmental Microbiology* 69(10), 5941–5949. https://doi.org/10.1128/AEM.69.10.5941-5949.2003

Jenul, C., Sieber, S., Daeppen, C., Mathew, A., Lardi, M., Pessi, G., ... Eberl, L. 2018. Biosynthesis of fragin is controlled by a novel quorum sensing signal. *Nature Communications* 9(1), 1297.

Kusari, P., Kusari, S., Lamshöft, M., Sezgin, S., Spiteller, M., and Kayser, O. 2014. Quorum quenching is an antivirulence strategy employed by endophytic bacteria. *Applied Microbiology and Biotechnology* 98, 7173–7183.

Kwan, J. C., Meickle, T., Ladwa, D., Teplitski, M., Paul, V., and Luesch, H. 2011. Lyngbyoic acid, a 'tagged' fatty acid from a marine Cyanobacterium, disrupts quorum sensing in *Pseudomonas aeruginosa*. *Molecular BioSystems* 7, 1205–1216.

LaSarre, B., and Federle, M. J. 2013. Exploiting quorum sensing to confuse bacterial pathogens. *Microbiology and Molecular Biology Reviews* 77(1), 73–111.

Lin, Y. H., Xu, J. L., Hu, J., Wang, L. H., Ong, S. L., Leadbetter, J. R., and Zhang, L. H. 2003. Acyl-homoserine lactone acylase from Ralstonia strain XJ12B represents a novel and potent class of quorum-quenching enzymes. *Molecular Microbiology* 47(3), 849–860. https://doi.org/10.1046/j.1365-2958.2003.03351.x

Lopes, R. B. M., de Oliveira Costa, L. E., Vanetti, M. C. D., de Araújo, E. F., and de Queiroz, M. V. 2015. Endophytic bacteria isolated from common bean (Phaseolus vulgaris) exhibiting high variability showed antimicrobial activity and quorum sensing inhibition. *Current Microbiology* 71, 509–516.

Marin, S. D. L., Xu, Y., Meijler, M. M., and Janda, K. D. 2007. Antibody catalyzed hydrolysis of a quorum sensing signal found in Gram-negative bacteria. *Bioorganic & Medicinal Chemistry Letters* 17(6), 1549–1552.

Micoli, F., Costantino, P., and Adamo, R. 2018. Potential targets for next generation antimicrobial glycoconjugate vaccines. *FEMS Microbiology Reviews* 42, 388–423. https://doi.org/10.1093/femsre/fuy011

Mookherjee, A., Singh, S., and Maiti, M. K. (2018). Quorum sensing inhibitors: Can endophytes be prospective sources?. *Archives of Microbiology* 200, 355–369.

Packiavathy, I. A. S. V., Priya, S., Pandian, S. K., and Ravi, A. V. 2014. Inhibition of biofilm development of uropathogens by curcumin–An anti-quorum sensing agent from Curcuma longa. *Food Chemistry* 148, 453–460.

Park, S.-Y., Kang, H.-O., Jang, H.-S., Lee, J.-K., Koo, B.-T., and Yum, D.-Y. 2005. Identification of extracellular N-acylhomoserine lactone acylase from a Streptomyces sp. and its application to quorum quenching. *Applied and Environmental Microbiology* 71(5), 2632–2641. https://doi.org/10.1128/AEM.71.5.2632-2641.2005

Qin, X., Kräft, T., and Goycoolea, F. M. 2018. Chitosan encapsulation modulates the effect of trans-cinnamaldehyde on AHL-regulated quorum sensing activity. *Colloids Surf B Biointerfaces* 169, 453–461. https://doi.org/10.1016/j.colsurfb.2018.05.054

Ramage, G., Saville, S. P., Wickes, B. L., and Lopez-Ribot, J. L. 2002. Inhibition of Candida albicans biofilm formation by farnesol, a quorum-sensing molecule. *Applied and Environmental Microbiology* 68, 5459–5463. https://doi.org/10.1128/aem.68.11.5459 -5463.2002

Rasmussen, T. B., Skindersoe, M. E., Bjarnsholt, T., Phipps, R. K., Christensen, K. B., Jensen, P. O., ... Givskov, M. (2005). Identity and effects of quorum-sensing inhibitors produced by Penicillium species. *Microbiology* 151(5), 1325–1340.

Reen, F. J., Gutiérrez-Barranquero, J. A., and Parages, M. L. 2018. Coumarin: A novel player in microbial quorum sensing and biofilm formation inhibition. *Applied Microbiology and Biotechnology* 102, 2063–2073.

Romero, M., Diggle, S. P., Heeb, S., Camara, M., and Otero, A. 2008. Quorum quenching activity in Anabaena sp. PCC 7120: Identification of AiiC, a novel AHL-acylase. *FEMS Microbiology Letters* 280(1), 73–80. https://doi.org/10.1111/j.1574-6968.2007.01046.x

Saipriya, K., Swathi, C. H., Ratnakar, K. S., and Sritharan, V. 2020. Quorumsensing system in Acinetobacter baumannii: A potential target for new drug development. *Journal of Applied Microbiology* 128, 15–27. https://doi.org/10.1111/jam.14330

Schipper, C., Hornung, C., Bijtenhoorn, P., Quitschau, M., Grond, S., and Streit, W. 2009. Metagenome-derived clones encoding two novel lactonase family proteins involved in biofilm inhibition in *Pseudomonas aeruginosa*. *Applied and Environmental Microbiology* 75, 224–233.

Shaaban, M., Elgaml, A., and Habib, E. E. 2019. Biotechnological applications of quorum sensing inhibition as novel therapeutic strategies for multidrug resistant pathogens. *Microbial Pathogenesis* 127, 138–143. https://doi.org/10.1016/j.micpath.2018.11.043

Shukla, A., Shukla, G., Parmar, P., Patel, B., Goswami, D., and Saraf, M. 2021. Exemplifying the next generation of antibiotic susceptibility intensifiers of phytochemicals by LasR-mediated quorum sensing inhibition. *Scientific Reports* 11(1), 22421.

Sifri, C. D. 2008. Quorum sensing: Bacteria talk sense. *Clinical Infectious Diseases* 47(8), 1070–1076. https://doi.org/10.1371/journal.pone.0134684

Sikdar, R., and Elias, M. 2020. Quorum quenching enzymes and their effects on virulence, biofilm, and microbiomes: A review of recent advances. *Expert Review of Anti-Infective Therapy* 18(12), 1221–1233.

Singh, P. B. R., Shoeb, M., Sharma, S., Naqvi, A., Gupta, V. K., and Singh, B. N. 2017. Scaffold of selenium nanovectors and honey phytochemicals for inhibition of *Pseudomonas aeruginosa* quorum sensing and biofilm formation. *Frontiers in Cellular and Infection Microbiology* 7, 93. https://doi.org/10.3389/fcimb.2017.00093.

Sio, C. F., Otten, L. G., Cool, R. H., Diggle, S. P., Braun, P. G., Bos, R., Daykin, M., Cámara, M., Williams, P., and Quax, W. J. 2006. Quorum quenching by an N-acyl-homoserine lactone acylase from *Pseudomonas aeruginosa* PAO1. *Infection and Immunity* 74(3), 1673–1682. https://doi.org/10.1128/ IAI.74.3.1673-1682.2006

Skindersoe, M. E., Alhede, M., Phipps, R., Yang, L., Jensen, P. O., Rasmussen, T. B., Bjarnsholt, T., Tolker-Nielsen, T., Høiby, N., and Givskov, M. 2008. Effects of antibiotics on quorum sensing in *Pseudomonas aeruginosa*. *Antimicrobial Agents and Chemotherapy* 52(10), 3648–3663. https://doi.org/10.1128/AAC.01230-07

Song, Y., Cai, Z. H., Lao, Y. M., Jin, H., Ying, K. Z., Lin, G. H., and Zhou, J. 2018. Antibiofilm activity substances derived from coral symbiotic bacterial extract inhibit biofouling by the model strain *Pseudomonas aeruginosa* PAO 1. *Microbial Biotechnology* 11(6), 1090–1105. https://doi.org/10.1111/1751-7915.13312

Teasdale, M. E., Donovan, K. A., Forschner-Dancause, S. R., and Rowley, D. C. 2011. Gram-positive marine bacteria as a potential resource for the discovery of quorum sensing inhibitors. *Marine Biotechnology* 13, 722–732. https://doi.org/10.1007/s10126-010-9334-7

Tommasi, R., Brown, D. G., Walkup, G. K., Manchester, J. I., and Miller, A. A. 2015. ESKAPEing the labyrinth of antibacterial discovery. *Nature Reviews Drug Discovery* 14, 529–542. https://doi.org/10.1038/nrd4572

Vandeputte, O. M., Kiendrebeogo, M., Rajaonson, S., Diallo, B., Mol, A., Jaziri, M. E., and Baucher, M. 2010. Identification of catechin as one of the flavonoids from Combretum albiflorum bark extract that reduces the production of quorum sensing-controlled virulence factors in *Pseudomonas aeruginosa* PAO1. *Applied and Environmental Microbiology* 76, 243–253. https://doi.org/10.1128/AEM.01059-09

von Bodman, S. B., Willey, J. M., and Diggle, S. P. 2008. Cell-cell communication in bacteria: United we stand. *Journal of Bacteriology* 190, 4377–4391. https://doi.org/10.1128/JB.00486-08

Wahjudi, M., Papaioannou, E., Hendrawati, O., van Assen, A. H. G., van Merkerk, R., Cool, R. H., Poelarends, G. J., and Quax, W. J. 2011. PA0305 of *Pseudomonas aeruginosa* is a quorum quenching acylhomoserine lactone acylase belonging to the Ntn hydrolase superfamily. *Microbiology* 157(7), 2042–2055.

Xavier, K. B., and Bassler, B. L. 2005. Interference with AI-2-mediated bacterial cell-cell communication. *Nature* 437, 750–753. https://doi.org/10.1038/nature03960

Zhang, L. H., and Dong, Y. H. 2004. Quorum sensing and signal interference: Diverse implications. *Molecular Microbiology* 53(6), 1563–1571. https://doi.org/10.1111/j.1365-2958.2004.04234.x

Zhang, M., Wang, M., Zhu, X., Yu, W., and Gong, Q. 2018. Equisetin as potential quorum sensing inhibitor of *Pseudomonas aeruginosa*. *Biotechnology Letters* 40, 865–870.

Zhang, J., Feng, T., Wang, J., Wang, Y., and Zhang, X. H. 2019. The mechanisms and applications of quorum sensing (QS) and quorum quenching (QQ). *Journal of Ocean University of China* 18, 1427–1442.

Index